The New Net Carb & Glycemic Index Counters: 7500+ Foods with Carb, Protein, Fat Contents & 4000+ foods with Glycemic Index

DR. H. MAHER

Table of Contents

INTRODUCTION

People struggle to lose weight or prevent weight gain, while trying to follow their dietary guidelines – eat low carb, eat more fat, eat more whole grains, eat complex carbohydrates, eat low fat, eat less meat, eat low glycemic index food, eat more protein, eat low calories, etc. However, the ketogenic diet and low-glycemic diet produce mid to long-term results and are more effective in promoting weight-loss, preventing weight gain, reversing some chronic disease, maintaining healthy condition and improving blood markers.

That's why more and more people from celebrities to ordinary people have turned to them as their primary diets to achieve a more efficient weight management or reach some health goals.

Literature is huge in the field, and you will find valuable books about how to quick start your keto diet, how to reset your metabolism, which new dietary guidelines to follow. And, at the end you will probably find yourself like millions of dieters with the same fundamental question: How to keep your macronutrients grams counts within the strict limits recommended by your diet? Here comes this keto macros counter book.

Data are available thanks to governmental agencies who have populated their databases with valuable, reliable and extensive information. The nature of data gets the redaction of a simple, easy-to-use, and comprehensive guidebook difficult, and a huge work of data processing was necessary in order to provide this volume of information in this compact format.

This Ketogenic food counting book is a necessary tool that all dieters need to have in order to track and keep their daily intake under control and take to full benefit of their low-carb diet in general, and keto diet in particular. We have also added the glycemic index values of 4000+ foods and the glycemic index and glycemic load of 700+ foods, providing you more data, and nearly everything you need to know to count macronutrients, glycemic index and glycemic load in your diet, and reach your goals, whether your objective is to lose weight, gain mass muscles, improve blood markers, prevent weight gain, maintain health condition, reverse diabetes, manage hypertension or simply eat healthy food.

The NEW Complete Guide provides the following:
    For more than 7500 foods commonly eaten:
- o Calorie counts
- o Carbohydrate grams
- o Net Carbohydrates grams
- o Protein grams
- o Fat grams

A complete list of 4000+ glycemic index of foods Foods are divided into three categories according to their glycemic index:
- o Low glycemic index food
- o Moderate glycemic index food

o   High glycemic index food

What can you expect by using this book?

This book will give you an extensive and authoritative collection of accurate data essential to quick start your keto diet or low carb-diet and achieve your goals in term of weight loss, weight management, diabetes management. Thus, you will be able to keep your daily carbohydrates intakes within the strict limits recommended by the diet you follow.

- The first part will give you an overview of the ketogenic diet, the hormones that play a key role in weight-loss diets, and the main recommendations to achieve your goals and reach your ideal weight.

- The second part is divided into four chapters and provides exhaustive tables of foods with their respective glycemic index (GI) values and Glycemic load (GL). Low GI foods, moderate GI foods and High GI foods are presented and sorted alphabetically. The last chapter provides the list of 4000+ of foods with their respective glycemic index values.

- The third part includes the keto macronutrients (total carb, net carb, fat and protein) values of 7,500 foods commonly eaten divided into eighteen categories including Dairy and Eggs Products, Beverages, Baked Products, Cereal Grains and Pasta, Fruits and Fruit Juices, Meals, Entrees, and Side Dishes; Nut and Seed Products, Vegetables...

All the data provided in this book come from the most authoritative organizations in the field:
- The US department of agriculture
- The UK Food Standards Agency (FSA)
- The Food Standards Australia New Zealand (FSANZ)
- The International Glycemic Index database

PART I: KETO DIET OVERVIEW

WHAT IS THE KETOGENIC DIET?

The ketogenic diet (keto diet, ketosis based diet) is a low carbohydrate, high-fat diet plan that has been used since the 19th century to control and treat specific diseases like diabetes, epilepsy, cancers, polycystic ovary.

However, the ketogenic diet is gaining significant consideration as a powerful weight-loss strategy due to its relative safety, potential and superiority when compared to others diet methods including Atkins, Dukan, Paleo, and South Beach diet methods that are all high in protein but moderate in fat. The ketogenic diet is characterized by its high-fat content, typically 75%, moderate in protein 20% and very low carb, usually 5%.

How It Works

The premise of the keto diet for weight loss is that if you drastically reduce your carbohydrate intake and replace it with fat, you will put your body in a safe metabolic condition experienced when fasting called ketosis.

Indeed, glucose, which is obtained by eating carbohydrate foods is the primary source of energy for all cells in your body.

So during low dietary carbohydrate intake, your body begins by using the glucose stored from your liver and release glucose by breaking down muscle.

If the deprivation state continues, the level of insulin in blood decreases and your body begins to use fat as its principal fuel. The liver produce ketone bodies from fat, to compensate for the reduction of glucose and your body enter into the ketosis metabolic state.

Additionally, the ketones preserve the proteins stored in the muscles from being used to produce energy.

It is important to notice that Ketosis is reached through both eating high-fat and very-low-carb, intermittent fasting, or a combination of both.

Ketogenic Diet is superior to other Diets in Weight Losing

A ketogenic diet is a powerful method to lose weight and lower risk factors for disease. In fact, research reveals that the ketogenic diet is far superior to the often promoted low-fat diet.

RESEARCH NOTICED that healthy fats could really drive weight loss, in addition to the benefits of heart health from consuming some suitable fats. Increased protein intake also provides numerous benefits for people on a Keto diet.

ADDITIONALLY, research reveals that the ketogenic diet is far superior to a Calorie-restricted low-fat diet. Studies found that Keto for Women 5 people on a keto diet lost 2.2 times more weight than those on a Calorie-restricted low-fat diet.

Different Types of Ketogenic Diets

The ketogenic diet has many variantes, including:

- Standard ketogenic diet (SKD): This is the most known diet method. It is characterized by a very low-carbohydrate, high-fat and moderate-protein. The usual ratio is 75% fat, 20% protein, and 5% carbohydrates.

- The cyclical ketogenic diet (CKD): This diet involves periods of higher-carb refeeds, such as five ketogenic days followed by two high-carbohydrates days. The Cyclical ketogenic diet is a more advanced method primarily used by bodybuilders or athletes.

- The targeted ketogenic diet (TKD): This diet permits you to add carbohydrates when you are doing workouts. The targeted ketogenic diet is a more advanced method primarily used by bodybuilders or athletes.

- High-protein ketogenic diet (HKD): This is similar to a stan- dard ketogenic diet, but includes more protein and less fat. The usual ratio is 60% fat, 35% protein, and 5% carbohydrates.

Ketogenic Diet Advantages

In the first few days of beginning the ketogenic diet, it's not unusual to experience a short period in which you may have fatigue, headaches, and nausea. These symptoms are the early sign that your body is switching from burning glucose for energy to burning fat and are called Keto Flu.

The changeover can provoke side effect for a short period, but once your body enters the fat-burning stage, you may notice that you gained greater endurance and much more energy.

Weight loss and hunger suppression

When the liver produces the ketones, it limits the secretion of Ghrelin, a hormone that induces the sensation of hunger while increasing the production of cholecystokinin the hormone responsible for the feeling of satiety.

Therefore, a loss of appetite makes it easier to lose more weight. The Keto Diet usually results in rapid and substantial weight loss associated with hunger suppression.

The Ketogenic Diet and diabetes

The keto diet substantially restricts your daily carbohydrates to less than twenty grams. It pushes the body to break down fats for energy and produces ketones as a fuel source.

The ketogenic diet allows the body to maintain glucose levels at a low but healthy level and thus may help people with type 2 diabetes to control long-term blood. A one-year study determined that placing people with type 2 diabetes into ketosis metabolic condition dramatically enhanced their blood sugar control.

Ketogenic Diet gets the liver healthier.

The accumulation of fats in the liver is associated with type 2 diabetes and prediabetes. In some cases, this fat accumulation can cause severe damages to the liver.

Studies noticed that Keto Diet is associated with fewer risk of developing fatty liver disease (fat accumulation), and help to maintains and gets the liver healthier.

Keto Diet may help treat cancer

Early researches suggest that the keto diet have a favorable effect on cancer and may slow down the development of cancerous tumors. The studies indicate that when the body enters the ketosis, ketone bodies supply energy for the body. In that case, the cancer cells.

Cancer cells manifest increased glucose metabolism compared with healthy cells and require a large amount of glucose to develop. With a shift toward ketone production, the body becomes less favorable for their development.

Keto may boost heart health

.

It may seem surprising that a high-fat diet could be positive for your heart. Studies suggest that the Keto diet is associated with a reduction of triglyceride level, increases in good HDL cholesterol, and notable decreases in both diastolic and systolic blood pressure.

Hormones That Regulate Body Weight

The Insulin hormone

Insulin is a polypeptide hormone that regulates the absorption of sugar by body cells and maintains the level of sugar present in the blood at a healthy level.. This hormone is produced by the β cells of the pancreas. When we eat, food travels to our stomach and intestines where it is broken down into micronutrients. These micronutrients are absorbed and transported by our bloodstream. The pancreas, which is the main regulator of our blood sugar, produces the insulin hormone, and releases it into the bloodstream when we eat. Insulin is a hormone that controls the level of glucose in the blood by controlling its production by the liver and its use by the muscle. Its primary function is to allow body cells, including muscles and other cells to absorb and transform sugar (glucose) into energy throughout the body.

Insulin sends also signals to liver, muscle, and adipocytes (fat cells) to store the excess of glucose for further use. Excess sugar is stored in 3 ways:

- In muscle tissues in the form of glycogen.

- In the liver in the form of glycogen.

- In adipose tissue (fat reserves of the body) in the form of triglycerides which are fat molecules that store energy

Weight gain and insulin

Weight gain is explained by the secretion of insulin. Insulin is the hormone responsible for weight gain secreted by the pancreas. If you do not secrete pancreas insulin, you do not gain weight.

Hyperglycemia is the abnormally high blood sugar level. Hyperglycemia is felt like a rush of adrenaline, a gain of energy, making us feel extremely good.

However, hyperglycemia lasts only a short time because when the blood sugar level is too high, the pancreas will secrete insulin to release the sugar in the blood and pass it to the cells.

As seen earlier, excess of sugar is stored in 3 ways, including in adipose tissue (fat reserves of the body) in the form of triglycerides which are fat molecules that store energy.

Refined sugar and starches consumption have also been associated with a higher risk of obesity, insulin resistance, fatty liver, metabolic syndrome, and a higher risk of chronic disease.

Insulin Resistance

Insulin resistance is a serious and silent health condition that occurs when cells in your muscles, liver and body fat start ignoring the signal that insulin hormone is sending out in order to transfer sugar (glucose) out of the bloodstream and put it into your body cells.

As insulin resistance develops, the body reacts by producing more and more insulin to lower the blood sugar.

Over time (months or years depending on the severity of the metabolic disfunction), the β cells in the pancreas that are working hard to make a higher supply of insulin, can no longer keep working to provide more and more insulin. Consequently, your blood sugar may reflect the pancreas failure to maintain the level in the healthy range, and your blood sugar begins to rise, indicating pre-diabetes or at worst diabetes type 2.

Symptoms of insulin resistance

Insulin resistance is silent and presents no symptoms in the first stage of its development. The symptoms start to appear later when the condition worsens, and the pancreas fails to produce enough amount of insulin to keep your blood sugar within the normal ranges. When this occurs, the symptoms may include:

- Excessive hunger Lethargy or tiredness Difficulty concentrating Brain fog

- Waist weight gain

- High blood pressure

Can insulin resistance be reduced or reversed?

Fortunately, It is possible to reduce the effects of insulin resis- tance and boost your insulin sensitivity by following a number of effective methods, including:

- Low carbohydrate diets

- Low carbohydrate and high-fat diet (ketogenic diets) Low glycemic diets

- Low-calorie diets

- Weight loss surgery

- Regular exercise in combination with healthy diets

These methods have a similar way of working in that they all reduce the daily glucose intake drastically, lower the body's need for insulin, reduce insulin spike in the bloodstream, promote weight loss and prevent weight gain.

The Cortisol hormone

Cortisol is the stress hormone, produced by the adrenal gland when the body is in stressful situations. The hypothalamus, via the pituitary gland, sends a chemical signal to the adrenal glands to produce and release both adrenaline and cortisol.

Cortisol is naturally released every day in small and regular quantities. However, like adrenaline, cortisol can also be secreted and released in reaction to physical and emotional stress and triggers the body's fight-or-flight response.

These two stress hormones work simultaneously: adrenaline produces a significant increase in strength, performance, awareness, and increases metabolism. It also let fat cells to release additional energy. Cortisol helps the body produce glucose from proteins, and increase the body's energy in times of stress quickly.

However, cortisol is also involved in a variety of essential function for your health. Most of the body cells have cortisol receptors to use this steroid hormone for a variety of critical functions, including:

- blood sugar regulation

- metabolism regulation

- inflammation reduction

- memory formulation

Cortisol is important for your health, but an excess of cortisol can harm your body and induce a variety of unwanted symptoms.

What cause high cortisol levels?

A high cortisol level can be caused by several things. High cortisol is known as Cushing syndrome. This health condition results from your body secreting and releasing too much cortisol.
Cushing syndrome causes many unwanted symptoms,

including:

- obesity

- weight gain

- fatty deposits, especially in the face, midsection, and between the shoulders

- purple stretch marks on the arms, breasts, thighs, and abdomen

- thinning skin

- slow-healing injuries

Being under stress, induce a constant state of excess cortisol production. And, as seen above, this cortisol drives excess glucose production in a non-fight-or-flight situation. This excess glucose is converted into fat and stored by the body.

Thus, high levels of produced cortisol increase the risk of obesity highly, induce abdominal obesity, and increased the amount of fat storage.

Other factors that cause peaks in cortisol production are carbohydrates deprivation (in low carb diet, for example) and overconsumption of simple carbohydrates.

In both cases, when blood sugar levels fall, this induces a surge of stress hormones, including cortisol and adrenaline.

Stress hormones and their role in the body

Stress hormones are released in reply to body stressors. Hormonal responses of the woman body to stress are essential provided they occur in less frequently. They may become damaging and unhealthy when they happen too often. Prolonged exposure to porn induce severe damages to the brain and presents evidence that porn is not a healthy stressor.

Stress is habitually accompanied by high energy demand. Consequently, a severe stress situation induces a fast glucose release into the blood, which provides the required energy to deal with the stressful situation.

The principal players in the stress mechanism are: The adreno-corticotropic hormone (ACTH), The glucocorticoids such as cortisol, adrenaline and noradrenaline.

When this happens, blood glucose levels rise, concurrently with heart rate and blood pressure.

So at its simplest, stress leads to an increase in blood glucose, heart rate, and blood pressure, which induces an increased insulin release.

The Leptin Hormone

Leptin referred to as the starvation, or "hunger hormone" is an hormone produced by fat tissues and is secreted into our bloodstream. It plays an important role in weight regulation by reducing a person's appetite.

The Leptin hormone was discovered in 1994 and has gained significant interest for its powerful function in weight regulation and obesity. Leptin communicates with specific centers of the brain to influence how the body manages its store of fat. It sends a signal to the brain that the body has enough amount of stored fat, producing the body to burn calories from stored fat and reducing appetite.

Indeed, leptin plays the key regulator of body fat, and send signals to the brain to burn stored fat. This powerful effect would normally prevent obesity, overweight. Early researches have seen in leptin the solution for obesity. A supplementation of leptin would induce body fat burning, weight loss, and weight gain prevention. However, experiments revealed an unknown phenomenon which became until now, not fully understood.

Leptin resistance

Because leptin is produced by fat tissues, it is released in the bloodstream proportionally to the weight of a person. Its levels are high for people who are in overweight or obese than in people having normal weight.

However, researches have shown that the benefit of leptin in appetite-reducing is very low for obese people suggesting that people in obesity condition aren't sensitive to the benefi- cial effect of leptin and have developed Leptin resistance.

Leptin resistance is an abnormal condition that is associated with more weight gain for people in overweight or obesity. Thus, obese people tend to eat more and more because the hormonal signal that normally send to the brain that the body has enough amount of stored fat seems to be ignored.

Ongoing researches are focusing on this kind of leptin resis- tance in obese people which stops the brain acknowledging the leptin's signal. Some studies, however, suggest that obesity induces multiple cellular processes that attenuate or prevent leptin signaling, amplifying the extent of weight gain. Leptin Resistance may arise from poor leptin transport across the blood-brain barrier (BBB), alteration of the leptin receptor, and defect of leptin signaling...

Ways to Improve Leptin Resistance and Promote Weight Loss

Strong evidence shows that Leptin resistance can be drastically reduced by following these guidelines:

- Avoid Ultra-processed food: the impact of Ultra-processed food is still under studies, but many pieces of evidence suggest that these kinds of foods compromise the integrity of your gut, the normal functioning and the production of gut hormones.

- Lower your triglycerides: Having high triglycerides level in your bloodstream can prevent the transport of leptin to your brain.

- Eat healthy protein: Eating healthy proteins can improve leptin sensitivity.

- Eat healthy fats and keep your ratio omega 6/ omega 3 inferior to 3.

- Avoid simple carbohydrates, starches, and eat healthy carbohydrates (complex carbs, fiber).

The Ghrelin Hormone

Ghrelin, known as the "hunger hormone," is an acyl-peptide responsible for stimulating hunger by sending a chemical signal to tells you when to eat. Ghrelin is secreted and released primarily by the stomach. Smaller amounts of this hormone are also secreted by the small intestine, and pancreas.

Ghrelin has various functions. It is known mainly as the hormone that triggers hunger by stimulating the appetite. It induces increases in food intake and promotes fat storage and weight gain.

These findings suggest that by controlling the level of gherkin and let it down, we can reduce appetite and food intake.

An experiment consisting of administering ghrelin to people concluded that food intake was increased by 30% in this population.

How is ghrelin controlled?

Ghrelin levels are mainly regulated by food intake. Levels of ghrelin in the bloodstream rise typically before eating and when fasting in line with increased hunger.

Experimental studies demonstrated that Ghrelin levels are lower in obese or overweight individuals. Conversely, lean indi- viduals have a high level of ghrelin.

Studies also found that some nutrients slow down the ghrelin release in the bloodstream and thus reduce the impact of the hormones of hunger.

Soluble and insoluble fibers inhibit ghrelin secretion, which implies that eating complex carbohydrates has a positive and significant effect in reducing the production and release of ghrelin.

Glucose also has the same effect as dietary fibers in inhibiting Ghrelin secretion. However, as seen earlier, glucose, starches, and simple carbohydrates must be prohibited due to their impact in rising insulin release.

Recent studies demonstrated that contrary to a common belief, proteins did not reduce the production or release of ghrelin.

The PYY family

The gut hormone peptide YY 3–36 (PYY3–36) is a polypeptide hormone released from L-cells found in large intestine and the intestinal mucosa of the ileum.

The hormone PYY is released proportionally to nutrient intake. Indeed, the amount of this hormone is strongly influ- enced by the number of calories consumed, the macronutrient and micronutrient composition of the eaten meal.

After eating, PYY levels rise within the fifteen first minutes and reach a peak level within ninety minutes. Its main role is to reduce appetite, the psychological driver for eating. It also plays an important role in regulating the energy balance in the body.

Higher levels of PYY results on reduced appetite and conse- quently reduced calorie intake, and help in weight loss.

Conversely, low levels of PYY induce strong feelings of hunger and cravings, while predisposing fatty tissue retention.

Keto Flu And How To Avoid It

WHAT IS KETO FLU?

Keto flu designs the set of symptoms generally occurring in the low-carb diets, , and it happens when you quickly jump into a ketogenic diet without observing some simple precautions.

The keto flu or carbs flu is a set of symptoms experienced by some persons when they first start the ketogenic diet.

These symptoms, which can appear similar to the flu symp- toms, are caused by the body which is experiencing and adapting to minimal carbohydrates intake.

REDUCING your carbohydrates intake forces the body to burn ketones for energy supply rather than glucose. Ketones, as you have seen earlier, are byproducts of the fat breakdown and become the primary fuel source in a ketogenic diet (ketosis stage).

THIS SEVERE AND abrupt reduction of carbs —in a keto diet, carbohydrates are reduced to under 30 grams per day.— provoke a huge stress to the body and produce withdrawal symptoms. The keto flu effects may vary from person to person, and range from mild to severe. While some persons may start a very low-carb diet without any side effects, others may experience one or more symptoms, including :

- Constipation

- Diarrhea

- Dizziness

- Headache

- Irritability

- Muscle cramps

- Nausea

- Reduced concentration

- Stomach pain

- Sleeping difficulties

- Sugar cravings

- General weakness

SYMPTOMS generally last about one week. However, some people may experience them for a more extended period of time.

How to avoid the Keto Flu

In addition to the physical symptoms associated with keto flu, you may experience strong demotivation and distress.

Fortunately, there are two proven methods to reduce these side effects and help your body get through the transition stage safely.

- Start smoothly and safely. A stepwise approach rather than switching to a 100% ketogenic diet will help you avoid the keto flu symptoms. We recommend a four- step proven approach to get rid of the side effects.

- Stay hydrated. Dehydration and loss of minerals associated with the keto diet. Your body will secrete much less insulin. You will eliminate a lot of sodium and fluids. As a result, you have to drink lots of water and add electrolytes, potassium, magnesium, and sodium to your diet.

Keto Diet And Type 1 & Type 2 Diabetes

DIABETES MELLITUS REFERS TO DISEASES IN WHICH BLOOD glucose levels are too high. Glucose comes from the foods eaten by a person. Insulin is a hormone produced by the pancreas that allows the glucose to get into body cells to provide them energy.

Diabetes refers to an abnormal rise in blood sugar (also called hyperglycemia) caused by pancreatic dysfunction. The pancreas is an essential organ responsible for producing insulin to metabolize sugar to a form that can get into body cells to feed them by energy. When the pancreas becomes unable to perform this fundamental function, the blood sugar level increases and sugar accumulates in the body and becomes toxic to the vital organs. In fact, having a high level of glucose in the blood can cause severe health prob- lems. It can damage eyes, kidneys, heart, and nerves irreversibly.

TYPE 1 DIABETES is an autoimmune disease: the body does not make insulin due to irreversible damages in the cells of the pancreas. The patient must then inject daily insulin doses and follow a strict diet to prevent the severe adverse effect. Unfortunately, Type 1 diabetes is an autoimmune disease and remains incurable. It represents, however, relatively few portions because it only affects 10% of people with diabetes.

TYPE 2 DIABETES, is the more common type; the body does not make sufficient amount of insulin or use insulin inefficiently. Without enough insulin, the glucose stays in your blood. Type 2 diabetes is caused by different factors, including lifestyle factors, some strict diets, overweight, obesity, Hyperthyroidism, and genes.

Pre-diabetes

Even if a person is not sick, it is possible that he suffers from pre-diabetes without knowing it. This term refers to an intermediate stage characterized by an abnormally higher level of blood glucose than usual. This represents a warning signal that informs people with pre-diabetes diagnosis that they are at high risk of developing type 2 diabetes if they don't take appropriate an urgent action, especially if those people have other risk factors: overweight, obesity, sedentary lifestyle, high blood pressure.

IN TYPE 2 DIABETES, the mechanism is different from type 1 diabetes: insulin is normally secreted by the pancreas, but with lower efficiency.

Prevent diabetes and prediabetes with the Keto method

One proven method to prevent diabetes type 2, is to limit your intake of "bad carbs". So, selecting foods based on their glycemic index (GI) or glycemic load (GL) value may help you reduce the risk of diabetes type 2 and manage your weight. The idea behind this method is that many foods that you may include in a low-carb, healthy, well-balanced diet with minimally processed and refined foods have low glycemic index values.

Macronutrient Ratio For Weight Loss

The calories intake matters

THE TWINKIE DIET REFERS TO AN EXPERIMENT CONDUCTED A few years ago by Mark Haub, Professor of nutrition at Kansas State University. Mark Haub set-out to discredit the claim of many diets' specialists, arguing that Calorie-counting is entirely irrelevant and unnecessary for weight-loss. Haub wasn't trying to claim that eating junk-food (cream cakes, cookies, chips, snacks) is beneficial to our health, but he does it only to demonstrate that if the Calories are deficient, weight-loss is possible despite the quality of what a person eats.

Mark Haub was limited to an intake of 1800 Calories a day while his daily requirements are about 2600 Calories, which made a daily caloric deficit of 800 Calories.

AT THE END of the experiment, Mark Haub lost weight as he expected.

- His bodyweight went from 207 down to 174 pounds.

- His body mass index (BMI) dropped from 28.8 (overweight) to 24.9 (normal).

- His LDL (bad cholesterol) dropped by 20%

- His HDL (good cholesterol) increased by 20% His triglycerides (a type of fat (lipid) found in the blood) dropped by 39 percent.

- His body fat went down from 33.4 to 24.9%

THE MAIN CONCLUSION of the experiment is obvious: the caloric deficit works. However, we have to notice that calories are not equal. You have to choose high quality foods and avoid bad carbohydrates.

Calculation of your keto macros

The calculation of your keto diet macros begins by establishing your TDEE (total daily energy expenditure) and setting a Calorie Deficit.

You can skip the explanation given below and use our "advanced keto calculator", which will give you your daily keto macronutrients.

Advanced Keto Calculator: https://www.easyketodiet.net/advanced-keto-calculator/

You can skip this paragraph and use the Advanced Keto Calculator

Before you calculate your ketogenic macros, you must start by setting a Calorie deficit target. We think that 10% is a safe starting point.

Take this example to bring clarity to the calculation method. A moderately active woman, Cherry, who is 30 years old, 5'5", and 180 pounds, will need 2120 Calories per day. That represents her total daily energy expenditure (TDEE).

Calculation of the WLTDE (Weight Loss TDEE) and Calorie deficit

In a 10% Calorie deficit plan, the Weight Loss TDEE (WLTDE) is 1908 Calories. This is calculated by multiplying 90% by her TDEE (2120 Calories) = 1908 Calories.

THE CALORIE DEFICIT equals then to 212 Calories per day. This is calculated by multiplying 10% by the TDEE (2120 Calories) = 212 Calories.

At this stade, Cherry can expect to have 1484 Calories deficit per week. This is calculated by multiplying 7 (days) by her daily Calorie deficit (212 Calories) = 1484 Calories.

She can expect to lose 0.424 pounds per week. This is calculated by dividing the Calorie deficit per week (1484) by 3500, which represent a loss of one pound.

Calculation of the Carbohydrates Quantity?

The ketogenic diet is a low-carb diet, and your daily carbo- hydrates intake must represent 5% of your total daily intake. That means that 5% of your total Calories must come from carbs. For the majority of people, this represents 20 to 30 grams of carbohydrate per day.

Let us pursue our example:

Your normal TDEE= 2120 Calories (This is what the woman' body will burn normally)

Her Calorie deficit= 212 Calories (10%)

Her weight loss TDEE =2120 - 212 = 1908 Calories (what she will eat)

How to calculate the quantity of carbohydrates:

The woman weight loss TDEE is 1.908, 5% of carbs means you should only consume 23.85 g per day. This is calculated by multiplying 5% by 1680 = 95.4. Then divide 95.4 by 4, because there are four calories per gram of carbs.

Calculation of the Proteins Quantity?

Some people on a ketogenic diet make a mistake and consume too much protein.

Your body will convert protein to energy for the body and prevent your body from burning extra fat, which is counterproductive. So to take the maximum advantage of the ketogenic diet, you must limit your daily intake in protein to 20%.

Protein should come mainly from animal meats, full-fat dairy, eggs, and whole food sources.

That means that 20% of your total Calories must come from protein.

Let us pursue our example:

The woman weight loss TDEE is 1.908, 20% of protein means she should only consume 95,4 g per day. This is calculated by multiplying 20% by 1908 = 381,6. Then divide 381,6 by 4, because there are four calories per gram of protein.

Calculation of the Fat Quantity?

The rest of your remaining daily Calories, i.e., 75% daily calories should come from fat.

It's essential that you eat healthy sources of fat and avoid processed fats and some vegetable oils.

The woman weight loss TDEE is 1.908, 75% of fat means she should consume 159 g per day. This is calculated by multiplying 75% by 1908 = 1431. Then divide 1,431 by nine because there are nine calories per gram of fat.

SO FOR A MODERATELY ACTIVE WOMAN, aged 30 years old, 5'5", 180 pounds with a weight loss TDEE of 1908 Calories. The

keto macros are:

Protein: 95,4 grams (20%) Fat: 159 grams (75%) Carbs: 23.85 grams (5%)

ONCE YOU GAIN A BETTER insight and understanding of your individual macronutrient breakdown and keep tracking your Keto macros, you'll see how fast you start to achieve your goals.

Additionally, counting your Keto macronutrients is crucial and will enable you to enter Ketosis much faster.

PART II: Glycemic Index & Glycemic Load

Glycemic index and glycemic load: Overview

Carbohydrate is an essential part of our diets, but not all carbs are equal. The Glycemic Index is an experimental ranking of carbohydrate in foods to measure how slowly or how quickly foods induce rises in blood glucose levels.

There are three classifications for GI:
Individual food portion:
Low: 55 or less
Mid: 56 – 69
High: 70+

How Is Glycemic Index Measured?
 Glycemic Index values of foods are measured using valid and proven scientific methods, and cannot be guessed just by looking at the composition of a given food or the nutrition facts on food packaging.

Thus, the GI calculation Follows the international standard method, and provides values that are commonly accepted. The Glycemic Index value of a food is calculated by feeding over than ten healthy people a portion of the food object of the study and containing fifty grams of digestible carbohydrate and then measuring the effect for each participant on his blood glucose levels (blood glucose response) over the next two hours.
The second part of the process consists of giving the same participants an equal carbohydrate portion of the glucose (used as the reference food) and measuring their blood glucose response over the next two hours.
 The Glycemic Index value for the food is then calculated for each participant by using a simple formula (dividing the blood glucose response for the food by their blood glucose response for the glucose (reference food)). The final value of the Glycemic Index for the food is the average Glycemic Index value for the participants (over 10).

Carbohydrates with a low GI value (55 or less) are more slowly digested, absorbed, and metabolized and cause a smaller and slower rise in blood glucose and, therefore, usually, insulin levels.

Low glycemic diet or foods are associated with reduced risk of chronic disease. Foods that have low glycemic index are known for their property to release glucose in the blood slowly and regularly. Conversely, Foods that have a high glycemic index are known for their property to release glucose rapidly. Researches suggest that foods with a low glycemic index (LGI foods) are ideal for weight loss diets and foster lasting weight loss, in addition to their positive effect on the pancreas (insulin release), eyes, and kidney.

The glycemic index (GI) is formed by scale from 1 to 100. Each food gets a score on this scale according to experimental data. **A lower score indicates that food takes longer time to raise the blood sugar levels.**

Glycemic Load is another critical tool to track carbohydrates quality and quantity. Glycemic Load (GL) combines both the quality and amount of carbohydrates following a simple formula:

Glycemic Load (GL) = GI x Carbohydrate (grams) content per portion ÷ 100

For example, an apple has a GI of 32 and contains 13 grams of carbohydrates.
GL= 32 x 13/100 = 3

Sweet potato has a GL of 11. So, We can predict that sweet potato will have the more glycemic effect of an apple (approximately four times).
Like the glycemic index, the glycemic load (GL) of a food can be classified as:
- **Low:** 10 or less
- **Medium:** 11 – 19
- **High:** 20 or more

For an effective Glycemic Index / Glycemic load diet, we recommend you to eat daily the equivalent of 100 in glycemic load. However, following this target can be struggling and sometimes impossible due to the lack of data. The Process of measuring the glycemic index is expensive, time-consuming, and complicated.

To bypass this difficulty, you must mainly use the Net carb grams tables provided for 7000 foods covering the majority of foods we eat. Thus, you can easily monitor your daily carb intake to keep it within the strict limits recommended by your diet.

The data provided in this book comes mainly from the international database of the glycemic index. This database is managed by the team of Dr Jennie Brand-Miller, the Australian researcher who has been since 1981 at the forefront of the glycemic index science.

The International database of the glycemic index is hosted by the University of Sydney and gathers all the data published in the scientific journals and the measurements carried out by the Australian researchers within the Department of Human Nutrition of the University of Sydney.

You can use our "glycemic index counter" if you want to have the GI & GL values for a given food, in the following address: https://www.easyketodiet.net/glycemic-index-counter/

Low Glycemic Index Foods Tables

Food Name	GI	Serving (g)	GL
3 Grain Bread, sprouted grains	55	30	5
45% oat bran and 50% wheat flour bread	50	30	9
50% oat bran bread	44	30	8
9-Grain Multi-Grain bread	43	30	6
American, easy-cook rice, consumed with 10 g margarine	49	150	22
Apple and blackcurrant juice, no added sugar	45	250	11
Apple and cherry juice, pure, unsweetened	43	250	14
Apple and mango juice, pure, unsweetened	47	250	16
Apple blueberry muffin	49	60	12
Apple juice, Granny Smith, unsweetened	44	250	13
Apple juice, pure, clear, unsweetened	44	250	13
Apple juice, pure, cloudy, unsweetened	37	250	11
Apple juice, unsweetened, reconstituted	39	250	10
Apple muffin, made with rolled oats and sugar	44	60	13
Apple muffin, made with rolled oats and without sugar	48	60	9
Apple, raw	36 ± 4	120	5
Apple, raw, Golden Delicious	39 ± 2	120	6
Apricot & apple fruit strips, gluten-free	29 ± 4	20	5
Apricot 100% Pure Fruit spread, no added sugar	43 ± 3	30	7
Apricot dried fruit snack	42 ± 4	15	5
Apricot fruit spread, reduced sugar	55 ± 2	30	7
Apricot halves canned in fruit juice	51 ± 4	120	6
Apricot, raw	34 ± 2	120	3
Apricots, dried	30 ± 2	60	8
Arepa, made from white corn meal flour	53 ± 2	100	19
Aussie Bodies Start the Day UHT, Choc Banana flavored drink	24 ± 3	250	4

Food Name	GI	Serving (g)	GL
Aussie Bodies Start the Day UHT, Chocolate flavored drink	26 ± 3	250	4
Aussie Bodies Trim Protein Shake, Chocolate flavoured beverage	39 ± 3	250	5
Aussie Bodies Trim Protein Shake, French Vanilla flavoured beverage	41 ± 2	250	5
Bakers Delight™ Hi Fibre Lo GI white bread	52 ± 2	30	8
Bakers Delight™ Wholemeal Country Grain bread	53 ± 2	30	6
Banana cake, made with sugar	47 ± 2	60	14
Banana cake, made without sugar	55 ± 2	60	12
Banana, over-ripe	52 ± 2	120	11
Banana, over-ripe (yellow flecked with brown)	48 ± 3	120	12
Banana, raw	47 ± 2	120	11
Banana, ripe (all yellow)	51 ± 2	120	13
Banana, slightly under-ripe (yellow with green sections)	42 ± 2	120	11
Banana, under-ripe	30 ± 2	120	6
Barley	23 ± 4	150	11
Barley kernels, high-amylose (covered), boiled in water for 25 min (kernel:water = 1:2)	26 ± 2	150	11
Barley kernels, high-amylose (hull-less) boiled in water for 25 min	20 ± 2	150	8
Barley kernels, waxy (hull-less), boiled in water for 25 min	22 ± 3	150	9
Barley, cracked (Malthouth, Tunisia)	50 ± 2	150	21
Barley, pearled	22 ± 3	150	9
Barley, pearled	29 ± 3	150	12
Barley, pearled, boiled 60 min	35 ± 2	150	15
Basmati, white rice, boiled 12 min	52 ± 2	150	15
Basmati, white rice, boiled, with 10 g margarine	43 ± 2	150	18
Blueberry muffin	50 ± 2	60	15
Breakfast Marmalade 100% Fruit Spread, Cottees™ brand	55 ± 3	30	10
Brown & Wild rice, Uncle Ben's® Ready Whole Grain Medley™ (pouch)	45 ± 3	150	18

Food Name	GI	Serving (g)	GL
Brown & Wild rice, Uncle Ben's® Ready Whole Grain Medley™ (pouch)	45 ± 2	150	18
Brown rice, steamed	50 ± 1	150	16
Brown Rice, Uncle Ben's® Ready Whole Grain (pouch)	48 ± 2	150	20
Buckwheat groats, hydrothermally treated, dehusked, boiled 12 min	45 ± 3	150	13
Buckwheat noodles, instant	53 ± 2	180	22
Build-Up™ nutrient-fortified drink, vanilla with fibre	41 ± 3	250	13
Butternut pumpkin, boiled	51 ± 2	80	3
Capellini pasta	45 ± 3	180	20
Capilano Premium Honey, blend of eucalypt & floral honeys	51 ± 2	25	11
Carrot cake, prepared with coconut flour	36 ± 2	60	8
Carrot juice, freshly made	43 ± 2	250	10
Carrot soup, President's Choice® Blue Menu™ Soupreme	35 ± 3	250	5
Carrots, peeled, boiled	33 ± 2	80	2
Carrots, raw, diced	35 ± 2	80	2
Carrots, raw, ground	39 ± 4	80	2
Cashew nut halves	27 ± 2	50	3
Cashew nuts	25 ± 2	50	3
Cashew nuts, organic, roasted and salted	25 ± 2	50	3
Cashew nuts, roasted and salted	27 ± 2	50	3
Cereal bar, cranberry flavor	42 ± 3	30	6
Cereal bar, hazelnut flavor	33 ± 3	30	4
Cereal bar, orange flavor	33 ± 3	30	5
Cereal biscuit (30 g), cocoa flavor wheat biscuits consumed with 125 mL skim milk	46 ± 3	155	12
Cereal biscuit (30 g), honey flavor wheat biscuits consumed with 125 mL skim milk	52 ± 3	155	14
Cereal biscuit (30 g), wheat based biscuits consumed with 125 mL skim milk	47 ± 3	155	12
Cherries, raw, sour	22 ± 2	120	3

Food Name	GI	Serving (g)	GL
Chicken Flavored Brown Rice, Uncle Ben's® Ready Whole Grain (pouch)	46 ± 3	150	18
Chicken Flavored Brown Rice, Uncle Ben's® Ready Whole Grain (pouch)	46 ± 3	150	18
Chicken McNuggets™ consumed with sweet Thai chilli sauce	55 ± 3	100	12
Chicken nuggets, frozen, reheated in microwave oven 5 min	46 ± 3	100	7
Chicken tikka masala and rice, convenience meal	34 ± 3	300	21
Chilli beef noodles, prepared convenience meal	42 ± 3	300	19
Chilli con carne, made from haricot beans	34 ± 3	300	12
Chocolate butterscotch muffin	53 ± 2	50	15
Chocolate cake made from packet mix with chocolate frosting	38 ± 3	111	20
Chocolate candy, sugar free, artificially sweetened, Dove®	23 ± 2	50	3
Chocolate chip muffin	52 ± 3	60	17
Chocolate crinkles, containing coconut flour	43 ± 3	50	10
Chocolate Daydream™ shake, fructose, Revival Soy®	33 ± 3	250	6
Chocolate Daydream™ shake, sucralose, Revival Soy®	25 ± 3	250	1
Chocolate pudding, instant, made from powder and whole milk	47 ± 2	100	7
Chocolate, dark with raisins, peanuts and jam	44 ± 3	50	12
Chocolate, dark, Dove®	23 ± 4	50	6
Chocolate, plain	42 ± 4	50	13
Chocolate, plain with sucrose	34 ± 3	50	7
Citrus, reduced-fat mousse, prepared from commercial mousse mix with water	47 ± 2	50	14
Coarse rye kernel bread, 80% intact kernels and 20% white wheat flour	41 ± 3	30	5
Coarse wheat kernel bread, 80% intact kernels and 20% white wheat flour	52 ± 2	30	10
Cocoavia™ Chocolate Covered Almonds, artificially sweetened	21 ± 3	30	2
Coconut sugar	54 ± 1	5	3
Continental fruit loaf, wheat bread with dried fruit	47 ± 2	30	7

Food Name	GI	Serving (g)	GL
Corn granules	52 ± 1	150	15
Corn tortilla	52 ± 1	50	12
Corn tortilla, made from white corn, Diego's brand	49 ± 3	50	11
Corn tortilla, served with refried mashed pinto beans and tomato sauce	39 ± 2	100	9
Country Grain Organic Rye bread	53 ± 2	30	5
Cranberry & Orange Soy muffin, President's Choice® Blue Menu™	48 ± 2	70	14
Cranberry juice cocktail	52 ± 1	250	16
Crème fraiche dessert, peach	28 ± 1	150	7
Crème fraiche dessert, raspberry	30 ± 1	150	5
Crusty malted wheat bread	52 ± 1	30	7
Double chocolate muffin	46 ± 2	60	16
English Muffin bread, Whole Grain Multigrain, President's Choice® Blue Menu™	45 ± 3	30	5
Fettucine, egg	32 ± 1	180	15
Fish fingers	38 ± 1	100	7
Fromage Frais, red fruit: blackcurrant	22 ± 1	100	2
Fromage Frais, red fruit: raspberry	31 ± 1	100	2
Fromage Frais, red fruit: red cherry	25 ± 1	100	2
Fructose, 25 g portion, Sweeten Less	11	10	1
Fructose, 50 g portion	20	10	2
Fructose, 50 g portion	23	10	2
Fructose, 50 g portion, Sweeten Less	12	10	1
Fruit and Spice Loaf bread, thick sliced	54 ± 1	30	8
Fusilli pasta twists, boiled 10 min in salted water, served with cheddar cheese	27 ± 2	0	0
Fusilli pasta twists, boiled 10 min in salted water, served with canned tuna	28 ± 2	0	0
Fusilli pasta twists, boiled 10 min in salted water, served with chilli con carne	40 ± 3	0	0

Food Name	GI	Serving (g)	GL
Fusilli pasta twists, dry pasta, boiled in 10 min in unsalted water	54 ± 1	180	26
Fusilli pasta twists, tricolour, dry pasta, boiled 10 min in unsalted water	51 ± 1	180	23
Fusilli pasta twists, wholewheat, dry pasta, boiled 10 min in unsalted water	55 ± 1	180	23
Gluten Free Low GI White bread	53	30	4
Gluten-free pasta, maize starch, boiled 8 min	54 ± 1	180	23
Gluten-free pasta, maize starch, boiled 8 min	54 ± 1	180	23
Golden Hearth™ Organic Heavy Wholegrain bread	53 ± 1	30	7
Grapefruit, raw	25 ± 2	120	3
Grapefruit, ruby red segments, canned in juice	47 ± 2	120	10
Grapes, raw	45 ± 4	120	7
Green banana, peeled, boiled 10 min	37 ± 2	120	10
Ground beef served with rice and an orange	31 ± 2	300	24
Haricot beans, home-cooked, soaked overnight, boiled 1h in water, baked in tomato sauce 2h	23 ± 2	150	7
Haricot/Navy beans	39 ± 2	150	12
Haricot/Navy beans, boiled	31 ± 2	150	9
Hazelnut, 2.4% fat mousse, prepared from commercial mousse mix with water	36 ± 2	50	4
Healthy Choice™ Hearty 7 Grain bread	55 ± 1	30	8
Honey Crunch cereal (30 g), consumed with 125 mL skim milk	54 ± 2	155	16
Honey, Iron Bark (34% fructose)	48 ± 1	25	7
Honey, Red Gum (35% fructose)	46 ± 1	25	8
Honey, Stringy Bark (52% fructose)	44 ± 1	25	9
Honey, Yapunya (42 % fructose)	52 ± 1	25	9
Honey, Yellow box (46% fructose)	35 ± 1	25	6
Hot oat cereal (30 g) prepared with 125 mL skim milk	47 ± 1	155	11
Hot oat cereal (30 g), berry flavor prepared with 125 mL skim milk	43 ± 1	155	11

Food Name	GI	Serving (g)	GL
Hot oat cereal (30 g), cocoa flavor prepared with 125 mL skim milk	40 ± 1	155	9
Hot oat cereal (30 g), fruit flavor prepared with 125 mL skim milk	47 ± 1	155	12
Hot oat cereal (30 g), honey flavor prepared with 125 mL skim milk	47 ± 1	155	12
Hot oat cereal (30 g), orchard fruit flavor prepared with 125 mL skim milk	50 ± 1	155	12
Ice cream, low-fat, Bulla Light Creamy vanilla	36 ± 1	50	7
Ice cream, low-fat, Bulla Light Real Dairy chocolate	27 ± 1	50	3
Ice cream, low-fat, Bulla Light Real Dairy mango	30	50	4
Ice cream, low-fat, Light & Creamy, Raspberry Ripple	55 ± 1	50	9
Ice cream, low-fat, vanilla, 'Light'	46 ± 2	50	7
Instant 'two-minute' noodles, Maggi® (Nestlé, Auckland, New Zealand)	48 ± 2	180	12
Instant 'two-minute' noodles, Maggi® (Nestlé, Australia) (1995)	46 ± 2	180	11
Instant 'two-minute' noodles, Maggi®, all flavors (Nestlé Australia) (2005)	52 ± 2	180	13
Instant noodles, all flavors (Woolworths Limited, Australia)	52 ± 2	180	11
Instant rice, white, cooked 3 min	46 ± 3	150	19
Kidney beans	29 ± 2	150	7
Kiwi fruit, Hayward	47 ± 2	120	6
Lasagne sheets, dry pasta, boiled in unsalted water for 10 min	55 ± 2	180	26
Lasagne, egg, dry pasta, boiled in unsalted water for 10 min	53 ± 2	180	23
Lasagne, egg, verdi, dry pasta, boiled in unsalted water for 10 min	52 ± 2	180	23
Lemonade, Scheweppes®, lemon soft drink	54 ± 4	250	15
Lentils, brown, canned, drained, Edgell's™ brand	42 ± 2	150	9
Lentils, green, dried, boiled	37 ± 2	150	5
Lentils, red, split, dried, boiled 25 min	21 ± 2	150	4
Lentils, raw	29 ± 2	150	5

Food Name	GI	Serving (g)	GL
Long Grain and Wild, Jasmine rice, Uncle Ben's® Ready Rice (pouch)	49 ± 3	150	21
Long Grain and Wild, Jasmine rice, Uncle Ben's® Ready Rice (pouch)	49 ± 3	150	21
Long grain rice quick-cooking variety, white, pre-cooked, microwaved 2 min, Express Rice, plain	52 ± 3	150	19
Long grain rice quick-cooking variety, white, pre-cooked, microwaved 2 min, Express Rice, plain	52 ± 3	150	19
Low-fat yoghurt, apricot	42 ± 1	200	12
Low-fat yoghurt, black cherry	41 ± 1	200	11
Low-fat yoghurt, hazelnut	53 ± 1	200	15
Low-fat yoghurt, Nestlé Diet Mixed Berry	28 ± 1	200	3
Low-fat yoghurt, Nestlé Diet Peaches & Cream	28 ± 1	200	3
Low-fat yoghurt, raspberry	34 ± 1	200	10
LU P'tit Déjeuner Chocolat cookies	42 ± 3	50	14
LU P'tit Déjeuner Miel et Pépites Chocolat cookies	45 ± 3	50	16
LU P'tit Déjeuner Miel et Pépites Chocolat cookies	49 ± 3	50	18
LU P'tit Déjeuner Miel et Pépites Chocolat cookies	52 ± 3	50	18
LU Petit Dejeuner Cereals & Chocolate Chips, low in sugar cookies	37 ± 3	50	13
LU Petit Dejeuner Chocolate & Cereals cookies	46 ± 3	50	16
LU Petit Dejeuner Coconut, nuts and chocolate cookies	51 ± 3	50	17
LU Petit Dejeuner Coconut, nuts and chocolate cookies	55 ± 3	50	19
LU Petit Dejeuner Fruits and Muesli cookies	45 ± 3	50	16
LU Petit Dejeuner Fruits and Muesli cookies	47 ± 3	50	17
LU Petit Dejeuner Fruits and Muesli cookies	49 ± 3	50	18
LU Petit Dejeuner Honey & Chocolate chips cookies	46 ± 3	50	16
LU Petit Dejeuner Honey & Chocolate chips cookies	47 ± 3	50	17
LU Petit Dejeuner Milk and Cereals cookies	39 ± 3	50	13
LU Petit Dejeuner Milk and Cereals cookies	55 ± 3	50	19
LU Petit Dejeuner Multicereals cookies	46 ± 3	50	16

Food Name	GI	Serving (g)	GL
LU Petit Dejeuner with Fruits and Figs cookies	41 ± 3	50	14
LU Petit Dejeuner with Prunes cookies	51 ± 3	50	17
LU Petit Dejeuner, Chocolate, low in sugar cookies	51 ± 3	50	18
Mandarin segments, canned in juice	47 ± 2	120	6
Mango, raw	41 ± 2	120	8
Mango, 1.8% fat mousse, prepared from commercial mousse mix with water	33 ± 2	50	4
Mango, low-fat frozen fruit dessert, Frutia™	42 ± 2	100	10
Marmalade, orange	48 ± 2	30	9
Marmalade, orange 100% Pure Fruit spread, no added sugar	27 ± 2	30	4
Mars Active® Energy Drink, flavored milk	46 ± 3	250	15
Milk, full-fat/whole	36 ± 4	250	4
Milk, reduced fat	30 ± 4	250	4
Milk, semi-skimmed	32 ± 2	250	4
Milk, skim	32 ± 2	250	4
Mixed berry, 2.2% fat mousse, prepared from commercial mousse mix with water	36 ± 2	50	4
Mixed nuts and raisins	21 ± 2	50	3
Mixed nuts, roasted and salted	24 ± 2	50	4
Moolgiri white rice	54 ± 2	150	17
Muesli, gluten-free with 1.5% fat milk (125 mL)	39 ± 2	30	7
Muesli, toasted	43 ± 2	30	7
Muesli, Wheat free, consumed with 150 mL semi-skimmed milk	49 ± 2	30	9
Muesli, yeast & wheat free	45 ± 2	30	4
Muffin, plain, made from wheat flour	46 ± 2	50	11
Muffin, reduced-fat, low-calorie, made from high-amylose corn starch and maltitol	37 ± 3	50	9
Multigrain (50% kibbled wheat grain) bread	43 ± 2	30	6
Multigrain Loaf bread, spelt wheat flour	54 ± 2	30	8

Food Name	GI	Serving (g)	GL
Multigrain porridge, containing rolled oats, wheat, triticale, rye, barley and rice, cooked with water	55 ± 2	250	19
Multiseed bread	54 ± 2	30	7
Nectarines, raw	43 ± 2	120	4
Oat porridge made from roasted thick (1.0 mm)	50 ± 1	250	14
Oat porridge made from steamed thick (1.0 mm) dehulled oat flakes	53 ± 1	250	14
Orange & Grapefruit segments, canned in juice	53 ± 2	120	10
Orange Delight Cocktail beverage with pulp, President's Choice® Blue Menu™	44 ± 2	250	7
Orange juice	46 ± 2	250	12
Orange juice, unsweetened, reconstituted concentrate, Commercial brand	54 ± 2	250	11
Orange, raw	38 ± 7	120	7
Original Long Grain, Jasmine rice, Uncle Ben's® Ready Rice (pouch)	48 ± 3	150	22
Original Long Grain, Jasmine rice, Uncle Ben's® Ready Rice (pouch)	48 ± 3	150	22
Pancakes, prepared with coconut flour	46 ± 3	80	10
Pasta bake, tomato and mozzarella	23 ± 3	300	10
Peach & Grapes, canned in natural fruit juice	46 ± 2	120	6
Peach & pear fruit strips, gluten-free	29 ± 2	20	3
Peach & Pineapple, canned in natural fruit juice	45 ± 2	120	6
Peach, canned in light syrup	52 ± 2	120	9
Peach, canned in natural juice	45 ± 2	120	5
Peach, dried	35 ± 2	60	8
Peach, raw	28 ± 2	120	4
Peanuts, crushed	7 ± 2	50	0
Pear halves, canned in natural juice	43 ± 2	120	5
Pear, dried	43 ± 2	60	12
Pear, raw	33 ± 4	120	4

Food Name	GI	Serving (g)	GL
Pineapple, raw	51 ± 2	120	8
Pineapple & Papaya pieces, canned in natural juice	53 ± 2	120	9
Pineapple pieces, canned in natural fruit juice	55 ± 2	120	10
Ploughman's™ Wholegrain bread, original recipe	47 ± 2	30	6
Plum, raw	40 ± 2	120	7
Popcorn	55 ± 2	20	6
Porridge oats, made from rolled oats	50 ± 2	250	10
Porridge, jumbo oats, consumed with 150 mL semi-skimmed milk	40 ± 2	250	9
Porridge, made from rolled oats	55 ± 2	250	13
Potato crisps, plain, salted	51 ± 2	50	12
Pound cake	38 ± 2	60	9
Proti pasta, protein-enriched, boiled in water	28 ± 2	180	14
Prune juice	43 ± 2	250	15
Prunes, pitted	29 ± 2	60	10
Quinoa, cooked, refrigerated, reheated in microwave for 1.5 min	53 ± 2	150	13
Raisin Bran Flax muffin, President's Choice® Blue Menu™	52 ± 3	70	17
Raisins	49 ± 2	28	10
Raspberry 100% Pure Fruit spread, no added sugar	26 ± 2	25	3
Seeded bread	49 ± 2	30	6
Sliced Apples, canned, solid packed without juice	42 ± 2	120	4
Slim Fast™ French Vanilla ready-to-drink shake	37 ± 2	250	10
Smoothie drink soy, banana	30 ± 4	250	7
Smoothie drink, banana	30 ± 4	250	8
Smoothie drink, banana and strawberry, V8 Splash®	44 ± 4	250	11
Smoothie drink, mango	32 ± 4	250	9
Smoothie drink, raspberry	33 ± 4	250	14
Soy Crunch Multi-Grain Cereal, President's Choice® Blue Menu™	47 ± 3	30	9

Food Name	GI	Serving (g)	GL
Soy milk, full-fat (3%), 120 mg calcium, Calciforte	41 ± 3	250	6
Soy milk, full-fat (3%), Calciforte, 120 mg calcium, with maltodextrin	36 ± 3	250	6
Soy milk, full-fat (3%), Original, 0 mg calcium, with maltodextrin	44 ± 3	250	8
Spaghetti bolognaise, home made	52 ± 2	360	25
Spaghetti, white, boiled	42 ± 3	180	18
Strawberries, fresh, raw	40 ± 3	120	1
Strawberry & wildberry dried fruit leather, Sunripe School Straps	40 ± 3	30	8
Strawberry & wildberry dried fruit leather, Sunripe School Straps	40 ± 3	30	8
Strawberry fruit leather	29 ± 3	30	7
SuperJuice Kickstart, containing apple juice, blueberry puree and banana puree	39 ± 3	250	11
Sushi, roasted sea algae, vinegar and rice	55 ± 3	100	20
Sushi, salmon	48 ± 3	100	17
Sweet and sour chicken with noodles, prepared convenience meal	41 ± 3	300	21
Sweet corn	55 ± 3	80	9
Sweet corn on the cob, boiled 20 min	48 ± 3	80	8
Sweet corn, cooked	52 ± 3	150	17
Sweet corn, frozen, reheated in microwave	47 ± 3	150	16
Sweet potato, boiled	44 ± 3	150	11
Tagliatelle, egg pasta, boiled in water for 7 min	46 ± 3	180	20
Tandoori chicken masala & rice convenience meal	45 ± 2	300	27
Tomato juice, no added sugar	33 ± 5	250	3
Tomato soup	38 ± 2	250	6
Tropical dried fruit snack	41 ± 4	15	5
Tuna fish bun	46 ± 4	87	14
V8 Splash®, tropical blend fruit drink	47 ± 3	250	13

Food Name	GI	Serving (g)	GL
V8® 100% vegetable juice	43 ± 3	250	4
Vanilla cake, made from packet mix with vanilla frosting	42 ± 3	111	24
Vanilla pudding, instant, made from powder and whole milk	40 ± 3	100	6
Vermicelli pasta, white, boiled	35 ± 3	180	16
White bread, homemade, frozen, defrosted and toasted	52 ± 2	30	7
White rice, boiled	43 ± 4	150	16
White wheat flour bread, butter, cheese, regular milk and fresh cucumber	55 ± 3	200	37
Whole-wheat bread with dried fruit	47 ± 3	30	7
Wholegrain water crackers with sesame seeds and rosemary	53 ± 3	25	8
Wholemeal (whole wheat) bread	50 ± 3	30	6
Wild berry dried fruit snack	35 ± 2	15	4
Wild Oats Cluster Crunch Hazelnut Chocolate breakfast cereal	43 ± 3	30	8
Xpress beverage, chocolate (soy bean, cereal and legume extract drink with fructose)	39 ± 3	250	13
Yam	51 ± 3	150	18

Moderate Glycemic Index Foods Tables

Food Name	GI	Serving (g)	GL
100% Whole wheat Burger Buns	62 ± 2	30	7
100% Whole wheat Hot Dog Rolls	62 ± 3	30	7
All-Bran Wheat Flakes™ breakfast cereal	60 ± 2	30	12
Apricot, coconut and honey muffin	60 ± 3	50	16
Apricot, raw	57 ± 2	120	5
Apricots, canned in light syrup	64 ± 3	120	12
Bagel, white bread	69 ± 3	70	24
Baked Beans in Tomato sauce, canned, reheated in microwave for 1.5 min	57 ± 2	150	13
Banana, oat and honey muffin	65 ± 2	50	17
Banana, raw	58 ± 2	120	13
Barley flakes breakfast cereal	69 ± 4	30	14
Barley flour bread, 100% barley flour	67 ± 3	30	9
Barley, rolled	66 ± 3	50	25
Basmati, easy cook white rice, boiled 9 min	67 ± 3	150	28
Basmati, easy-cook white rice, consumed with 10 g margarine	68 ± 3	150	28
Basmati, white rice, organic, boiled 10 min	57 ± 3	150	23
Beer, Toohey's New	66 ± 3	250	5
Blueberry (Wild) 10-Grain muffin, President's Choice® Blue Menu™	57 ± 3	70	22
Blueberry muffin	59 ± 3	57	17
Bran Flakes breakfast cereal	65 ± 3	30	12
Bran muffin	60 ± 3	57	14
Bread, flax, made from flax meal & wheat flour	67 ± 3	30	8
Breadfruit, raw	68 ± 2	120	18
Brown rice	66 ± 3	150	22
Buckwheat bread	67 ± 3	30	13

Food Name	GI	Serving (g)	GL
Carrot muffin	62 ± 3	57	20
Cereal biscuit (30 g), fruit flavor wheat biscuits consumed with 125 mL skim milk	56 ± 2	155	15
Cherries, dark, raw, pitted	63 ± 3	120	9
Chicken and mushroom soup	69 ± 2	250	13
Chickpea flour bread, made from extruded chickpea flour	67 ± 2	30	8
Classic French baguette bread with 10 g butter and 2 slices of ham (25 g)	59 ± 3	100	25
Clover honey, ratio of fructose: glucose, 1.09	69 ± 2	25	15
Coarse oat kernel bread, 80% intact oat kernels and 20% white wheat flour	65 ± 3	30	13
Coca Cola®, soft drink	63 ± 3	250	16
Coco yam (Xanthosoma spp.), peeled, cubed, boiled 30 min	61 ± 3	150	28
Cocoa Crunch cereal (30 g), consumed with 125 mL skim milk	58 ± 3	155	16
Cordial, orange, reconstituted	66 ± 2	250	13
Corn pasta, gluten-free, Orgran brand	68 ± 3	180	31
Cornmeal + margarine	69 ± 3	150	8
Cornmeal porridge	68 ± 3	150	9
Cornmeal, boiled in salted water 2 min	68 ± 2	150	9
Cottage pie	65 ± 2	300	22
Couscous, boiled 5 min	63 ± 4	150	21
Cranberry juice cocktail	68 ± 3	250	24
Cranberry juice drink	56 ± 3	250	16
Creamed rice porridge	59 ± 3	75	5
Dates	62 ± 3	60	21
Digestives, cookies	59 ± 2	25	9
Fanta®, orange soft drink	68 ± 3	250	23
Fibre First Multi-Bran Cereal, President's Choice® Blue Menu™	56 ± 3	30	6
Figs, dried, tenderised, Dessert Maid brand	61 ± 3	60	16

Food Name	GI	Serving (g)	GL
Fillet-O-Fish™ burger (fish patty, cheese and tartare sauce on a burger bun)	66 ± 3	128	20
Flan cake (Weston's Bakery, Toronto, Canada)	65 ± 3	70	31
French baguette bread with butter and strawberry jam	62 ± 3	70	26
Fruit and Fibre breakfast cereal	68 ± 3	30	13
Fruit loaf bread, sliced	57 ± 3	30	9
Fruit punch beverage	67 ± 3	250	19
Fruity-Bix™ bar, wheat biscuit cereal with dried fruit and nuts with yoghurt coating	56 ± 3	30	11
Fusilli pasta twists, boiled 10 min in salted water	61 ± 3	180	29
Glucose, 50 g portion, consumed with 14.5 g guar gum	62	10	6
Gnocchi, type not specified (Latina, Pillsbury Australia Ltd, Mt. Waverley, Australia)	68 ± 4	180	33
Granola Clusters breakfast cereal, Original, low fat, President's Choice® Blue Menu™	63 ± 2	30	14
Grany Rush Apricot, digestive cookies	62 ± 2	30	12
Grapes, black, Waltham Cross	59 ± 2	120	11
Hamburger (beef patty, ketchup, pickle, onion and mustard on a burger bun)	66 ± 4	95	17
Hamburger bun	61 ± 3	30	9
Happiness™ bread, cinnamon, raisin, pecan bread	63 ± 2	30	9
Healthwise™ for bowel health breakfast cereal	66 ± 2	30	12
Honey, Commercial Blend (38% fructose)	62 ± 2	25	11
Honey, Pure	58 ± 3	25	12
Honey, Pure	58 ± 3	25	12
Honey, Salvation Jane (32% fructose)	64 ± 3	25	10
Hunger Filler™, whole grain bread	59 ± 2	30	7
Ice cream (half vanilla, half chocolate), regular/type not specified	57 ± 2	50	6
Instant porridge	69 ± 2	250	14
Kiwi fruit	58 ± 2	120	7

Food Name	GI	Serving (g)	GL
Lean beef burger (lean beef patty, tomato, mixed lettuce, cheese, onion and sauce on a burger bun)	66 ± 4	164	17
Lentil and cauliflower cury with rice	60 ± 2	300	25
Low-fat yoghurt, peach melba	56 ± 2	200	16
Low-fat yoghurt, strawberry	61 ± 2	200	18
LU Petit Dejeuner Chocolate & Cereals cookies	58 ± 3	50	20
Macaroni, boiled	56 ± 2	180	27
Mars Bar® (M&M / Mars, USA)	68 ± 3	60	27
Marshmallows	62 ± 2	30	15
McChicken™ burger (chicken patty, lettuce, mayonnaise on a burger bun)	66 ± 2	186	26
Oro cookies	61 ± 3	40	21
Pastry	59 ± 3	57	15
Peach, canned in heavy syrup	64 ± 3	120	12
Peach, raw	56 ± 2	120	5
Pineapple, raw	66 ± 2	120	6
Pita bread, white	67 ± 2	30	10
Pita bread, white (Sainsbury's, UK), with 5 g margarine	67 ± 2	30	10
Pita bread, wholemeal	56 ± 2	30	8
Pizza, cheese	60 ± 2	100	16
Porridge, made from rolled oats	63 ± 2	250	19
Potato, type not specified, boiled	66 ± 2	150	13
Potato, white with skin, baked, consumed with 10 g margarine	69 ± 2	150	19
Potato, white, cooked	61 ± 2	150	16
Probiotic yoghurt drink, cranberry	56 ± 2	250	17
Raisins	66 ± 2	60	28
Soy Tasty™ breakfast cereal (flaked grains, soy nuts, dried fruit)	60 ± 2	30	12
Spaghetti, white, durum wheat, boiled 20 min	58 ± 3	180	26
Special K™ breakfast cereal	69 ± 3	30	14

Food Name	GI	Serving (g)	GL
Sugar (Sucrose), 100 g portion	65	10	7
Sunflower and barley bread	57 ± 2	30	6
Sweet corn	62 ± 2	80	11
Sweet corn, boiled	60 ± 2	80	11
Traditional French baguette (prepared with wheat flour, water, salt and 20 g yeast)	69 ± 2	30	12
Vegetable soup	60 ± 2	250	11
White bread with added wheatgerm and fiber	59 ± 2	30	6
White bread with butter	59 ± 2	100	28
White bread, fresh, toasted	63 ± 2	30	8
White bread, homemade, fresh, toasted	66 ± 2	30	9
White bread, wheat flour	69 ± 2	30	10
White bread, wheat flour, frozen, defrosted and toasted	64 ± 2	30	8
Wholemeal bread, stoneground flour	59 ± 1	30	7
Yoghurt, black cherry	67 ± 3	200	8
Yoghurt, bourbon vanilla	64 ± 3	200	20
Yoghurt, lemon curd	67 ± 3	200	30
Yoghurt, peach melba	57 ± 3	200	18

High Glycemic Index Foods Tables

Food Name	GI	Serving (g)	GL
15 g Oat bran (containing 2 g ß-glucan), consumed as a drink mixed with 41g glucose and water	84 ± 3	10	2
Bagel, white, frozen (Lender's Bakery, Montreal, Canada)	72 ± 3	70	25
Baguette, white, plain	95 ± 2	30	14
Barley flour bread, made from 50% wheat flour and 50% coarse sieved barley flour	74 ± 3	30	12
Barquette Abricot cookies	71 ± 4	40	23
Blackbread, Riga	76 ± 3	30	10
Bran Flakes™ breakfast cereal	74 ± 4	30	13
Bread stuffing, Paxo	74 ± 3	30	16
Breadfruit roasted on preheated charcoal	72 ± 3	120	20
Broken rice, white, cooked in rice cooker	86 ± 3	150	37
Brown rice	87 ± 2	150	29
Brown rice, boiled in excess water for 25 min, SunRice brand	72 ± 3	150	29
Brown rice, boiled in excess water for 25 min, SunRice brand	72 ± 3	150	29
Cheerios™ breakfast cereal	74 ± 4	30	15
Chicken Tandoori Deli Choice white French roll white bread	78 ± 3	270	44
Chocapic™ breakfast cereal, wheat-based flaked cereal	70 ± 4	30	17
Coco Pops™ breakfast cereal (cocoa flavored puffed rice)	77 ± 4	30	20
Corn Bran™ breakfast cereal	75 ± 4	30	15
Corn Chex™ breakfast cereal	83 ± 4	30	21
Corn pasta, gluten-free, Orgran brand	78 ± 2	180	32
Corn Pops™ breakfast cereal	80 ± 4	30	21
Cornflakes breakfast cereal	79 ± 4	30	20
Cornflakes breakfast cereal (Kellogg's, France)	93 ± 4	30	25
Cornflakes breakfast cereal consumed with 150 mL semi-skimmed milk	93 ± 4	30	23
Cornflakes, Crunchy Nut™ breakfast cereal	72 ± 4	30	17

Food Name	GI	Serving (g)	GL
Cornflakes™ breakfast cereal	77 ± 4	30	19
Cornflakes™ breakfast cereal	80 ± 4	30	21
Cornflakes™ breakfast cereal (Kellogg's Inc., Canada)	86 ± 4	30	22
Cornflakes™ breakfast cereal (Kellogg's, USA)	92 ± 4	30	24
Cotton honey, ratio of fructose:glucose, 1.03	74 ± 2	25	16
Crunchy Nut Cornflakes™ bar	72 ± 4	30	19
Crunchy Nut Cornflakes™ bar	72 ± 3	30	19
Cupcake, strawberry-iced, Squiggles	73 ± 3	38	19
Doughnut, wheat dough, deep-fried	75 ± 2	50	15
Fiber White™ bread	77 ± 2	30	11
French baguette bread with chocolate spread	72 ± 3	70	27
French bread, fermented with yeast	81 ± 2	30	13
Fruit and cinnamon bread	71 ± 3	30	11
Fruit and cinnamon bread	71 ± 2	30	11
Gluten Free Multigrain bread	79 ± 3	30	10
Gluten-free buckwheat bread, made with buckwheat meal & rice flour	72 ± 2	30	8
Gluten-free white bread, unsliced (gluten-free wheat starch)	71 ± 3	30	10
Golden Wheats™ breakfast cereal	71 ± 2	30	16
Granola Clusters breakfast cereal, Raisin & Almond, low fat, President's Choice® Blue Menu™	70 ± 4	30	15
Grapenuts™ breakfast cereal	75 ± 4	30	16
Honey Goldies™ wheat biscuits with additional ingredients	72 ± 4	30	15
Honey Rice Bubbles™ breakfast cereal	77 ± 3	30	20
Honey Smacks™ breakfast cereal	71 ± 4	30	16
Honey, Commercial Blend (28% fructose), NSW blend	72 ± 3	25	9
Instant oat cereal porridge prepared with water	83 ± 3	250	30
Instant oat porridge, cooked in microwave with water	82 ± 3	250	20
Japanese Wasabi & Honey Rice & Corn Crisps,	82 ± 3	50	32
Jelly beans, assorted colors (Allen's, Nestlé, Australia)	80 ± 4	30	22

Food Name	GI	Serving (g)	GL
Jelly beans, assorted colors (Savings, Grocery Holdings, Tooronga, Australia)	76 ± 3	30	21
Morning Coffee™ cookies	79 ± 4	25	15
Muesli	86 ± 4	30	18
Multigrain bread, with 5 g maragrine	80 ± 3	30	8
Pancakes, prepared from wheat flour	80 ± 3	80	16
Pikelets, Golden brand	85 ± 3	40	18
Pizza, plain baked dough, served with parmesan cheese and tomato sauce	80 ± 2	100	22
Potato, type not specified, boiled in salted water	76 ± 2	150	26
Potato, type not specified, peeled, boiled	85 ± 2	150	26
Pumpkin Soup, creamy, Heinz® Very Special™, with pumpkin, cream, potatoes	76 ± 2	250	14
Pumpkin, boiled in salted water	75 ± 2	80	3
Raspberry Fruit bar, fat-free, President's Choice® Blue Menu™ (Loblaw Brands Limited, Canada)	74 ± 2	40	23
Real Fruit Bars, strawberry (Uncle Toby's, Australia)	90 ± 3	30	23
Rice milk drink, low-fat, Australia's Own Natural™	92 ± 3	250	29
Rice Pops™, with 125 mL semi-skimmed milk	80 ± 4	30	20
Rice porridge	88 ± 3	150	13
Rockmelon/Cantaloupe, raw	70 ± 2	120	4
Special K™ breakfast cereal, made from rice	84 ± 4	30	20
Strawberry processed fruit bars, Real Fruit Bars	90 ± 2	30	23
Watermelon, raw	80 ± 2	120	5
Wheat based cereal biscuit, wheat biscuits (plain flaked wheat)	72 ± 4	30	14
Wheat-bites™ breakfast cereal	72 ± 3	30	18
White bread, wheat flour	78 ± 3	30	12
Wholemeal (whole wheat) bread	71 ± 2	30	9

Glycemic index Of 4000+ food

Food are sorted alphabetically. Low glycemic food have their GI below 55, moderate glycemic food have their GI in the range of 55 and 69. Food that have a GI higher than 70 are considered as high GI food and must be avoided.

Reminder: **How Is Glycemic Index Measured?**
Glycemic Index values of foods are measured using valid and proven scientific methods, and cannot be guessed just by looking at the composition of a given food or the nutrition facts on food packaging.

Thus, the GI calculation Follows the international standard method, and provides values that are commonly accepted. The Glycemic Index value of a food is calculated by feeding over than ten healthy people a portion of the food object of the study and containing fifty grams of digestible carbohydrate and then measuring the effect for each participant on his blood glucose levels (blood glucose response) over the next two hours.
The second part of the process consists of giving the same participants an equal carbohydrate portion of the glucose (used as the reference food) and measuring their blood glucose response over the next two hours.
The Glycemic Index value for the food is then calculated for each participant by using a simple formula (dividing the blood glucose response for the food by their blood glucose response for the glucose (reference food)). The final value of the Glycemic Index for the food is the average Glycemic Index value for the participants (over 10).

The tables below are divided into 14 categories and sorted alphabetically.

Beef, Lamp, Veal, Pork & Poultry

Food Name	Glycemic Index
Beef brisket, cooked, lean only eaten	0.0
Beef brisket, cooked, lean only eaten	0.0
Beef brisket, cooked, NS as to fat eaten	0.0
Beef brisket, cooked, NS as to fat eaten	0.0
Beef liver, battered, fried	95.0
Beef liver, braised	50.0
Beef liver, breaded, fried	95.0
Beef liver, cooked, NS as to cooking method	50.0
Beef liver, fried or broiled, no coating	50.0
Beef steak, battered, fried, lean and fat eaten	50.0
Beef steak, battered, fried, lean only eaten	50.0
Beef steak, battered, fried, NS as to fat eaten	50.0
Beef steak, braised, lean and fat eaten	0.0
Beef steak, braised, lean only eaten	0.0
Beef steak, braised, NS as to fat eaten	0.0
Beef steak, breaded or floured, baked or fried, lean and fat eaten	50.0
Beef steak, breaded or floured, baked or fried, lean only eaten	50.0
Beef steak, breaded or floured, baked or fried, NS as to fat eaten	50.0
Beef steak, broiled or baked, lean and fat eaten	0.0
Beef steak, broiled or baked, lean only eaten	0.0
Beef steak, broiled or baked, NS as to fat eaten	0.0
Beef steak, fried, lean and fat eaten	0.0
Beef steak, fried, lean only eaten	0.0
Beef steak, fried, NS as to fat eaten	0.0
Beef steak, NS as to cooking method, lean and fat eaten	0.0

Food Name	Glycemic Index
Beef steak, NS as to cooking method, lean only eaten	0.0
Beef steak, NS as to cooking method, NS as to fat eaten	0.0
Beef, dried, chipped, cooked in fat	0.0
Beef, dried, chipped, uncooked	50.0
Beef, NS as to cut, cooked, lean only eaten	0.0
Beef, NS as to cut, cooked, lean only eaten	0.0
Beef, NS as to cut, cooked, NS as to fat eaten	0.0
Beef, NS as to cut, cooked, NS as to fat eaten	0.0
Beef, NS as to cut, fried, NS to fat eaten	0.0
Beef, pastrami (beef, smoked, spiced)	50.0
Beef, pickled	50.0
Beef, pot roast, braised or boiled, lean and fat eaten	0.0
Beef, pot roast, braised or boiled, lean only eaten	0.0
Beef, pot roast, braised or boiled, lean only eaten	0.0
Beef, pot roast, braised or boiled, NS as to fat eaten	0.0
Beef, pot roast, braised or boiled, NS as to fat eaten	0.0
Beef, roast, canned	0.0
Beef, roast, roasted, lean and fat eaten	0.0
Beef, roast, roasted, lean and fat eaten	0.0
Beef, roast, roasted, lean only eaten	0.0
Beef, roast, roasted, lean only eaten	0.0
Beef, roast, roasted, NS as to fat eaten	0.0
Beef, roast, roasted, NS as to fat eaten	0.0
Beef, shortribs, barbecued, with sauce, lean and fat eaten	50.0
Beef, shortribs, barbecued, with sauce, lean only eaten	50.0
Beef, shortribs, barbecued, with sauce, NS as to fat eaten	50.0
Beef, shortribs, cooked, lean and fat eaten	0.0
Beef, shortribs, cooked, lean only eaten	0.0

Food Name	Glycemic Index
Beef, shortribs, cooked, NS as to fat eaten	0.0
Beef, sliced, prepackaged or deli, luncheon meat	50.0
Beef, stew meat, cooked, lean and fat eaten	0.0
Beef, stew meat, cooked, lean only eaten	0.0
Beef, stew meat, cooked, lean only eaten	0.0
Beef, stew meat, cooked, NS as to fat eaten	0.0
Beef, stew meat, cooked, NS as to fat eaten	0.0
Calves liver, breaded, fried	95.0
Calves liver, cooked, NS as to cooking method	95.0
Calves liver, fried or broiled, no coating	50.0
Chicken breast, with or without bone, battered, fried, prepared skinless, coating not eaten	95.0
Chicken breast, with or without bone, breaded, baked or fried, prepared skinless, coating not eaten	95.0
Chicken liver, battered, fried	95.0
Chicken liver, braised	50.0
Chicken liver, breaded, fried	95.0
Chicken liver, cooked, NS as to cooking method	95.0
Chicken liver, fried or sauteed, no coating	50.0
Chicken nuggets	95.0
Chicken or turkey cake, patty, or croquette	95.0
Chicken or turkey loaf, prepackaged or deli, luncheon meat	50.0
Chicken patty, fillet, or tenders, breaded, cooked	95.0
Chicken, baby food, strained	50.0
Chicken, back, with or without bone, battered, fried, prepared with skin, skin/coating eaten	95.0
Chicken, back, with or without bone, breaded, baked or fried, prepared with skin, skin/coating eaten	95.0
Chicken, back, with or without bone, broiled, skin eaten	0.0
Chicken, back, with or without bone, floured, baked or fried, prepared with skin, NS as to skin/coating eaten	95.0
Chicken, back, with or without bone, floured, baked or fried, prepared with skin, skin/coating eaten	95.0

Food Name	Glycemic Index
Chicken, back, with or without bone, floured, baked or fried, prepared with skin, skin/coating not eaten	95.0
Chicken, back, with or without bone, fried, no coating, NS as to skin eaten	0.0
Chicken, back, with or without bone, fried, no coating, skin eaten	0.0
Chicken, back, with or without bone, fried, no coating, skin not eaten	0.0
Chicken, back, with or without bone, NS as to cooking method, skin eaten	0.0
Chicken, back, with or without bone, roasted, skin eaten	0.0
Chicken, back, with or without bone, roasted, skin not eaten	0.0
Chicken, back, with or without bone, stewed, skin eaten	0.0
Chicken, back, with or without bone, stewed, skin not eaten	0.0
Chicken, boneless, NS as to part and cooking method, light or dark meat, NS as to skin eaten	0.0
Chicken, boneless, NS as to part and cooking method, light or dark meat, skin not eaten	0.0
Chicken, boneless, NS as to part, battered, fried, light or dark meat, prepared with skin, NS as to skin/coating eaten	95.0
Chicken, boneless, NS as to part, battered, fried, light or dark meat, prepared with skin, skin/coating eaten	95.0
Chicken, boneless, NS as to part, breaded, baked or fried, light or dark meat, prepared skinless, coating eaten	95.0
Chicken, boneless, NS as to part, breaded, baked or fried, light or dark meat, prepared skinless, NS as to coating eaten	95.0
Chicken, boneless, NS as to part, breaded, baked or fried, light or dark meat, prepared with skin, NS as to skin/coating eaten	95.0
Chicken, boneless, NS as to part, broiled, light or dark meat, NS as to skin eaten	0.0
Chicken, boneless, NS as to part, broiled, light or dark meat, skin not eaten	0.0
Chicken, boneless, NS as to part, floured, baked or fried, light or dark meat, prepared with skin, NS as to skin/coating eaten	95.0
Chicken, boneless, NS as to part, floured, baked or fried, light or dark meat, prepared with skin, skin/coating eaten	95.0
Chicken, boneless, NS as to part, floured, baked or fried, light or dark meat, prepared with skin, skin/coating not eaten	95.0
Chicken, boneless, NS as to part, fried, no coating, light or dark meat, NS as to skin eaten	0.0
Chicken, boneless, NS as to part, fried, no coating, light or dark meat, skin eaten	0.0

Food Name	Glycemic Index
Chicken, boneless, NS as to part, fried, no coating, light or dark meat, skin not eaten	0.0
Chicken, boneless, NS as to part, roasted, light or dark meat, NS as to skin eaten	0.0
Chicken, boneless, NS as to part, roasted, light or dark meat, skin eaten	0.0
Chicken, boneless, NS as to part, roasted, light or dark meat, skin not eaten	0.0
Chicken, boneless, NS as to part, stewed, light or dark meat, NS as to skin eaten	0.0
Chicken, boneless, NS as to part, stewed, light or dark meat, skin eaten	0.0
Chicken, boneless, NS as to part, stewed, light or dark meat, skin not eaten	0.0
Chicken, breast, with or without bone, battered, fried, prepared skinless, coating eaten	95.0
Chicken, breast, with or without bone, battered, fried, prepared skinless, NS as to coating eaten	95.0
Chicken, breast, with or without bone, battered, fried, prepared with skin, NS as to skin/coating eaten	95.0
Chicken, breast, with or without bone, battered, fried, prepared with skin, skin/coating eaten	95.0
Chicken, breast, with or without bone, battered, fried, prepared with skin, skin/coating not eaten	95.0
Chicken, breast, with or without bone, breaded, baked or fried, prepared skinless, coating eaten	95.0
Chicken, breast, with or without bone, breaded, baked or fried, prepared with skin, NS as to skin/coating eaten	95.0
Chicken, breast, with or without bone, breaded, baked or fried, prepared with skin, skin/coating eaten	95.0
Chicken, breast, with or without bone, breaded, baked or fried, prepared with skin, skin/coating not eaten	95.0
Chicken, breast, with or without bone, broiled, NS as to skin eaten	0.0
Chicken, breast, with or without bone, broiled, skin eaten	0.0
Chicken, breast, with or without bone, broiled, skin not eaten	0.0
Chicken, breast, with or without bone, floured, baked or fried, prepared skinless, NS as to coating eaten	95.0
Chicken, breast, with or without bone, floured, baked or fried, prepared with skin, NS as to skin/coating eaten	95.0
Chicken, breast, with or without bone, floured, baked or fried, prepared with skin, skin/coating eaten	95.0
Chicken, breast, with or without bone, floured, baked or fried, prepared with skin, skin/coating not eaten	95.0

Food Name	Glycemic Index
Chicken, breast, with or without bone, fried, no coating, NS as to skin eaten	0.0
Chicken, breast, with or without bone, fried, no coating, skin eaten	0.0
Chicken, breast, with or without bone, fried, no coating, skin not eaten	0.0
Chicken, breast, with or without bone, NS as to cooking method, NS as to skin eaten	0.0
Chicken, breast, with or without bone, NS as to cooking method, skin eaten	0.0
Chicken, breast, with or without bone, NS as to cooking method, skin not eaten	0.0
Chicken, breast, with or without bone, roasted, NS as to skin eaten	0.0
Chicken, breast, with or without bone, roasted, skin eaten	0.0
Chicken, breast, with or without bone, roasted, skin not eaten	0.0
Chicken, breast, with or without bone, stewed, NS as to skin eaten	0.0
Chicken, breast, with or without bone, stewed, skin eaten	0.0
Chicken, breast, with or without bone, stewed, skin not eaten	0.0
Chicken, canned, meat only, dark meat	0.0
Chicken, canned, meat only, light and dark meat	50.0
Chicken, canned, meat only, light meat	0.0
Chicken, canned, meat only, NS as to light or dark meat	50.0
Chicken, chicken roll, roasted, NS as to light or dark meat	50.0
Chicken, drumstick, with or without bone, battered, fried, prepared with skin, NS as to skin/coating eaten	95.0
Chicken, drumstick, with or without bone, battered, fried, prepared with skin, skin/coating eaten	95.0
Chicken, drumstick, with or without bone, battered, fried, prepared with skin, skin/coating not eaten	0.0
Chicken, drumstick, with or without bone, breaded, baked or fried, prepared skinless, coating eaten	95.0
Chicken, drumstick, with or without bone, breaded, baked or fried, prepared skinless, coating not eaten	95.0
Chicken, drumstick, with or without bone, breaded, baked or fried, prepared with skin, NS as to skin/coating eaten	95.0
Chicken, drumstick, with or without bone, breaded, baked or fried, prepared with skin, skin/coating eaten	95.0
Chicken, drumstick, with or without bone, breaded, baked or fried, prepared with skin, skin/coating not eaten	0.0

Food Name	Glycemic Index
Chicken, drumstick, with or without bone, broiled, skin eaten	0.0
Chicken, drumstick, with or without bone, broiled, skin not eaten	0.0
Chicken, drumstick, with or without bone, floured, baked or fried, prepared skinless, coating eaten	95.0
Chicken, drumstick, with or without bone, floured, baked or fried, prepared with skin, NS as to skin/coating eaten	95.0
Chicken, drumstick, with or without bone, floured, baked or fried, prepared with skin, skin/coating eaten	95.0
Chicken, drumstick, with or without bone, floured, baked or fried, prepared with skin, skin/coating not eaten	0.0
Chicken, drumstick, with or without bone, fried, no coating, NS as to skin eaten	0.0
Chicken, drumstick, with or without bone, fried, no coating, skin eaten	0.0
Chicken, drumstick, with or without bone, fried, no coating, skin not eaten	0.0
Chicken, drumstick, with or without bone, NS as to cooking method, NS as to skin eaten	0.0
Chicken, drumstick, with or without bone, NS as to cooking method, skin eaten	0.0
Chicken, drumstick, with or without bone, NS as to cooking method, skin not eaten	0.0
Chicken, drumstick, with or without bone, roasted, NS as to skin eaten	0.0
Chicken, drumstick, with or without bone, roasted, skin eaten	0.0
Chicken, drumstick, with or without bone, roasted, skin not eaten	0.0
Chicken, drumstick, with or without bone, stewed, NS as to skin eaten	0.0
Chicken, drumstick, with or without bone, stewed, skin eaten	0.0
Chicken, drumstick, with or without bone, stewed, skin not eaten	0.0
Chicken, ground	0.0
Chicken, leg (drumstick and thigh), with or without bone, battered, fried, prepared with skin, NS as to skin/coating eaten	95.0
Chicken, leg (drumstick and thigh), with or without bone, battered, fried, prepared with skin, skin/coating eaten	95.0
Chicken, leg (drumstick and thigh), with or without bone, battered, fried, prepared with skin, skin/coating not eaten	95.0
Chicken, leg (drumstick and thigh), with or without bone, breaded, baked or fried, prepared with skin, NS as to skin/coating eaten	95.0
Chicken, leg (drumstick and thigh), with or without bone, breaded, baked or fried, prepared with skin, skin/coating eaten	95.0

Food Name	Glycemic Index
Chicken, leg (drumstick and thigh), with or without bone, breaded, baked or fried, prepared with skin, skin/coating not eaten	95.0
Chicken, leg (drumstick and thigh), with or without bone, broiled, NS as to skin eaten	0.0
Chicken, leg (drumstick and thigh), with or without bone, broiled, skin eaten	0.0
Chicken, leg (drumstick and thigh), with or without bone, broiled, skin not eaten	0.0
Chicken, leg (drumstick and thigh), with or without bone, floured, baked or fried, prepared with skin, NS as to skin/coating eaten	95.0
Chicken, leg (drumstick and thigh), with or without bone, floured, baked or fried, prepared with skin, skin/coating eaten	95.0
Chicken, leg (drumstick and thigh), with or without bone, floured, baked or fried, prepared with skin, skin/coating not eaten	95.0
Chicken, leg (drumstick and thigh), with or without bone, fried, no coating, NS as to skin eaten	0.0
Chicken, leg (drumstick and thigh), with or without bone, fried, no coating, skin eaten	0.0
Chicken, leg (drumstick and thigh), with or without bone, fried, no coating, skin not eaten	0.0
Chicken, leg (drumstick and thigh), with or without bone, NS as to cooking method, NS as to skin eaten	0.0
Chicken, leg (drumstick and thigh), with or without bone, NS as to cooking method, skin not eaten	0.0
Chicken, leg (drumstick and thigh), with or without bone, roasted, NS as to skin eaten	0.0
Chicken, leg (drumstick and thigh), with or without bone, roasted, skin eaten	0.0
Chicken, leg (drumstick and thigh), with or without bone, roasted, skin not eaten	0.0
Chicken, leg (drumstick and thigh), with or without bone, stewed, NS as to skin eaten	0.0
Chicken, leg (drumstick and thigh), with or without bone, stewed, skin eaten	0.0
Chicken, leg (drumstick and thigh), with or without bone, stewed, skin not eaten	0.0
Chicken, neck or ribs, with or without bone, floured, baked or fried, prepared with skin, skin/coating not eaten	95.0
Chicken, neck or ribs, with or without bone, NS as to cooking method, NS as to skin eaten	0.0
Chicken, thigh, with or without bone, battered, fried, prepared skinless, coating not eaten	95.0
Chicken, thigh, with or without bone, battered, fried, prepared with skin, NS as to skin/coating eaten	95.0

Food Name	Glycemic Index
Chicken, thigh, with or without bone, battered, fried, prepared with skin, skin/coating eaten	95.0
Chicken, thigh, with or without bone, battered, fried, prepared with skin, skin/coating not eaten	95.0
Chicken, thigh, with or without bone, breaded, baked or fried, prepared skinless, coating eaten	95.0
Chicken, thigh, with or without bone, breaded, baked or fried, prepared skinless, coating not eaten	95.0
Chicken, thigh, with or without bone, breaded, baked or fried, prepared with skin, NS as to skin/coating eaten	95.0
Chicken, thigh, with or without bone, breaded, baked or fried, prepared with skin, skin/coating eaten	95.0
Chicken, thigh, with or without bone, broiled, NS as to skin eaten	0.0
Chicken, thigh, with or without bone, broiled, skin eaten	0.0
Chicken, thigh, with or without bone, broiled, skin not eaten	0.0
Chicken, thigh, with or without bone, floured, baked or fried, prepared with skin, NS as to skin/coating eaten	95.0
Chicken, thigh, with or without bone, floured, baked or fried, prepared with skin, skin/coating eaten	95.0
Chicken, thigh, with or without bone, floured, baked or fried, prepared with skin, skin/coating not eaten	95.0
Chicken, thigh, with or without bone, fried, no coating, NS as to skin eaten	0.0
Chicken, thigh, with or without bone, fried, no coating, skin eaten	0.0
Chicken, thigh, with or without bone, fried, no coating, skin not eaten	0.0
Chicken, thigh, with or without bone, NS as to cooking method, NS as to skin eaten	0.0
Chicken, thigh, with or without bone, NS as to cooking method, skin eaten	0.0
Chicken, thigh, with or without bone, NS as to cooking method, skin not eaten	0.0
Chicken, thigh, with or without bone, roasted, NS as to skin eaten	0.0
Chicken, thigh, with or without bone, roasted, skin eaten	0.0
Chicken, thigh, with or without bone, roasted, skin not eaten	0.0
Chicken, thigh, with or without bone, smoked, skin eaten	0.0
Chicken, thigh, with or without bone, stewed, NS as to skin eaten	0.0
Chicken, thigh, with or without bone, stewed, skin eaten	0.0
Chicken, thigh, with or without bone, stewed, skin not eaten	0.0

Food Name	Glycemic Index
Chicken, wing, with or without bone, battered, fried, prepared with skin, NS as to skin/coating eaten	95.0
Chicken, wing, with or without bone, battered, fried, prepared with skin, skin/coating eaten	95.0
Chicken, wing, with or without bone, battered, fried, prepared with skin, skin/coating not eaten	0.0
Chicken, wing, with or without bone, breaded, baked or fried, prepared with skin, NS as to skin/coating eaten	95.0
Chicken, wing, with or without bone, breaded, baked or fried, prepared with skin, skin/coating eaten	95.0
Chicken, wing, with or without bone, breaded, baked or fried, prepared with skin, skin/coating not eaten	0.0
Chicken, wing, with or without bone, broiled, NS as to skin eaten	0.0
Chicken, wing, with or without bone, broiled, skin eaten	0.0
Chicken, wing, with or without bone, broiled, skin not eaten	0.0
Chicken, wing, with or without bone, floured, baked or fried, prepared with skin, NS as to skin/coating eaten	95.0
Chicken, wing, with or without bone, floured, baked or fried, prepared with skin, skin/coating eaten	95.0
Chicken, wing, with or without bone, floured, baked or fried, prepared with skin, skin/coating not eaten	0.0
Chicken, wing, with or without bone, fried, no coating, NS as to skin eaten	0.0
Chicken, wing, with or without bone, fried, no coating, skin eaten	0.0
Chicken, wing, with or without bone, fried, no coating, skin not eaten	0.0
Chicken, wing, with or without bone, NS as to cooking method, NS as to skin eaten	0.0
Chicken, wing, with or without bone, NS as to cooking method, skin eaten	0.0
Chicken, wing, with or without bone, NS as to cooking method, skin not eaten	0.0
Chicken, wing, with or without bone, roasted, NS as to skin eaten	0.0
Chicken, wing, with or without bone, roasted, skin eaten	0.0
Chicken, wing, with or without bone, roasted, skin not eaten	0.0
Chicken, wing, with or without bone, stewed, NS as to skin eaten	0.0
Chicken, wing, with or without bone, stewed, skin eaten	0.0
Chicken, wing, with or without bone, stewed, skin not eaten	0.0

Food Name	Glycemic Index
Chicken, with bone, NS as to part and cooking method, light or dark meat, NS as to skin eaten	0.0
Chicken, with bone, NS as to part, battered, fried, light or dark meat, prepared with skin, skin/coating eaten	95.0
Chicken, with bone, NS as to part, breaded, baked or fried, light or dark meat, prepared with skin, skin/coating eaten	95.0
Chicken, with bone, NS as to part, broiled, light or dark meat, NS as to skin eaten	0.0
Chicken, with bone, NS as to part, broiled, light or dark meat, skin eaten	0.0
Chicken, with bone, NS as to part, broiled, light or dark meat, skin not eaten	0.0
Chicken, with bone, NS as to part, floured, baked or fried, light or dark meat, prepared with skin, skin/coating not eaten	95.0
Chicken, with bone, NS as to part, roasted, light or dark meat, NS as to skin eaten	0.0
Chicken, with bone, NS as to part, roasted, light or dark meat, skin eaten	0.0
Chicken, with bone, NS as to part, roasted, light or dark meat, skin not eaten	0.0
Chicken, with bone, NS as to part, stewed, light or dark meat, NS as to skin eaten	0.0
Chicken, with bone, NS as to part, stewed, light or dark meat, skin not eaten	0.0
Corned beef, canned, ready-to-eat	0.0
Corned beef, canned, ready-to-eat	0.0
Corned beef, cooked, lean only eaten	0.0
Corned beef, cooked, lean only eaten	0.0
Corned beef, cooked, NS as to fat eaten	50.0
Corned beef, pressed	0.0
Cornish game hen, cooked, skin not eaten	0.0
Cornish game hen, roasted, NS as to skin eaten	0.0
Cornish game hen, roasted, skin eaten	0.0
Cornish game hen, roasted, skin not eaten	0.0
Dove, fried	95.0
Ground beef or patty, cooked, NS as to regular, lean, or extra lean	0.0
Ground beef, extra lean, cooked	0.0
Ground beef, lean, cooked	0.0

Food Name	Glycemic Index
Ground beef, raw	0.0
Ground beef, regular, cooked	0.0
Ground meat, NFS	0.0
Ham, fresh, cooked, lean and fat eaten	0.0
Ham, fresh, cooked, lean only eaten	0.0
Ham, fresh, cooked, NS as to fat eaten	0.0
Ham, fried, lean only eaten	0.0
Ham, smoked or cured, canned, lean only eaten	0.0
Ham, smoked or cured, canned, NS as to fat eaten	0.0
Ham, smoked or cured, cooked, lean only eaten	0.0
Lamb chop, NS as to cut, cooked, lean and fat eaten	0.0
Lamb chop, NS as to cut, cooked, lean only eaten	0.0
Lamb chop, NS as to cut, cooked, NS as to fat eaten	0.0
Lamb, ground or patty, cooked	0.0
Lamb, loin chop, cooked, lean only eaten	0.0
Lamb, NS as to cut, cooked	0.0
Lamb, ribs, cooked, NS as to fat eaten	0.0
Lamb, roast, cooked, lean only eaten	0.0
Beef brisket, cooked, lean and fat eaten	0.0
Lamb, roast, cooked, NS as to fat eaten	0.0
Liver dumpling	50.0
Liver paste or pate, chicken	50.0
Liver, beef or calves, and onions	50.0
Liver, NS as to type, cooked	50.0
Liverwurst	50.0
Meat spread or potted meat, NFS	50.0
Meat, NFS	0.0
Meat, NFS	0.0

Food Name	Glycemic Index
Pheasant, cooked	0.0
Pork chop, battered, fried, lean and fat eaten	95.0
Pork chop, battered, fried, lean only eaten	95.0
Pork chop, battered, fried, NS as to fat eaten	95.0
Pork chop, breaded or floured, broiled or baked, lean and fat eaten	95.0
Pork chop, breaded or floured, broiled or baked, lean only eaten	95.0
Pork chop, breaded or floured, broiled or baked, NS as to fat eaten	95.0
Pork chop, breaded or floured, fried, lean and fat eaten	95.0
Pork chop, breaded or floured, fried, lean only eaten	95.0
Pork chop, breaded or floured, fried, NS as to fat eaten	95.0
Pork chop, broiled or baked, lean and fat eaten	0.0
Pork chop, broiled or baked, lean only eaten	0.0
Pork chop, broiled or baked, NS as to fat eaten	0.0
Pork chop, fried, lean and fat eaten	0.0
Pork chop, fried, lean only eaten	0.0
Pork chop, fried, NS as to fat eaten	0.0
Pork chop, NS as to cooking method, lean and fat eaten	0.0
Pork chop, NS as to cooking method, lean only eaten	0.0
Pork chop, NS as to cooking method, NS as to fat eaten	0.0
Pork chop, smoked or cured, cooked, lean and fat eaten	0.0
Pork chop, smoked or cured, cooked, lean only eaten	0.0
Pork chop, smoked or cured, cooked, NS as to fat eaten	0.0
Pork chop, stewed, lean and fat eaten	0.0
Pork chop, stewed, lean only eaten	0.0
Pork chop, stewed, NS as to fat eaten	0.0
Pork ears, tail, head, snout, miscellaneous parts, cooked	50.0
Pork liver, braised	50.0
Pork liver, breaded, fried	95.0

Food Name	Glycemic Index
Pork liver, cooked, NS as to cooking method	50.0
Pork roast, loin, cooked, lean and fat eaten	0.0
Pork roast, loin, cooked, lean only eaten	0.0
Pork roast, loin, cooked, NS as to fat eaten	0.0
Pork roast, NS as to cut, cooked, lean and fat eaten	0.0
Pork roast, NS as to cut, cooked, lean only eaten	0.0
Pork roast, NS as to cut, cooked, NS as to fat eaten	0.0
Pork roast, smoked or cured, cooked, lean only eaten	0.0
Pork roast, smoked or cured, cooked, NS as to fat eaten	50.0
Pork skin, rinds, deep-fried	0.0
Pork steak or cutlet, battered, fried, NS as to fat eaten	95.0
Pork steak or cutlet, breaded or floured, broiled or baked, lean and fat eaten	95.0
Pork steak or cutlet, breaded or floured, broiled or baked, lean only eaten	95.0
Pork steak or cutlet, breaded or floured, broiled or baked, NS as to fat eaten	95.0
Pork steak or cutlet, breaded or floured, fried, lean only eaten	95.0
Pork steak or cutlet, breaded or floured, fried, NS as to fat eaten	95.0
Pork steak or cutlet, broiled or baked, lean and fat eaten	0.0
Pork steak or cutlet, broiled or baked, lean only eaten	0.0
Pork steak or cutlet, broiled or baked, NS as to fat eaten	0.0
Pork steak or cutlet, fried, lean and fat eaten	0.0
Pork steak or cutlet, fried, lean only eaten	0.0
Pork steak or cutlet, fried, NS as to fat eaten	0.0
Pork steak or cutlet, NS as to cooking method, lean only eaten	0.0
Pork steak or cutlet, NS as to cooking method, NS as to fat eaten	0.0
Pork, ground or patty, breaded, cooked	95.0
Pork, ground or patty, cooked	0.0
Pork, neck bones, cooked	0.0
Pork, NS as to cut, cooked, lean only eaten	0.0

Food Name	Glycemic Index
Pork, NS as to cut, cooked, NS as to fat eaten	0.0
Pork, NS as to cut, fried, lean and fat eaten	0.0
Pork, NS as to cut, fried, lean only eaten	0.0
Pork, NS as to cut, fried, NS as to fat eaten	0.0
Pork, pig's feet, cooked	0.0
Pork, pig's feet, pickled	32.0
Pork, pig's hocks, cooked	0.0
Pork, spareribs, barbecued, with sauce, lean and fat eaten	50.0
Pork, spareribs, barbecued, with sauce, lean only eaten	50.0
Pork, spareribs, barbecued, with sauce, NS as to fat eaten	50.0
Pork, spareribs, cooked, lean and fat eaten	0.0
Pork, spareribs, cooked, lean only eaten	0.0
Pork, spareribs, cooked, NS as to fat eaten	0.0
Pork, tenderloin, baked	0.0
Pork, tenderloin, battered, fried	95.0
Pork, tenderloin, braised	0.0
Pork, tenderloin, breaded, fried	95.0
Pork, tenderloin, cooked, NS as to cooking method	0.0
Quail, cooked	0.0
Seasoned shredded soup meat (Ropa vieja, sopa de carne ripiada)	50.0
Steak, NS as to type of meat, cooked, lean and fat eaten	0.0
Steak, NS as to type of meat, cooked, lean only eaten	0.0
Steak, NS as to type of meat, cooked, NS as to fat eaten	0.0
Swiss steak	50.0
Turkey ham	50.0
Turkey ham, sliced, extra lean, prepackaged or deli, luncheon meat	50.0
Turkey or chicken breast, prepackaged or deli, luncheon meat	0.0
Turkey pastrami	50.0

Food Name	Glycemic Index
Turkey salami	28.0
Turkey, baby food, strained	50.0
Turkey, back, cooked	0.0
Turkey, canned	0.0
Turkey, dark meat, roasted, NS as to skin eaten	0.0
Turkey, dark meat, roasted, skin eaten	0.0
Turkey, dark meat, roasted, skin not eaten	0.0
Turkey, drumstick, cooked, NS as to skin eaten	0.0
Turkey, drumstick, cooked, skin eaten	0.0
Turkey, drumstick, cooked, skin not eaten	0.0
Turkey, drumstick, roasted, NS as to skin eaten	0.0
Turkey, drumstick, roasted, skin eaten	0.0
Turkey, drumstick, roasted, skin not eaten	0.0
Turkey, drumstick, smoked, cooked, skin eaten	0.0
Turkey, ground	0.0
Turkey, light and dark meat, roasted, NS as to skin eaten	0.0
Turkey, light and dark meat, roasted, skin eaten	0.0
Turkey, light and dark meat, roasted, skin not eaten	0.0
Turkey, light meat, breaded, baked or fried, skin not eaten	95.0
Turkey, light meat, cooked, NS as to skin eaten	0.0
Turkey, light meat, cooked, skin eaten	0.0
Turkey, light meat, cooked, skin not eaten	0.0
Turkey, light meat, roasted, NS as to skin eaten	0.0
Turkey, light meat, roasted, skin eaten	0.0
Turkey, light meat, roasted, skin not eaten	0.0
Turkey, light or dark meat, smoked, cooked, NS as to skin eaten	0.0
Turkey, light or dark meat, smoked, cooked, skin not eaten	0.0
Turkey, neck, cooked	0.0

Food Name	Glycemic Index
Turkey, NFS	0.0
Turkey, rolled roast, light or dark meat, cooked	50.0
Turkey, thigh, cooked, NS as to skin eaten	0.0
Turkey, thigh, cooked, skin eaten	0.0
Turkey, thigh, cooked, skin not eaten	0.0
Turkey, wing, cooked, NS as to skin eaten	0.0
Turkey, wing, cooked, skin eaten	0.0
Turkey, wing, cooked, skin not eaten	0.0
Veal chop, broiled, lean only eaten	0.0
Veal chop, broiled, NS as to fat eaten	0.0
Veal chop, fried, lean and fat eaten	50.0
Veal chop, fried, lean only eaten	50.0
Veal cutlet or steak, broiled, lean only eaten	0.0
Veal cutlet or steak, fried, lean only eaten	0.0
Veal cutlet or steak, fried, NS as to fat eaten	50.0
Veal cutlet or steak, NS as to cooking method, lean only eaten	0.0
Veal cutlet or steak, NS as to cooking method, NS as to fat eaten	0.0
Veal patty, breaded, cooked	50.0
Veal, ground or patty, cooked	0.0
Veal, NS as to cut, cooked, lean only eaten	0.0
Veal, NS as to cut, cooked, NS as to fat eaten	0.0
Veal, roasted, lean and fat eaten	0.0
Veal, roasted, lean only eaten	0.0
Venison/deer jerky	50.0
Venison/deer ribs, cooked	0.0
Venison/deer steak, breaded or floured, cooked, NS as to cooking method	50.0
Venison/deer steak, cooked, NS as to cooking method	0.0
Venison/deer, NFS	0.0

Food Name	Glycemic Index
Venison/deer, roasted	0.0
Venison/deer, stewed	0.0

Beverages

Food Name	Glycemic Index
Apple cider-flavored drink, made from powdered mix, low calorie, with vitamin C added	50.0
Apple juice	40.0
Apple juice, with added vitamin C	40.0
Apple-cherry juice	43.0
Apple-grape juice	40.0
Apple-grape-raspberry juice	40.0
Apple-pear juice	40.0
Apple-raspberry juice	40.0
Apple-white grape juice drink, low calorie, with vitamin C added	50.0
Apricot-orange juice	50.0
Beer	36.0
Beer, lite	36.0
Apple cider	40.0
Brandy	0.0
Carbonated citrus juice drink	63.0
Cereal beverage	50.0
Cereal beverage with beet roots, from powdered instant	50.0
Chocolate syrup, skim milk added	37.5
Chocolate syrup, whole milk added	36.0
Chocolate-flavored drink, whey- and milk-based	37.5
Chocolate-flavored soda, sugar-free	50.0
Citrus juice drink, low calorie	50.0
Cocoa and sugar mixture, lowfat milk added	37.5
Cocoa and sugar mixture, milk added, NS as to type of milk	37.0
Cocoa and sugar mixture, skim milk added	37.5
Cocoa and sugar mixture, whole milk added	36.0
Cocoa, hot chocolate, not from dry mix, made with whole milk	36.0

Food Name	Glycemic Index
Cocoa, sugar, and dry milk mixture, water added	37.5
Cocoa, sugar, and dry milk mixture, water added	37.5
Coffee and chicory, made from ground	50.0
Coffee and chicory, NS as to ground or instant	50.0
Coffee, acid neutralized, from powdered instant	50.0
Coffee, decaffeinated, and chicory, made from powdered instant	50.0
Coffee, decaffeinated, made from ground	50.0
Coffee, decaffeinated, made from powdered instant	50.0
Coffee, decaffeinated, NS as to ground or instant	50.0
Coffee, decaffeinated, with cereal	50.0
Coffee, espresso	50.0
Coffee, espresso, decaffeinated	50.0
Coffee, made from ground, equal parts regular and decaffeinated	50.0
Coffee, made from ground, regular	50.0
Coffee, made from ground, regular, flavored	50.0
Coffee, made from liquid concentrate	50.0
Coffee, made from powdered instant, 50% less caffeine	50.0
Coffee, made from powdered instant, regular	50.0
Coffee, NS as to type	50.0
Coffee, regular, NS as to ground or instant	50.0
Cola with fruit or vanilla flavor	58.0
Cola with fruit or vanilla flavor, sugar-free	50.0
Cordial or liqueur	50.0
Corn beverage	50.0
Cranberry juice drink with vitamin C added	58.7
Cranberry juice drink, low calorie, with vitamin C added	50.0
Cranberry juice, unsweetened	68.0
Cranberry-apple juice drink with vitamin C added	48.0

Food Name	Glycemic Index
Cranberry-apple juice drink, low calorie, with vitamin C added	50.0
Cranberry-white grape juice mixture, unsweetened	68.0
Cream soda, sugar-free	0.0
Diet beverage, liquid, canned	26.0
Flavored milk drink, whey- and milk-based, flavors other than chocolate	35.0
Fruit drink	58.7
Fruit drink, low calorie	50.0
Fruit juice blend, 100% juice, with added Vitamin C	40.0
Fruit juice, NFS	50.0
Fruit-flavored drink, made from powdered mix, mainly sugar, with high vitamin C added	68.0
Fruit-flavored drink, made from sweetened powdered mix (fortified with vitamin C)	68.0
Fruit-flavored drink, made from unsweetened powdered mix (fortified with vitamin C), with sugar added in preparation	68.0
Fruit-flavored drink, non-carbonated, made from low calorie powdered mix	50.0
Fruit-flavored drinks, punches, ades, low calorie, with vitamin C added	50.0
Fruit-flavored thirst quencher beverage	78.0
Fruit-flavored thirst quencher beverage, low calorie	50.0
Gin	0.0
Ginger ale, sugar-free	0.0
Grape juice, NS as to added sweetener	46.0
Grape juice, unsweetened	46.0
Grape juice, unsweetened, with added vitamin C	46.0
Grape-tangerine-lemon juice	50.0
Grapefruit and orange juice, canned, unsweetened	49.0
Grapefruit and orange juice, fresh	49.0
Grapefruit and orange juice, NFS	49.0
Grapefruit juice drink, low calorie, with vitamin C added	50.0
Grapefruit juice, canned, bottled or in a carton, unsweetened	48.0

Food Name	Glycemic Index
Grapefruit juice, canned, bottled or in a carton, with sugar	48.0
Grapefruit juice, canned, bottled, or in a carton, sweetened with low calorie sweetener	48.0
Grapefruit juice, freshly squeezed	48.0
Grapefruit juice, frozen, unsweetened (reconstituted with water)	48.0
Grapefruit juice, NFS	48.0
Grapefruit juice, unsweetened, NS as to form	48.0
Ice cream soda, chocolate	59.5
Ice cream soda, flavors other than chocolate	64.5
Ice pop	68.0
Instant breakfast, fluid, canned	26.0
Instant breakfast, powder, milk added	26.0
Juice drink, low calorie	50.0
Lemonade	68.0
Lemonade-flavored drink, made from powdered mix, low calorie, with vitamin C added	50.0
Lemonade, low calorie	50.0
Milk beverage, made with whole milk, flavors other than chocolate	35.0
Milk shake with malt	53.0
Milk-based fruit drink	42.5
Milk, chocolate, NFS	37.0
Milk, chocolate, reduced fat milk-based (formerly "lowfat")	37.5
Milk, chocolate, reduced fat milk-based (formerly "lowfat")	37.5
Milk, chocolate, skim milk-based	37.5
Milk, chocolate, whole milk-based	36.0
Milk, flavors other than chocolate, whole milk-based	35.0
Milk, malted, fortified, chocolate, made with milk	45.0
Milk, malted, fortified, natural flavor, made with milk	45.0
Milk, malted, fortified, NS as to flavor, made with milk	45.0
Milk, malted, unfortified, NS as to flavor, made with milk	45.0

Food Name	Glycemic Index
Nonalcoholic malt beverage	36.0
Orange and banana juice	50.0
Orange breakfast drink	68.0
Orange breakfast drink, low calorie	50.0
Orange breakfast drink, made from frozen concentrate	68.0
Orange juice, canned, bottled or in a carton, unsweetened	50.0
Orange juice, canned, bottled or in a carton, with sugar	50.0
Orange juice, freshly squeezed	50.0
Orange juice, frozen, unsweetened (reconstituted with water)	50.0
Orange juice, frozen, unsweetened, not reconstituted	50.0
Orange juice, frozen, with calcium added (reconstituted with water)	50.0
Orange juice, frozen, with sugar (reconstituted with water)	50.0
Orange juice, NFS	50.0
Orange juice, with calcium added, canned, bottled or in a carton, unsweetened	50.0
Orange-cranberry juice drink, low calorie, with vitamin C added	50.0
Orange-white grape-peach juice	50.0
Pineapple juice-non-citrus juice blend, unsweetened, with added vitamin C	46.0
Pineapple juice, NS as to sweetened or unsweetened	46.0
Pineapple juice, unsweetened	46.0
Pineapple juice, unsweetened, with added Vitamin C	46.0
Pineapple juice, with sugar	46.0
Pineapple-apple-guava juice, with added vitamin C	43.0
Pineapple-grapefruit juice, canned, bottled or in a carton, unsweetened	47.0
Pineapple-orange juice, canned, NS as to sweetened or unsweetened; sweetened, NS as to type of sweetener	48.0
Pineapple-orange juice, canned, unsweetened	48.0
Pineapple-orange juice, frozen (reconstituted with water)	48.0
Pineapple-orange juice, NFS	48.0
Pineapple-orange-banana juice	48.0

Food Name	Glycemic Index
Postum	50.0
Prune juice, unsweetened	29.0
Rice beverage	50.0
Rice beverage	50.0
Root beer, sugar-free	0.0
Rum	0.0
Sangria	50.0
Soft drink, cola-type	58.0
Soft drink, cola-type, decaffeinated	58.0
Soft drink, cola-type, decaffeinated, sugar-free	50.0
Soft drink, cola-type, sugar-free	50.0
Soft drink, cola-type, with higher caffeine	58.0
Soft drink, fruit flavored, caffeine containing	63.0
Soft drink, fruit flavored, caffeine containing, sugar-free	0.0
Soft drink, fruit-flavored, caffeine free	63.0
Soft drink, fruit-flavored, sugar free, caffeine free	0.0
Soft drink, NFS	58.0
Soft drink, NFS, sugar-free	50.0
Soft drink, pepper-type, decaffeinated, sugar-free	50.0
Soft drink, pepper-type, sugar-free	50.0
Strawberry-banana-orange juice	50.0
Tea, chamomile	50.0
Tea, herbal	50.0
Tea, leaf, decaffeinated, unsweetened	50.0
Tea, leaf, unsweetened	50.0
Tea, made from frozen concentrate, unsweetened	50.0
Tea, made from powdered instant, decaffeinated, unsweetened	50.0
Tea, made from powdered instant, unsweetened	50.0

Food Name	Glycemic Index
Tea, NS as to type, decaffeinated, unsweetened	50.0
Tea, NS as to type, unsweetened	50.0
Tomato and vegetable juice, mostly tomato	38.0
Tomato and vegetable juice, mostly tomato, low sodium	38.0
Tomato juice	38.0
Vodka	0.0
Whiskey	50.0
Wine cooler	50.0
Wine, dessert, sweet	50.0
Wine, light	50.0
Wine, light, nonalcoholic	50.0
Wine, rice	50.0
Wine, table, dry	50.0

Breads & Bakery Products

Food Name	Glycemic Index
Air filled fritter or fried puff, without syrup, Puerto Rican style (Bunuelos de viento)	59.0
Bagel	72.0
Bagel, multigrain	43.0
Bagel, multigrain, toasted	43.0
Bagel, multigrain, with raisins	43.0
Bagel, multigrain, with raisins, toasted	43.0
Bagel, oat bran	47.0
Bagel, oat bran, toasted	47.0
Bagel, pumpernickel	50.0
Bagel, pumpernickel, toasted	50.0
Bagel, toasted	72.0
Bagel, wheat	71.0
Bagel, wheat, toasted	71.0
Bagel, wheat, with fruit and nuts	71.0
Bagel, wheat, with fruit and nuts, toasted	71.0
Bagel, wheat, with raisins	71.0
Bagel, wheat, with raisins, toasted	71.0
Bagel, whole wheat, 100%	71.0
Bagel, whole wheat, 100%, toasted	71.0
Bagel, whole wheat, 100%, with raisins	71.0
Bagel, whole wheat, 100%, with raisins, toasted	71.0
Bagel, whole wheat, other than 100% or NS as to 100%	71.0
Bagel, whole wheat, other than 100% or NS as to 100%, toasted	71.0
Bagel, with fruit other than raisins	72.0
Bagel, with fruit other than raisins, toasted	72.0
Bagel, with raisins	72.0

Food Name	Glycemic Index
Bagel, with raisins, toasted	72.0
Baklava	59.0
Bread stick, hard, low sodium	70.0
Bread stick, NS as to hard or soft	70.0
Bread stick, soft	70.0
Bread stick, soft, prepared with garlic and parmesan cheese	70.0
Bread stuffing	74.0
Bread stuffing made with egg	74.0
Bread, barley	67.0
Bread, black	76.0
Bread, black, toasted	76.0
Bread, cinnamon	70.0
Bread, cinnamon, toasted	73.0
Bread, Cuban	95.0
Bread, Cuban, toasted	95.0
Bread, dough, fried	66.0
Bread, French or Vienna	95.0
Bread, French or Vienna, toasted	95.0
Bread, French or Vienna, whole wheat, other than 100% or NS as to 100%, made from home recipe or purchased at bakery	71.0
Bread, French or Vienna, whole wheat, other than 100% or NS as to 100%, made from home recipe or purchased at bakery, toasted	71.0
Bread, fruit and nut	57.9
Bread, fruit, without nuts	57.9
Bread, garlic	95.0
Bread, garlic, toasted	95.0
Bread, Italian, Grecian, Armenian	70.0
Bread, Italian, Grecian, Armenian, toasted	73.0
Bread, lowfat, 98% fat free	95.0
Bread, lowfat, 98% fat free, toasted	95.0

Food Name	Glycemic Index
Bread, made from home recipe or purchased at a bakery, NS as to major flour	70.0
Bread, made from home recipe or purchased at a bakery, toasted, NS as to major flour	73.0
Bread, marble rye and pumpernickel	50.0
Bread, marble rye and pumpernickel, toasted	50.0
Bread, multigrain	43.0
Bread, multigrain, reduced calorie and/or high fiber	43.0
Bread, multigrain, reduced calorie and/or high fiber, toasted	43.0
Bread, multigrain, toasted	43.0
Bread, multigrain, with raisins	43.0
Bread, multigrain, with raisins, toasted	43.0
Bread, Native, Puerto Rican style (Pan Criollo)	70.0
Bread, Native, Puerto Rican style, toasted (Pan Criollo)	73.0
Bread, NS as to major flour	70.0
Bread, nut	57.9
Bread, oat bran	31.0
Bread, oat bran, reduced calorie and/or high fiber	31.0
Bread, oat bran, reduced calorie and/or high fiber, toasted	31.0
Bread, oat bran, toasted	31.0
Bread, oatmeal	55.0
Bread, oatmeal, toasted	55.0
Bread, pita	57.0
Bread, pita, toasted	57.0
Bread, pita, wheat or cracked wheat	53.0
Bread, pita, wheat or cracked wheat, toasted	53.0
Bread, pita, whole wheat, 100%	71.0
Bread, pita, whole wheat, 100%, toasted	71.0
Bread, pita, whole wheat, other than 100% or NS as to 100%	71.0
Bread, pita, whole wheat, other than 100% or NS as to 100%, toasted	71.0

Food Name	Glycemic Index
Bread, pumpernickel	50.0
Bread, pumpernickel, toasted	50.0
Bread, pumpkin	57.9
Bread, raisin	63.0
Bread, raisin, toasted	63.0
Bread, reduced calorie and/or high fiber, Italian	68.0
Bread, reduced calorie and/or high fiber, Italian, toasted	68.0
Bread, reduced calorie and/or high fiber, white or NFS	68.0
Bread, reduced calorie and/or high fiber, white or NFS, toasted	68.0
Bread, reduced calorie and/or high fiber, white or NFS, with fruit and/or nuts	68.0
Bread, reduced calorie and/or high fiber, white or NFS, with fruit and/or nuts, toasted	68.0
Bread, rice, toasted	66.5
Bread, rye	58.0
Bread, rye, reduced calorie and/or high fiber	68.0
Bread, rye, reduced calorie and/or high fiber, toasted	68.0
Bread, rye, toasted	58.0
Bread, sour dough	54.0
Bread, sour dough, toasted	54.0
Bread, sprouted wheat, toasted	53.0
Bread, sunflower meal	57.0
Bread, wheat bran	71.0
Bread, wheat bran, toasted	71.0
Bread, wheat or cracked wheat	71.0
Bread, wheat or cracked wheat, made from home recipe or purchased at bakery	53.0
Bread, wheat or cracked wheat, made from home recipe or purchased at bakery, toasted	53.0
Bread, wheat or cracked wheat, reduced calorie and/or high fiber	71.0
Bread, wheat or cracked wheat, reduced calorie and/or high fiber, toasted	71.0

Food Name	Glycemic Index
Bread, wheat or cracked wheat, toasted	71.0
Bread, wheat or cracked wheat, with raisins	53.0
Bread, wheat or cracked wheat, with raisins, toasted	53.0
Bread, white	70.0
Bread, white with whole wheat swirl	70.0
Bread, white with whole wheat swirl, toasted	70.0
Bread, white, low sodium or no salt	70.0
Bread, white, low sodium or no salt, toasted	73.0
Bread, white, made from home recipe or purchased at a bakery	70.0
Bread, white, made from home recipe or purchased at a bakery, toasted	73.0
Bread, white, special formula, added fiber	68.0
Bread, white, toasted	73.0
Bread, whole wheat, 100%	71.0
Bread, whole wheat, 100%, made from home recipe or purchased at bakery	71.0
Bread, whole wheat, 100%, made from home recipe or purchased at bakery, toasted	71.0
Bread, whole wheat, 100%, toasted	71.0
Bread, whole wheat, 100%, with raisins	71.0
Bread, whole wheat, 100%, with raisins, toasted	71.0
Bread, whole wheat, NS as to 100%, with raisins	71.0
Bread, whole wheat, NS as to 100%, with raisins, toasted	71.0
Bread, whole wheat, other than 100% or NS as to 100%	71.0
Bread, whole wheat, other than 100% or NS as to 100%, made from home recipe or purchased at bakery	71.0
Bread, whole wheat, other than 100% or NS as to 100%, made from home recipe or purchased at bakery, toasted	71.0
Bread, whole wheat, other than 100% or NS as to 100%, toasted	71.0
Bread, zucchini	57.9
Breakfast pastry, NFS	59.0
Breakfast tart	70.0

Food Name	Glycemic Index
Breakfast tart, lowfat	70.0
Brioche	67.0
Cake made with glutinous rice	64.0
Cake, angel food, NS as to icing	67.0
Cake, angel food, with fruit and icing or filling	67.0
Cake, angel food, with icing	67.0
Cake, angel food, without icing	67.0
Cake, applesauce, NS as to icing	44.0
Cake, applesauce, with icing	44.0
Cake, applesauce, without icing	44.0
Cake, banana, NS as to icing	47.0
Cake, banana, with icing	47.0
Cake, banana, without icing	47.0
Cake, black forest (chocolate-cherry)	38.0
Cake, butter, with icing	42.0
Cake, butter, without icing	42.0
Cake, carrot, NS as to icing	62.0
Cake, carrot, with icing	62.0
Cake, carrot, without icing	62.0
Cake, chocolate, devil's food, or fudge, made from home recipe or purchased ready-to-eat, NS as to icing	38.0
Cake, chocolate, devil's food, or fudge, pudding type mix, made by "cholesterol free" recipe (water, oil and egg whites added to dry mix), with "light" icing, coating or filling	38.0
Cake, chocolate, devil's food, or fudge, pudding-type mix (oil, eggs, and water added to dry mix), NS as to icing	38.0
Cake, chocolate, devil's food, or fudge, pudding-type mix (oil, eggs, and water added to dry mix), with icing, coating, or filling	38.0
Cake, chocolate, devil's food, or fudge, pudding-type mix (oil, eggs, and water added to dry mix), without icing or filling	38.0
Cake, chocolate, devil's food, or fudge, pudding-type mix, made by "Lite" recipe (eggs and water added to dry mix, no oil added to dry mix), with icing, coating, or filling	38.0

Food Name	Glycemic Index
Cake, chocolate, devil's food, or fudge, standard-type mix (eggs and water added to dry mix), with icing, coating, or filling	38.0
Cake, chocolate, devil's food, or fudge, standard-type mix (eggs and water added to dry mix), without icing or filling	38.0
Cake, chocolate, devil's food, or fudge, with icing, coating, or filling, made from home recipe or purchased ready-to-eat	38.0
Cake, chocolate, devil's food, or fudge, without icing or filling, made from home recipe or purchased ready-to-eat	38.0
Cake, chocolate, with icing, diet	38.0
Cake, coconut, with icing	42.0
Cake, cupcake, chocolate, NS as to icing	38.0
Cake, cupcake, chocolate, with icing or filling	38.0
Cake, cupcake, chocolate, with or without icing, fruit filling or cream filling, lowfat, cholesterol free	38.0
Cake, cupcake, chocolate, without icing or filling	38.0
Cake, cupcake, not chocolate, NS as to icing	57.5
Cake, cupcake, not chocolate, with fruit and cream filling	57.5
Cake, cupcake, not chocolate, with icing or filling	57.5
Cake, cupcake, not chocolate, with icing or filling, lowfat, cholesterol free	73.0
Cake, cupcake, not chocolate, without icing or filling	57.5
Cake, cupcake, NS as to type or icing	42.0
Cake, cupcake, NS as to type, with icing	42.0
Cake, Dobos Torte (non-chocolate layer cake with chocolate filling and icing)	38.0
Cake, frozen yogurt and cake layer, chocolate, with icing	49.5
Cake, fruit cake, light or dark, holiday type cake	57.9
Cake, German chocolate, with icing and filling	38.0
Cake, gingerbread, without icing	57.9
Cake, ice cream and cake roll, chocolate	49.5
Cake, ice cream and cake roll, not chocolate	51.5
Cake, lemon, lowfat, with icing	42.0
Cake, lemon, lowfat, without icing	42.0
Cake, lemon, NS as to icing	42.0

Food Name	Glycemic Index
Cake, lemon, with icing	42.0
Cake, lemon, without icing	42.0
Cake, marble, with icing	40.0
Cake, marble, without icing	40.0
Cake, NS as to type, with or without icing	42.0
Cake, nut, NS as to icing	42.0
Cake, nut, with icing	42.0
Cake, nut, without icing	42.0
Cake, plum pudding	57.9
Cake, poppyseed, without icing	42.0
Cake, pound, chocolate	54.0
Cake, pound, chocolate, fat free, cholesterol free	54.0
Cake, pound, fat free, cholesterol free	54.0
Cake, pound, reduced fat, cholesterol free	54.0
Cake, pound, with icing	54.0
Cake, pound, without icing	54.0
Cake, pumpkin, NS as to icing	62.0
Cake, pumpkin, with icing	62.0
Cake, pumpkin, without icing	62.0
Cake, raisin-nut, without icing	54.0
Cake, spice, NS as to icing	42.0
Cake, spice, with icing	42.0
Cake, spice, without icing	42.0
Cake, sponge, chocolate, with icing	87.0
Cake, sponge, with icing	46.0
Cake, sponge, without icing	46.0
Cake, upside down (all fruits)	44.0
Cake, white, made from home recipe or purchased ready-to-eat, NS as to icing	42.0

Food Name	Glycemic Index
Cake, white, pudding-type mix (oil, egg whites, and water added to dry mix), NS as to icing	42.0
Cake, white, pudding-type mix (oil, egg whites, and water added to dry mix), with icing	42.0
Cake, white, pudding-type mix (oil, egg whites, and water added to dry mix), without icing	42.0
Cake, white, standard-type mix (egg whites and water added to mix), with icing	42.0
Cake, white, standard-type mix (egg whites and water added to mix), without icing	42.0
Cake, white, standard-type mix (egg whites and water added), NS as to icing	42.0
Cake, white, with icing, made from home recipe or purchased ready-to-eat	42.0
Cake, white, without icing, made from home recipe or purchased ready-to-eat	42.0
Cake, yellow, made from home recipe or purchased ready-to- eat, NS as to icing	42.0
Cake, yellow, pudding-type mix (oil, eggs, and water added to dry mix), NS as to icing	42.0
Cake, yellow, pudding-type mix (oil, eggs, and water added to dry mix), with icing	42.0
Cake, yellow, pudding-type mix (oil, eggs, and water added to dry mix), without icing	42.0
Cake, yellow, standard-type mix (eggs and water added to dry mix), NS as to icing	42.0
Cake, yellow, standard-type mix (eggs and water added to dry mix), with icing	42.0
Cake, yellow, standard-type mix (eggs and water added to dry mix), without icing	42.0
Cake, yellow, with icing, made from home recipe or purchased ready-to-eat	42.0
Cake, yellow, without icing, made from home recipe or purchased ready-to-eat	42.0
Cake, zucchini, with icing	57.9
Cake, zucchini, without icing	57.9
Cheesecake	50.0
Cheesecake with fruit	50.0
Cheesecake, chocolate	50.0
Cheesecake, chocolate, reduced fat	50.0
Cheesecake, diet	50.0

Food Name	Glycemic Index
Cheesecake, diet, with fruit	50.0
Cherry pie filling	48.0
Churros	76.0
Cobbler, apple	46.0
Cobbler, berry	59.0
Cobbler, cherry	55.0
Cobbler, peach	55.0
Cobbler, pineapple	59.0
Coffee cake, crumb or quick-bread type	57.9
Coffee cake, crumb or quick-bread type, cheese-filled	57.9
Coffee cake, crumb or quick-bread type, custard filled	57.9
Coffee cake, crumb or quick-bread type, reduced fat, cholesterol free	57.9
Coffee cake, crumb or quick-bread type, with fruit	57.9
Coffee cake, crumb or quick-bread type, with icing	57.9
Coffee cake, NFS	57.9
Coffee cake, yeast type	57.9
Coffee cake, yeast type, fat free, cholesterol free, with fruit	57.9
Coffee cake, yeast type, made from home recipe or purchased at a bakery	57.9
Corn flour patty or tart, fried	75.5
Corn pone, baked	75.5
Cornbread muffin, stick, round	75.5
Cornbread muffin, stick, round, made from home recipe	75.5
Cornbread muffin, stick, round, toasted	75.5
Cornbread stuffing	75.5
Cornbread, made from home recipe	75.5
Cornbread, prepared from mix	75.5
Cornmeal dumpling	75.5
Cornmeal sticks, boiled	75.5

Food Name	Glycemic Index
Cream puff, eclair, custard or cream filled, iced	59.0
Cream puff, eclair, custard or cream filled, iced, reduced fat	59.0
Cream puff, eclair, custard or cream filled, not iced	59.0
Cream puff, eclair, custard or cream filled, NS as to icing	59.0
Crepe, plain	67.0
Crisp, apple, apple dessert	48.7
Crisp, cherry	59.0
Crisp, peach	59.0
Crisp, rhubarb	59.0
Croissant	67.0
Croissant, cheese	67.0
Croissant, chocolate	67.0
Croissant, fruit	67.0
Cruller, NFS	76.0
Crumpet	69.0
Crumpet, toasted	69.0
Danish pastry, plain or spice	59.0
Danish pastry, with cheese	59.0
Danish pastry, with cheese, fat free, cholesterol free	59.0
Danish pastry, with fruit	59.0
Danish pastry, with nuts	59.0
Doughnut, cake type	76.0
Doughnut, cake type, chocolate	76.0
Doughnut, cake type, chocolate covered	76.0
Doughnut, cake type, chocolate covered, dipped in peanuts	76.0
Doughnut, cake type, chocolate, with chocolate icing	76.0
Doughnut, chocolate cream-filled	76.0
Doughnut, custard-filled	76.0

Food Name	Glycemic Index
Doughnut, custard-filled, with icing	76.0
Doughnut, jelly	76.0
Doughnut, NS as to cake or yeast	76.0
Doughnut, oriental	76.0
Doughnut, raised or yeast	76.0
Doughnut, raised or yeast, chocolate	76.0
Doughnut, raised or yeast, chocolate covered	76.0
Doughnut, raised or yeast, chocolate, with chocolate icing	76.0
Doughnut, wheat	76.0
Empanada, Mexican turnover, pumpkin	59.0
French cruller	76.0
French toast sticks, plain	67.0
French toast, plain	67.0
Fritter, apple	59.0
Funnel cake	76.0
Hush puppy	75.5
Injera (American-style Ethiopian bread)	72.0
Lemon pie filling	48.0
Muffin, bran with fruit, lowfat	60.0
Muffin, bran with fruit, no fat, no cholesterol	60.0
Muffin, carrot	62.0
Muffin, chocolate	53.0
Muffin, chocolate chip	53.0
Muffin, English	77.0
Muffin, English, multigrain	43.0
Muffin, English, multigrain, toasted	43.0
Muffin, English, oat bran, toasted	47.0
Muffin, English, toasted	77.0

Food Name	Glycemic Index
Muffin, English, wheat bran	71.0
Muffin, English, wheat bran, toasted	71.0
Muffin, English, wheat or cracked wheat	71.0
Muffin, English, wheat or cracked wheat, toasted	71.0
Muffin, English, wheat or cracked wheat, with raisins, toasted	71.0
Muffin, English, whole wheat, 100%, toasted	71.0
Muffin, English, whole wheat, 100%, with raisins, toasted	71.0
Muffin, English, whole wheat, other than 100% or NS as to 100%, toasted	71.0
Muffin, English, whole wheat, other than 100% or NS as to 100%, with raisins, toasted	71.0
Muffin, English, with fruit other than raisins, toasted	77.0
Muffin, English, with raisins	77.0
Muffin, English, with raisins, toasted	77.0
Muffin, fruit and/or nuts	59.0
Muffin, fruit, fat free, cholesterol free	59.0
Muffin, multigrain, with nuts	64.5
Muffin, NFS	61.1
Muffin, oat bran	60.0
Muffin, oat bran with fruit and/or nuts	60.0
Muffin, oatmeal	69.0
Muffin, plain	44.0
Muffin, pumpkin	62.0
Muffin, wheat	60.0
Muffin, wheat bran	60.0
Muffin, whole wheat	60.0
Muffin, zucchini	57.9
Pancakes, buckwheat	102.0
Pancakes, cornmeal	67.0
Pancakes, plain	67.0

Food Name	Glycemic Index
Pancakes, reduced calorie, high fiber	67.0
Pancakes, sour dough	67.0
Pancakes, whole wheat	67.0
Pancakes, with fruit	67.0
Pastry, fruit-filled	59.0
Pastry, Italian, with cheese	59.0
Pastry, mainly flour and water, fried	59.0
Pastry, Oriental, made with bean or lotus seed paste filling (baked)	59.0
Pastry, Oriental, made with bean paste and salted egg yolk filling (baked)	59.0
Pastry, puff	59.0
Pastry, puff, custard or cream filled, iced or not iced	59.0
Pie, apple, diet	59.0
Pie, apple, fried pie	59.0
Pie, apple, individual size or tart	59.0
Pie, apple, one crust	59.0
Pie, apple, two crust	59.0
Pie, apricot, fried pie	59.0
Pie, apricot, two crust	59.0
Pie, banana cream	59.0
Pie, berry, not blackberry, blueberry, boysenberry, huckleberry, raspberry, or strawberry, individual size or tart	59.0
Pie, berry, not blackberry, blueberry, boysenberry, huckleberry, raspberry, or strawberry; one crust	59.0
Pie, berry, not blackberry, blueberry, boysenberry, huckleberry, raspberry, or strawberry; two crust	59.0
Pie, blackberry, two crust	59.0
Pie, blueberry, individual size or tart	59.0
Pie, blueberry, one crust	59.0
Pie, blueberry, two crust	59.0
Pie, buttermilk	59.0
Pie, cherry, fried pie	59.0

Food Name	Glycemic Index
Pie, cherry, individual size or tart	59.0
Pie, cherry, made with cream cheese and sour cream	59.0
Pie, cherry, one crust	59.0
Pie, cherry, two crust	59.0
Pie, chess	59.0
Pie, chocolate cream	59.0
Pie, chocolate cream, individual size or tart	59.0
Pie, chocolate-marshmallow	59.0
Pie, coconut cream	59.0
Pie, coconut cream, individual size or tart	59.0
Pie, custard	59.0
Pie, custard, individual size or tart	59.0
Pie, individual size or tart, NFS	59.0
Pie, lemon (not cream or meringue)	59.0
Pie, lemon (not cream or meringue), individual size or tart	59.0
Pie, lemon cream	59.0
Pie, lemon cream, individual size or tart	59.0
Pie, lemon meringue	59.0
Pie, mince, individual size or tart	59.0
Pie, mince, two crust	59.0
Pie, NFS	59.0
Pie, oatmeal	59.0
Pie, peach, fried pie	59.0
Pie, peach, individual size or tart	59.0
Pie, peach, one crust	59.0
Pie, peach, two crust	59.0
Pie, peanut butter cream	59.0
Pie, pecan	59.0

Food Name	Glycemic Index
Pie, pecan, individual size or tart	59.0
Pie, pineapple cream	59.0
Pie, pineapple, individual size or tart	59.0
Pie, pineapple, two crust	59.0
Pie, plum, two crust	59.0
Pie, praline mousse, with nuts	59.0
Pie, prune, one crust	59.0
Pie, pudding, flavors other than chocolate	59.0
Pie, pudding, flavors other than chocolate, with chocolate coating, individual size	59.0
Pie, pumpkin	59.0
Pie, raisin, individual size or tart	59.0
Pie, raisin, two crust	59.0
Pie, raspberry, one crust	59.0
Pie, raspberry, two crust	59.0
Pie, rhubarb, one crust	59.0
Pie, rhubarb, two crust	59.0
Pie, squash	59.0
Pie, strawberry cream	59.0
Pie, strawberry-rhubarb, two crust	59.0
Pie, strawberry, individual size or tart	59.0
Pie, strawberry, one crust	59.0
Pie, sweetpotato	59.0
Pie, Toll house chocolate chip	59.0
Pie, vanilla cream	59.0
Roll, French or Vienna	95.0
Roll, French or Vienna, toasted	95.0
Roll, garlic	73.0
Roll, hard, NS as to major flour	73.0

Food Name	Glycemic Index
Roll, hoagie, submarine	73.0
Roll, hoagie, submarine, toasted	73.0
Roll, made from home recipe or purchased at a bakery, NS as to major flour	70.0
Roll, Mexican, bolillo	73.0
Roll, multigrain	43.0
Roll, multigrain, toasted	43.0
Roll, NS as to major flour	70.0
Roll, NS as to major flour, toasted	73.0
Roll, pumpernickel	50.0
Roll, pumpernickel, toasted	50.0
Roll, rye	58.0
Roll, sour dough	54.0
Roll, sweet	57.9
Roll, sweet, cinnamon bun, frosted	57.9
Roll, sweet, cinnamon bun, no frosting	57.9
Roll, sweet, crumb topping, Mexican (Pan Dulce)	59.0
Roll, sweet, no topping, Mexican (Pan Dulce)	59.0
Roll, sweet, sugar topping, Mexican (Pan Dulce)	59.0
Roll, sweet, toasted	57.9
Roll, sweet, with fruit and nuts, frosted	57.9
Roll, sweet, with fruit, frosted	57.9
Roll, sweet, with fruit, frosted, diet	57.9
Roll, sweet, with fruit, frosted, fat free	57.9
Roll, sweet, with fruit, no frosting	57.9
Roll, sweet, with nuts, frosted	57.9
Roll, sweet, with nuts, no frosting	57.9
Roll, wheat or cracked wheat	71.0
Roll, wheat or cracked wheat, made from home recipe or purchased at bakery	71.0

Food Name	Glycemic Index
Roll, white, hard	73.0
Roll, white, hard, toasted	73.0
Roll, white, soft	70.0
Roll, white, soft, made from home recipe or purchased at a bakery	70.0
Roll, white, soft, reduced calorie and/or high fiber	68.0
Roll, white, soft, reduced calorie and/or high fiber, toasted	68.0
Roll, white, soft, toasted	70.0
Roll, whole wheat, 100%	71.0
Roll, whole wheat, 100%, made from home recipe or purchased at bakery	71.0
Roll, whole wheat, 100%, toasted	71.0
Roll, whole wheat, NS as to 100%	71.0
Roll, whole wheat, NS as to 100%, toasted	71.0
Roll, whole wheat, other than 100% or NS as to 100%, made from home recipe or purchased at bakery	71.0
Roll, whole wheat, other than 100% or NS as to 100%, made from home recipe or purchased at bakery, toasted	71.0
Rolls, wheat or cracked wheat, toasted	71.0
Sopaipilla, without syrup or honey	59.0
Spoonbread	75.5
Strudel, apple	59.0
Strudel, berry	59.0
Strudel, cherry	59.0
Tamale, sweet, with fruit	59.0
Toast, NS as to major flour	73.0
Turnover or dumpling, apple	59.0
Turnover or dumpling, berry	59.0
Turnover or dumpling, cherry	59.0
Turnover or dumpling, lemon	59.0
Turnover or dumpling, peach	59.0
Turnover, guava	59.0

Food Name	Glycemic Index
Waffle, 100% whole wheat or 100% whole grain	76.0
Waffle, fruit	76.0
Waffle, multi-bran	76.0
Waffle, nut and honey	76.0
Waffle, oat bran	76.0
Waffle, plain	76.0
Waffle, plain, fat free	76.0
Waffle, plain, lowfat	76.0
Waffle, wheat, bran, or multigrain	76.0

Breakfast Cereals & Grains

Food Name	Glycemic Index
100% Bran	42.0
All-Bran	42.0
All-Bran Bran Buds, Kellogg's (formerly Bran Buds)	58.0
All-Bran with Extra Fiber	42.0
Apple Cinnamon Cheerios	74.0
Apple Cinnamon Oh's Cereal	74.0
Apple Cinnamon Rice Krispies	82.0
Apple Cinnamon Squares Mini-Wheats, Kellogg's (formerly Apple Cinnamon Squares)	58.0
Barley, cooked, fat not added in cooking	25.0
Barley, cooked, NS as to fat added in cooking	25.0
Berry Berry Kix	113.0
Bran Chex	58.0

Food Name	Glycemic Index
Bran Flakes, NFS (formerly 40% Bran Flakes, NFS)	74.0
Breakfast bar, cake-like	57.0
Breakfast bar, cereal crust with fruit filling, fat free	72.0
Breakfast bar, cereal crust with fruit filling, lowfat	72.0
Breakfast bar, date, with yogurt coating	53.5
Breakfast bar, diet meal type	39.3
Breakfast bar, NFS	57.0
Buckwheat groats, cooked, fat added in cooking	45.0
Buckwheat groats, cooked, fat not added in cooking	45.0
Bulgur, cooked or canned, fat added in cooking	48.0
Bulgur, cooked or canned, fat not added in cooking	48.0
Bulgur, cooked or canned, NS as to fat added in cooking	48.0
Cereal, NFS	74.6
Cereal, ready-to-eat, NFS	74.6
Cheerios	74.0
Chex cereal, NFS	58.0
Chicken rice soup, Puerto Rican style (Sopa de pollo con arroz)	64.0
Chocolate flavored frosted puffed corn cereal	80.0
Cocoa Krispies	77.0
Cocoa Pebbles	77.0
Cocoa Puffs	80.0
Common Sense Oat Bran, plain	77.0
Common Sense Oat Bran, with raisins	77.0
Complete Wheat Bran Flakes, Kellogg's (formerly 40% Bran Flakes)	74.0
Corn Chex	83.0
Corn flakes, Kellogg	81.0
Corn flakes, NFS	81.0
Corn Pops	80.0

Food Name	Glycemic Index
Corn Puffs	81.0
Corn, cooked, from canned, NS as to color, fat not added in cooking	46.0
Corn, cooked, from fresh, NS as to color, fat not added in cooking	53.5
Corn, cooked, from frozen, NS as to color, fat not added in cooking	47.0
Corn, cooked, NS as to form, NS as to color, fat not added in cooking	53.5
Corn, from canned, NS as to color, cream style	46.0
Corn, NS as to form, NS as to color, cream style	53.5
Corn, raw	53.5
Corn, white, cooked, from canned, fat not added in cooking	46.0
Corn, white, cooked, from fresh, fat not added in cooking	53.5
Corn, white, cooked, from frozen, fat not added in cooking	47.0
Corn, white, cooked, NS as to form, fat not added in cooking	53.5
Corn, white, from canned, cream style	46.0
Corn, yellow and white, cooked, from canned, fat not added in cooking	46.0
Corn, yellow and white, cooked, from fresh, fat not added in cooking	53.5
Corn, yellow and white, cooked, from frozen, fat not added in cooking	47.0
Corn, yellow and white, cooked, NS as to form, fat not added in cooking	53.5
Corn, yellow, canned, low sodium, fat not added in cooking	46.0
Corn, yellow, cooked, from canned, fat not added in cooking	46.0
Corn, yellow, cooked, from fresh, fat not added in cooking	53.5
Corn, yellow, cooked, from frozen, fat not added in cooking	47.0
Corn, yellow, cooked, NS as to form, fat not added in cooking	53.5
Corn, yellow, from canned, cream style	46.0
Corn, yellow, NS as to form, cream style	53.5
Cornmeal mush, made with milk	56.2
Cornmeal mush, made with water	89.0
Cornmeal, lime-treated, cooked (Masa harina)	69.0
Cracklin' Oat Bran	77.0

Food Name	Glycemic Index
Crispix	87.0
Crispy Brown Rice Cereal	82.0
Crispy Rice	82.0
Crispy Wheats'n Raisins	61.0
Crunchy Corn Bran, Quaker	75.0
Dirty rice	55.8
Double Chex	86.0
Fiber 7 Flakes, Health Valley	74.0
Fiber One	42.0
Flavored rice mixture	54.7
Flavored rice, brown and wild	54.0
Flavored rice, white and wild	54.0
Froot Loops	69.0
Frosted Cheerios	74.0
Frosted corn flakes, NFS	55.0
Frosted Flakes, Kellogg	55.0
Frosted Mini-Wheats	58.0
Frosted Wheat Bites	72.0
Fruit & Fibre (fiber) with peaches, raisins, almonds and oat clusters	42.0
Fruit & Fibre (fiber), NFS	42.0
Fruit Rings, NFS	69.0
Fruit Wheats	72.0
Golden Crisp (Formerly called Super Golden Crisp)	71.0
Golden Grahams	71.0
Grape-Nut Flakes	80.0
Grape-Nuts	71.0
Grits, cooked, corn or hominy, instant, fat not added in cooking	69.0
Grits, cooked, corn or hominy, instant, NS as to fat added in cooking	69.0

Food Name	Glycemic Index
Grits, cooked, corn or hominy, NS as to regular, quick or instant, NS as to fat added in cooking	69.0
Grits, cooked, corn or hominy, NS as to regular, quick, or instant, fat not added in cooking	69.0
Grits, cooked, corn or hominy, NS as to regular, quick, or instant, NS as to fat added in cooking, made with milk	69.0
Grits, cooked, corn or hominy, quick, fat not added in cooking	69.0
Grits, cooked, corn or hominy, quick, NS as to fat added in cooking	69.0
Grits, cooked, corn or hominy, regular, fat not added in cooking	69.0
Grits, cooked, corn or hominy, regular, NS as to fat added in cooking	69.0
Grits, cooked, flavored, corn or hominy, instant, fat not added in cooking	69.0
Grits, cooked, flavored, corn or hominy, instant, NS as to fat added in cooking	69.0
Healthy Choice Almond Crunch with raisins, Kellogg's	68.0
Healthy Choice Multi-Grain Flakes, Kellogg's	68.0
Healthy Choice Multi-Grain Squares, Kellogg's	70.0
High protein bar, candy-like, soy and milk base	56.0
Hominy, cooked, fat not added in cooking	40.0
Honey Bran	72.0
Honey Bunches of Oats	77.0
Honey Bunches of Oats with Almonds, Post	77.0
Honey Crunch Corn Flakes, Kellogg's	72.0
Honey Nut Cheerios	74.0
Honey Smacks	71.0
Just Right	60.0
Just Right Fruit and Nut (formerly Just Right with raisins, dates, and nuts)	60.0
Kashi cereal, NS as to ready to eat or cooked	74.0
Kashi, Puffed	74.0
Kix	81.0
Life (plain and cinnamon)	66.0
Malt-O-Meal Coco-Roos	77.0

Food Name	Glycemic Index
Malt-O-Meal Crispy Rice	82.0
Malt-O-Meal Golden Puffs (formerly Sugar Puffs)	71.0
Malt-O-Meal Honey and Nut Toasty O's	74.0
Malt-O-Meal Puffed Rice	87.0
Malt-O-Meal Puffed Wheat	74.0
Malt-O-Meal Toasted Oat Cereal	74.0
Malt-O-Meal Toasty O's	74.0
Malt-O-meal Tootie Fruities	69.0
Meal replacement bar	39.3
Millet, cooked, fat not added in cooking	71.0
Millet, puffed	107.0
Muesli with apples and almonds, Ralston Purina	49.0
Muesli with raisins, dates, and almonds	49.0
Muesli with raisins, peaches, and pecans	49.0
Mueslix cereal, NFS	48.0
Mueslix Crispy Blend (formerly Mueslix Five Grain Muesli Cereal)	48.0
Mueslix golden crunch cereal	48.0
Mueslix with raisins, walnuts, and cranberries	49.0
Multi Bran Chex	58.0
Multi Grain Cheerios	74.0
Multigrain cereal, cooked, fat not added in cooking	36.5
Natural Bran Flakes, Post (formerly called 40% Bran Flakes, Post)	74.0
Noodles, chow mein	50.0
Nut and Honey Crunch (flakes)	77.0
Nutri-Grain Almond Raisin	66.0
Nutri-Grain Biscuits, Whole Grain Shredded Wheat Cereal	72.5
Nutri-Grain Golden Wheat (formerly Nutri-Grain Wheat)	66.0
Nutty Nuggets, Ralston Purina	71.0

Food Name	Glycemic Index
Oat bran cereal, cooked, fat not added in cooking	55.0
Oat bran cereal, cooked, made with milk, fat not added in cooking	44.2
Oat bran cereal, cooked, NS as to fat added in cooking	55.0
Oat Bran Flakes, Health Valley	67.0
Oat cereal, NFS	74.0
Oat flakes, fortified	67.0
Oat Flakes, Post	67.0
Oatmeal Crisp with Almonds	77.0
Oatmeal with fruit, cooked	58.0
Oatmeal with maple flavor, cooked	58.0
Oatmeal, cooked, instant, fat not added in cooking	58.0
Oatmeal, cooked, instant, NS as to fat added in cooking	58.0
Oatmeal, cooked, NS as to regular, quick or instant, fat not added in cooking	58.0
Oatmeal, cooked, NS as to regular, quick or instant; NS as to fat added in cooking	58.0
Oatmeal, cooked, quick (1 or 3 minutes), fat not added in cooking	58.0
Oatmeal, cooked, quick (1 or 3 minutes), NS as to fat added in cooking	58.0
Oatmeal, cooked, regular, fat not added in cooking	58.0
Oatmeal, cooked, regular, NS as to fat added in cooking	58.0
Oatmeal, fortified, cooked, instant, fat not added in cooking	58.0
Oatmeal, multigrain, cooked, fat not added in cooking	58.0
Oatmeal, NS as to regular, quick, or instant, made with milk, fat not added in cooking	48.4
Oatmeal, with oat bran, fortified, cooked, instant, fat not added in cooking	58.0
Oh's, Honey Graham	71.0
PowerBar (fortified high energy bar)	56.0
Product 19	76.0
Pudding, rice	54.0
Pudding, rice flour, with nuts (Indian dessert)	54.0

Food Name	Glycemic Index
Quaker Oat Bran Cereal	55.0
Quaker Oatmeal Squares (formerly Quaker Oat Squares)	77.0
Raisin Bran, Kellogg	61.0
Raisin bran, NFS	61.0
Raisin Bran, Post	61.0
Raisin Bran, Ralston Purina	61.0
Raisin Bran, Total	61.0
Raisin Grape-Nuts	71.0
Raisin Squares Mini-Wheats, Kellogg's (formerly Raisin Squares)	65.0
Rice Chex	89.0
Rice dressing	64.0
Rice Krispies	82.0
Rice Krispies Treats Cereal (Kellogg's)	82.0
Rice pilaf	64.0
Rice, brown and wild, cooked, fat added in cooking	54.0
Rice, brown and wild, cooked, fat not added in cooking	54.0
Rice, brown and wild, cooked, NS as to fat added in cooking	54.0
Rice, brown, cooked, instant, fat added in cooking	64.0
Rice, brown, cooked, instant, fat not added in cooking	64.0
Rice, brown, cooked, instant, NS as to fat added in cooking	55.0
Rice, brown, cooked, regular, fat added in cooking	55.0
Rice, brown, cooked, regular, fat not added in cooking	55.0
Rice, brown, cooked, regular, NS as to fat added in cooking	55.0
Rice, cooked, NFS	64.0
Rice, cooked, NS as to type, fat added in cooking	64.0
Rice, cream of, cooked, fat not added in cooking	64.0
Rice, puffed	87.0
Rice, white and wild, cooked, fat added in cooking	54.0

Food Name	Glycemic Index
Rice, white and wild, cooked, fat not added in cooking	54.0
Rice, white and wild, cooked, NS as to fat added in cooking	54.0
Rice, white, cooked with (fat) oil, Puerto Rican style (Arroz blanco)	64.0
Rice, white, cooked, converted, fat added in cooking	47.0
Rice, white, cooked, converted, fat not added in cooking	47.0
Rice, white, cooked, converted, NS as to fat added in cooking	47.0
Rice, white, cooked, glutinous	98.0
Rice, white, cooked, instant, fat added in cooking	69.0
Rice, white, cooked, instant, fat not added in cooking	69.0
Rice, white, cooked, instant, NS as to fat added in cooking	69.0
Rice, white, cooked, regular, fat added in cooking	64.0
Rice, white, cooked, regular, fat not added in cooking	64.0
Rice, white, cooked, regular, NS as to fat added in cooking	64.0
Rice, wild, 100%, cooked, fat not added in cooking	57.0
Ripple Crisp Golden Corn	80.0
Shredded Wheat, 100%	75.0
Shredded Wheat'N Bran	61.0
Special K	69.0
Strawberry muesli with pecans and raisins, Ralston	49.0
Strawberry Squares Mini-Wheats, Kellogg's (formerly Strawberry Squares)	72.0
Team	82.0
Toasted oat cereal	74.0
Toasted Oatmeal, Honey Nut (Quaker)	77.0
Total	76.0
Total Corn Flakes	81.0
Uncle Sam's Hi Fiber Cereal	42.0
Weetabix Whole Wheat Cereal	70.0
Wheat Chex	58.0

Food Name	Glycemic Index
Wheat, cream of, cooked, instant, fat not added in cooking	74.0
Wheat, cream of, cooked, instant, NS as to fat added in cooking	74.0
Wheat, cream of, cooked, made with milk	49.8
Wheat, cream of, cooked, NS as to regular, quick, or instant, fat not added in cooking	66.0
Wheat, cream of, cooked, NS as to regular, quick, or instant, NS as to fat added in cooking	66.0
Wheat, cream of, cooked, quick, fat not added in cooking	66.0
Wheat, cream of, cooked, quick, NS as to fat added in cooking	66.0
Wheat, cream of, cooked, regular, fat not added in cooking	66.0
Wheat, cream of, cooked, regular, NS as to fat added in cooking	66.0
Wheat, puffed, plain	74.0
Wheat, puffed, presweetened with sugar	71.0
Wheaties	37.0
Wheaties, Honey Frosted (formerly Wheaties Honey Gold)	72.0
Whole wheat cereal, cooked, fat not added in cooking	48.0
Whole wheat cereal, cooked, NS as to fat added in cooking	48.0
Whole wheat cereal, wheat and barley, cooked, fat not added in cooking	36.5
Whole wheat cereal, wheat and barley, cooked, NS as to fat added in cooking	36.5
Yellow rice, cooked, regular, fat added in cooking	64.0
Yellow rice, cooked, regular, fat not added in cooking	64.0
Yellow rice, cooked, regular, NS as to fat added in cooking	64.0

Dairy Products and Alternatives

Food Name	Glycemic Index
Alfredo sauce	27.0
Blue or roquefort cheese dressing	50.0
Butter-margarine blend, stick, salted	50.0
Butter-margarine blend, stick, salted	50.0
Butter-margarine blend, stick, salted	50.0
Butter-margarine blend, stick, salted	50.0
Butter, NFS	50.0
Butter, NFS	50.0
Butter, NFS	50.0
Butter, NFS	50.0
Butter, NFS	50.0
Butter, stick, salted	50.0
Butter, stick, salted	50.0
Butter, stick, salted	50.0
Butter, stick, salted	50.0
Butter, stick, salted	50.0
Butter, stick, unsalted	50.0
Butter, stick, unsalted	50.0
Butter, stick, unsalted	50.0
Butter, stick, unsalted	50.0
Butter, stick, unsalted	50.0
Butter, whipped, tub, salted	50.0
Butter, whipped, tub, salted	50.0
Butter, whipped, tub, salted	50.0
Butter, whipped, tub, salted	50.0
Butter, whipped, tub, salted	50.0
Butter, whipped, tub, unsalted	50.0

Food Name	Glycemic Index
Butter, whipped, tub, unsalted	50.0
Butter, whipped, tub, unsalted	50.0
Butter, whipped, tub, unsalted	50.0
Butter, whipped, tub, unsalted	50.0
Buttermilk, fluid, 2% fat	29.5
Buttermilk, fluid, 2% fat	29.5
Buttermilk, fluid, nonfat	32.0
Caesar dressing	50.0
Canola, soybean and sunflower oil	0.0
Carry-out milk shake, chocolate	44.0
Carry-out milk shake, flavors other than chocolate	44.0
Cheese sauce	27.0
Cheese sauce made with lowfat cheese	27.0
Cheese spread, American or Cheddar cheese base	27.0
Cheese spread, American or Cheddar cheese base, lowfat, low sodium	27.0
Cheese spread, cream cheese or Neufchatel base	27.0
Cheese spread, NFS	27.0
Cheese spread, pressurized can	27.0
Cheese spread, Swiss cheese base	27.0
Cheese with nuts	27.0
Cheese, Blue or Roquefort	27.0
Cheese, Brick	27.0
Cheese, Brie	27.0
Cheese, Camembert	27.0
Cheese, Cheddar or American type, dry, grated	27.0
Cheese, Cheddar or American type, NS as to natural or processed	27.0
Cheese, Cheddar or Colby, low sodium	27.0
Cheese, Cheddar or Colby, low sodium, lowfat	27.0

Food Name	Glycemic Index
Cheese, Cheddar or Colby, lowfat	27.0
Cheese, Colby	27.0
Cheese, Colby Jack	27.0
Cheese, cottage cheese, with gelatin dessert and fruit	42.5
Cheese, cottage, creamed, large or small curd	27.0
Cheese, cottage, dry curd	27.0
Cheese, cottage, low sodium	27.0
Cheese, cottage, lowfat (1-2% fat)	32.0
Cheese, cottage, lowfat, low sodium	32.0
Cheese, cottage, lowfat, with fruit	45.0
Cheese, cottage, lowfat, with vegetables	32.0
Cheese, cottage, NFS	29.5
Cheese, cottage, salted, dry curd	32.0
Cheese, cottage, with fruit	42.5
Cheese, cream	27.0
Cheese, cream, lowfat	27.0
Cheese, Feta	27.0
Cheese, Fontina	27.0
Cheese, goat	27.0
Cheese, Gouda or Edam	27.0
Cheese, Gruyere	27.0
Cheese, Limburger	27.0
Cheese, Monterey	27.0
Cheese, Monterey, lowfat	27.0
Cheese, Mozzarella, low sodium	27.0
Cheese, Mozzarella, NFS	27.0
Cheese, Mozzarella, nonfat or fat free	32.0
Cheese, Mozzarella, part skim	27.0

Food Name	Glycemic Index
Cheese, Muenster	27.0
Cheese, Muenster, lowfat	27.0
Cheese, natural, Cheddar or American type	27.0
Cheese, natural, NFS	27.0
Cheese, NFS	27.0
Cheese, Parmesan, dry grated	27.0
Cheese, Parmesan, hard	27.0
Cheese, Parmesan, low sodium	27.0
Cheese, processed cheese food	27.0
Cheese, processed cheese product, American or Cheddar type, reduced fat	27.0
Cheese, processed cheese product, American or Cheddar type, reduced fat, reduced sodium	27.0
Cheese, processed cheese product, Swiss, reduced fat	27.0
Cheese, processed cream cheese product, nonfat or fat free	32.0
Cheese, processed, American and Swiss blends	27.0
Cheese, processed, American or Cheddar type	27.0
Cheese, processed, American or Cheddar type, low sodium	27.0
Cheese, processed, American or Cheddar type, lowfat	27.0
Cheese, processed, American or Cheddar type, nonfat or fat free	32.0
Cheese, processed, American, Cheddar, or Colby, lowfat, low sodium	27.0
Cheese, processed, Mozzarella, low sodium	27.0
Cheese, processed, Swiss	27.0
Cheese, processed, Swiss, low sodium	27.0
Cheese, processed, Swiss, lowfat	27.0
Cheese, processed, Swiss, lowfat, low sodium	27.0
Cheese, processed, with vegetables	27.0
Cheese, Provolone	27.0
Cheese, Provolone, reduced fat, reduced sodium	27.0
Cheese, Ricotta	27.0

Food Name	Glycemic Index
Cheese, Semi-soft, low sodium	27.0
Cheese, Swiss	27.0
Cheese, Swiss, low sodium	27.0
Cheese, Swiss, lowfat	27.0
Cheese, yogurt, NFS	27.0
Clam sauce, white	27.0
Cocoa with nonfat dry milk and low calorie sweetener, mixture, water added	24.0
Cocoa with nonfat dry milk and low calorie sweetener, mixture, water added	24.0
Cocoa, whey, and low-calorie sweetener mixture, lowfat milk added	24.0
Coconut custard, Puerto Rican style (Flan de coco)	38.0
Coleslaw dressing, reduced calorie	50.0
Corn oil	0.0
Cottage cheese, farmer's	27.0
Cream substitute, frozen	27.0
Cream substitute, light, liquid	27.0
Cream substitute, light, powdered	27.0
Cream substitute, liquid	27.0
Cream substitute, NS as to frozen, liquid, or powdered	27.0
Cream substitute, powdered	27.0
Cream, half and half	27.0
Cream, heavy, fluid	27.0
Cream, light, fluid	27.0
Cream, light, whipped, unsweetened	27.0
Cream, NS as to light, heavy, or half and half	27.0
Creamy dressing, made with sour cream and/or buttermilk and oil	50.0
Creamy dressing, made with sour cream and/or buttermilk and oil, reduced calorie	50.0
Creamy dressing, made with sour cream and/or buttermilk and oil, reduced calorie, fat-free, cholesterol-free	50.0

Food Name	Glycemic Index
Custard	38.0
Custard, Puerto Rican style (Flan)	38.0
Dip, cheese base other than cream cheese	27.0
Dip, cheese with chili pepper (chili con queso)	27.0
Dip, cream cheese base	27.0
Dip, sour cream base	27.0
Dip, sour cream base, reduced calorie	27.0
Flaxseed oil	0.0
French dressing	50.0
French dressing, reduced calorie	50.0
French dressing, reduced calorie, fat-free, cholesterol-free	50.0
Ghee, clarified butter	0.0
Ghee, clarified butter	0.0
Honey butter	55.0
Honey butter	55.0
Honey butter	55.0
Honey mustard dressing	50.0
Ice cream bar or stick, not chocolate covered or cake covered	61.0
Ice cream with sherbet	51.5
Ice cream, NFS	61.0
Ice cream, regular, chocolate	61.0
Ice cream, regular, flavors other than chocolate	61.0
Ice cream, rich, chocolate	37.0
Ice cream, rich, flavors other than chocolate	38.0
Ice cream, soft serve, chocolate	61.0
Ice cream, soft serve, flavors other than chocolate	61.0
Ice cream, soft serve, NS as to flavor	61.0
Imitation cheese, American or cheddar type	27.0

Food Name	Glycemic Index
Imitation cheese, American or cheddar type, low cholesterol	27.0
Imitation mozzarella cheese	27.0
Italian dressing, low calorie	50.0
Italian dressing, made with vinegar and oil	50.0
Italian dressing, reduced calorie	50.0
Italian dressing, reduced calorie, fat-free	50.0
Light butter, stick, salted	0.0
Light butter, stick, salted	0.0
Light butter, stick, salted	0.0
Light butter, stick, salted	0.0
Light butter, stick, salted	0.0
Light ice cream, chocolate (formerly ice milk)	50.0
Light ice cream, flavors other than chocolate (formerly ice milk)	50.0
Light ice cream, fudgesicle (formerly ice milk)	50.0
Light ice cream, NFS (formerly ice milk)	50.0
Light ice cream, premium, chocolate (formerly ice milk)	50.0
Light ice cream, premium, flavors other than chocolate (formerly ice milk)	50.0
Light ice cream, soft serve, chocolate (formerly ice milk)	50.0
Light ice cream, soft serve, flavors other than chocolate (formerly ice milk)	50.0
Light ice cream, soft serve, NS as to flavor (formerly ice milk)	50.0
Light ice cream, with sherbet or ice cream (formerly ice milk)	46.0
Margarine-like spread, fat free, liquid, salted	50.0
Margarine-like spread, fat free, liquid, salted	50.0
Margarine-like spread, fat free, liquid, salted	50.0
Margarine-like spread, fat free, liquid, salted	50.0
Margarine-like spread, fat free, liquid, salted	50.0
Margarine-like spread, fat free, tub, salted	50.0
Margarine-like spread, fat free, tub, salted	50.0

Food Name	Glycemic Index
Margarine-like spread, fat free, tub, salted	50.0
Margarine-like spread, fat free, tub, salted	50.0
Margarine-like spread, fat free, tub, salted	50.0
Margarine-like spread, liquid, salted	0.0
Margarine-like spread, liquid, salted	0.0
Margarine-like spread, liquid, salted	0.0
Margarine-like spread, liquid, salted	0.0
Margarine-like spread, liquid, salted	0.0
Margarine-like spread, reduced calorie, about 20% fat, tub, unsalted	0.0
Margarine-like spread, reduced calorie, about 20% fat, tub, unsalted	0.0
Margarine-like spread, reduced calorie, about 20% fat, tub, unsalted	0.0
Margarine-like spread, reduced calorie, about 20% fat, tub, unsalted	0.0
Margarine-like spread, reduced calorie, about 40% fat, stick, salted	0.0
Margarine-like spread, reduced calorie, about 40% fat, stick, salted	0.0
Margarine-like spread, reduced calorie, about 40% fat, stick, salted	0.0
Margarine-like spread, reduced calorie, about 40% fat, stick, salted	0.0
Margarine-like spread, reduced calorie, about 40% fat, stick, salted	0.0
Margarine-like spread, reduced calorie, about 40% fat, tub, salted	50.0
Margarine-like spread, reduced calorie, about 40% fat, tub, salted	50.0
Margarine-like spread, reduced calorie, about 40% fat, tub, salted	50.0
Margarine-like spread, reduced calorie, about 40% fat, tub, salted	50.0
Margarine-like spread, reduced calorie, about 40% fat, tub, salted	50.0
Margarine-like spread, stick, salted	0.0
Margarine-like spread, stick, salted	0.0
Margarine-like spread, stick, salted	0.0
Margarine-like spread, stick, salted	0.0
Margarine-like spread, stick, salted	0.0
Margarine-like spread, stick, unsalted	0.0

Food Name	Glycemic Index
Margarine-like spread, stick, unsalted	0.0
Margarine-like spread, stick, unsalted	0.0
Margarine-like spread, stick, unsalted	0.0
Margarine-like spread, stick, unsalted	0.0
Margarine-like spread, tub, salted	0.0
Margarine-like spread, tub, salted	0.0
Margarine-like spread, tub, salted	0.0
Margarine-like spread, tub, salted	0.0
Margarine-like spread, tub, salted	0.0
Margarine-like spread, whipped, tub, salted	0.0
Margarine-like spread, whipped, tub, salted	0.0
Margarine-like spread, whipped, tub, salted	0.0
Margarine-like spread, whipped, tub, salted	0.0
Margarine-like spread, whipped, tub, salted	0.0
Margarine, liquid, salted	0.0
Margarine, liquid, salted	0.0
Margarine, liquid, salted	0.0
Margarine, liquid, salted	0.0
Margarine, NFS	0.0
Margarine, NFS	0.0
Margarine, NFS	0.0
Margarine, NFS	0.0
Margarine, NFS	0.0
Margarine, stick, salted	50.0
Margarine, stick, salted	50.0
Margarine, stick, salted	50.0
Margarine, stick, salted	50.0
Margarine, stick, salted	50.0

Food Name	Glycemic Index
Margarine, stick, unsalted	50.0
Margarine, stick, unsalted	50.0
Margarine, stick, unsalted	50.0
Margarine, stick, unsalted	50.0
Margarine, stick, unsalted	50.0
Margarine, tub, salted	50.0
Margarine, tub, salted	50.0
Margarine, tub, salted	50.0
Margarine, tub, salted	50.0
Margarine, tub, salted	50.0
Margarine, tub, unsalted	50.0
Margarine, tub, unsalted	50.0
Margarine, tub, unsalted	50.0
Margarine, tub, unsalted	50.0
Margarine, tub, unsalted	50.0
Margarine, whipped, tub, salted	50.0
Margarine, whipped, tub, salted	50.0
Margarine, whipped, tub, salted	50.0
Margarine, whipped, tub, salted	50.0
Margarine, whipped, tub, salted	50.0
Margarine, whipped, tub, unsalted	50.0
Margarine, whipped, tub, unsalted	50.0
Mayonnaise-type salad dressing	50.0
Mayonnaise-type salad dressing	50.0
Mayonnaise-type salad dressing, cholesterol-free	50.0
Mayonnaise-type salad dressing, fat-free	50.0
Mayonnaise-type salad dressing, fat-free	50.0
Mayonnaise-type salad dressing, low-calorie or diet	50.0

Food Name	Glycemic Index
Mayonnaise-type salad dressing, low-calorie or diet	50.0
Mayonnaise-type salad dressing, low-calorie or diet, cholesterol-free	50.0
Mayonnaise-type salad dressing, low-calorie or diet, cholesterol-free	50.0
Mayonnaise, low-calorie or diet	50.0
Mayonnaise, low-calorie or diet	50.0
Mayonnaise, low-calorie or diet, low sodium	50.0
Mayonnaise, reduced calorie or diet, cholesterol-free	50.0
Mayonnaise, reduced calorie or diet, cholesterol-free	50.0
Mayonnaise, regular	50.0
Mayonnaise, regular	50.0
Milk beverage with nonfat dry milk and low calorie sweetener, high calcium, water added, chocolate	24.0
Milk dessert, frozen, chocolate (no butterfat)	61.0
Milk dessert, frozen, flavors other than chocolate (no butterfat)	61.0
Milk dessert, frozen, lowfat, flavors other than chocolate	50.0
Milk dessert, frozen, made with low-calorie sweetener, flavors other than chocolate	50.0
Milk shake, homemade or fountain-type, chocolate	44.0
Milk shake, homemade or fountain-type, flavors other than chocolate	44.0
Milk shake, made with skim milk, chocolate	46.5
Milk shake, made with skim milk, flavors other than chocolate	46.5
Milk shake, NS as to flavor or type	44.0
Milk, calcium fortified, cow's, fluid, 1% fat	32.0
Milk, calcium fortified, cow's, fluid, skim or nonfat	32.0
Milk, calcium fortified, cow's, fluid, skim or nonfat	32.0
Milk, calcium fortified, cow's, fluid, skim or nonfat	32.0
Milk, condensed, sweetened, NS as to dilution	61.0
Milk, condensed, sweetened, undiluted	61.0
Milk, cow's, fluid, 1% fat	32.0
Milk, cow's, fluid, 1% fat	32.0

Food Name	Glycemic Index
Milk, cow's, fluid, 1% fat	32.0
Milk, cow's, fluid, 2% fat	29.5
Milk, cow's, fluid, 2% fat	29.5
Milk, cow's, fluid, 2% fat	29.5
Milk, cow's, fluid, acidophilus, 1% fat	32.0
Milk, cow's, fluid, acidophilus, 1% fat	32.0
Milk, cow's, fluid, acidophilus, 1% fat	32.0
Milk, cow's, fluid, lactose reduced, 1% fat	32.0
Milk, cow's, fluid, lactose reduced, 1% fat	32.0
Milk, cow's, fluid, lactose reduced, 1% fat	32.0
Milk, cow's, fluid, lactose reduced, 2% fat	29.5
Milk, cow's, fluid, lactose reduced, 2% fat	29.5
Milk, cow's, fluid, lactose reduced, 2% fat	29.5
Milk, cow's, fluid, lactose reduced, nonfat	32.0
Milk, cow's, fluid, lactose reduced, nonfat	32.0
Milk, cow's, fluid, lactose reduced, nonfat	32.0
Milk, cow's, fluid, other than whole, NS as to 2%, 1%, or skim (formerly milk, cow's, fluid, "lowfat", NS as to percent fat)	32.0
Milk, cow's, fluid, other than whole, NS as to 2%, 1%, or skim (formerly milk, cow's, fluid, "lowfat", NS as to percent fat)	32.0
Milk, cow's, fluid, other than whole, NS as to 2%, 1%, or skim (formerly milk, cow's, fluid, "lowfat", NS as to percent fat)	32.0
Milk, cow's, fluid, skim or nonfat, 0.5% or less butterfat	32.0
Milk, cow's, fluid, skim or nonfat, 0.5% or less butterfat	32.0
Milk, cow's, fluid, skim or nonfat, 0.5% or less butterfat	32.0
Milk, cow's, fluid, whole	27.0
Milk, cow's, fluid, whole	27.0
Milk, cow's, fluid, whole	27.0
Milk, dry, reconstituted, lowfat	32.0
Milk, dry, reconstituted, lowfat	32.0
Milk, dry, reconstituted, lowfat	32.0

Food Name	Glycemic Index
Milk, dry, reconstituted, NFS	32.0
Milk, dry, reconstituted, NFS	32.0
Milk, dry, reconstituted, nonfat	32.0
Milk, dry, reconstituted, nonfat	32.0
Milk, dry, reconstituted, nonfat	32.0
Milk, dry, reconstituted, whole	27.0
Milk, dry, reconstituted, whole	27.0
Milk, dry, reconstituted, whole	27.0
Milk, evaporated, NS as to fat content and dilution	27.0
Milk, evaporated, NS as to fat content and dilution, used in coffee or tea (assume undiluted)	27.0
Milk, evaporated, NS as to fat content, undiluted	27.0
Milk, evaporated, whole, undiluted	27.0
Milk, goat's, fluid, whole	27.0
Milk, NFS	29.5
Milk, NFS	29.5
Milk, NFS	29.5
Milk, soy, dry, reconstituted, not baby's	40.0
Milk, soy, dry, reconstituted, not baby's	40.0
Milk, soy, ready-to-drink, not baby's	40.0
Milk, soy, ready-to-drink, not baby's	40.0
Milk, soy, ready-to-drink, not baby's	40.0
Mousse, chocolate	34.0
Mousse, not chocolate	34.0
Olive oil	0.0
Parmesan cheese topping, fat free	32.0
Peanut oil	0.0
Pudding pops, chocolate	44.0
Pudding, canned, chocolate	44.0

Food Name	Glycemic Index
Pudding, canned, chocolate and non-chocolate flavors combined	44.0
Pudding, canned, chocolate, fat free	44.0
Pudding, canned, chocolate, reduced fat	44.0
Pudding, canned, flavors other than chocolate	44.0
Pudding, canned, flavors other than chocolate, fat free	44.0
Pudding, canned, flavors other than chocolate, reduced fat	44.0
Pudding, canned, low calorie, containing artificial sweetener, chocolate	44.0
Pudding, canned, low calorie, containing artificial sweetener, flavors other than chocolate	44.0
Pudding, canned, tapioca	62.5
Pudding, canned, tapioca, fat free	62.5
Pudding, chocolate, prepared from dry mix, low calorie, containing artificial sweetener, milk added	44.0
Pudding, chocolate, prepared from dry mix, milk added	44.0
Pudding, chocolate, ready-to-eat, low calorie, containing artificial sweetener, NS as to from dry mix or canned	44.0
Pudding, chocolate, ready-to-eat, NS as to from dry mix or canned	44.0
Pudding, coconut	44.0
Pudding, flavors other than chocolate, prepared from dry mix, low calorie, containing artificial sweetener, milk added	44.0
Pudding, flavors other than chocolate, prepared from dry mix, milk added	44.0
Pudding, flavors other than chocolate, ready-to-eat, low calorie, containing artificial sweetener, NS as to from dry mix or canned	44.0
Pudding, flavors other than chocolate, ready-to-eat, NS as to from dry mix or canned	44.0
Pudding, Indian (milk, molasses and cornmeal-based pudding)	44.0
Pudding, NFS	44.0
Pudding, pumpkin	44.0
Pudding, tapioca, made from dry mix, made with milk	62.5
Pudding, tapioca, made from home recipe, made with milk	62.5
Puerto Rican white cheese (queso del pais, blanco)	27.0
Queso Anejo (aged Mexican cheese)	27.0

Food Name	Glycemic Index
Queso Asadero	27.0
Queso Chihuahua	27.0
Queso Fresco	27.0
Rapeseed oil	0.0
Rice beverage	50.0
Russian dressing	50.0
Russian dressing, low-calorie	50.0
Safflower oil	0.0
Salad dressing, NFS	50.0
Sandwich spread	50.0
Sesame oil	0.0
Sherbet, all flavors	42.0
Shrimp dip, cream cheese base	27.0
Sorbet and ice cream	51.5
Sour cream	27.0
Sour cream, fat free	32.0
Sour cream, half and half	27.0
Sour cream, light	27.0
Sour cream, reduced fat	27.0
Soybean oil	0.0
Spinach dip, sour cream base	27.0
Sweet and sour dressing	50.0
Thousand Island dressing	50.0
Thousand Island dressing, reduced calorie, fat-free, cholesterol-free	50.0
Tofu, frozen dessert, chocolate	115.0
Vegetable oil-butter spread, reduced calorie, stick, salted	0.0
Vegetable oil-butter spread, reduced calorie, stick, salted	0.0
Vegetable oil-butter spread, reduced calorie, stick, salted	0.0

Food Name	Glycemic Index
Vegetable oil-butter spread, reduced calorie, tub, salted	50.0
Vegetable oil-butter spread, reduced calorie, tub, salted	50.0
Vegetable oil-butter spread, reduced calorie, tub, salted	50.0
Vegetable oil-butter spread, tub, salted	50.0
Vegetable oil-butter spread, tub, salted	50.0
Vegetable oil-butter spread, tub, salted	50.0
Vegetable oil-butter spread, tub, salted	50.0
Vegetable oil-butter spread, tub, salted	50.0
Vegetable oil, NFS	0.0
Vinegar, sugar, and water dressing	50.0
Welsh rarebit	27.0
White sauce, milk sauce	27.0
Yogurt dressing	50.0
Yogurt, chocolate, nonfat milk	32.0
Yogurt, chocolate, NS as to type of milk	33.0
Yogurt, frozen, chocolate, lowfat milk	50.0
Yogurt, frozen, chocolate, nonfat milk	50.0
Yogurt, frozen, chocolate, nonfat milk, with low-calorie sweetener	50.0
Yogurt, frozen, chocolate, NS as to type of milk	50.0
Yogurt, frozen, chocolate, whole milk	50.0
Yogurt, frozen, flavors other than chocolate, lowfat milk	50.0
Yogurt, frozen, flavors other than chocolate, nonfat milk	50.0
Yogurt, frozen, flavors other than chocolate, nonfat milk, with low-calorie sweetener	50.0
Yogurt, frozen, flavors other than chocolate, NS as to type of milk	50.0
Yogurt, frozen, flavors other than chocolate, whole milk	50.0
Yogurt, frozen, flavors other than chocolate, with sorbet or sorbet-coated	50.0
Yogurt, frozen, NS as to flavor, lowfat milk	50.0
Yogurt, frozen, NS as to flavor, nonfat milk	50.0

Food Name	Glycemic Index
Yogurt, frozen, NS as to flavor, NS as to type of milk	50.0
Yogurt, fruit variety, lowfat milk	31.0
Yogurt, fruit variety, nonfat milk	32.0
Yogurt, fruit variety, nonfat milk, sweetened with low-calorie sweetener	19.0
Yogurt, fruit variety, NS as to type of milk	33.0
Yogurt, fruit variety, whole milk	33.0
Yogurt, NS as to type of milk or flavor	33.0
Yogurt, plain, lowfat milk	36.0
Yogurt, plain, nonfat milk	36.0
Yogurt, plain, NS as to type of milk	31.5
Yogurt, plain, whole milk	36.0
Yogurt, vanilla, lemon, maple, or coffee flavor, lowfat milk	27.0
Yogurt, vanilla, lemon, maple, or coffee flavor, nonfat milk	32.0
Yogurt, vanilla, lemon, maple, or coffee flavor, nonfat milk, sweetened with low calorie sweetener	19.0
Yogurt, vanilla, lemon, or coffee flavor, NS as to type of milk	27.0
Yogurt, vanilla, lemon, or coffee flavor, whole milk	27.0

Soups, Pasta and Noodles

Food Name	Glycemic Index
Asparagus soup, cream of, NS as to made with milk or water	27.0
Asparagus soup, cream of, prepared with milk	27.0
Bean and ham soup, chunky style	64.0
Bean and ham soup, home recipe	64.0
Bean and rice soup	42.2
Bean soup with vegetables and rice, canned, reduced sodium, prepared with water or ready-to-serve	55.3
Bean soup, home recipe	64.0
Bean soup, mixed beans	64.0
Bean soup, NFS	64.0
Bean soup, with macaroni	37.8
Bean soup, with macaroni and meat	38.3
Bean with bacon or pork soup	64.0
Beef and rice noodle soup, Oriental style (Vietnamese Pho Bo)	53.0
Beef broth, with tomato, home recipe	38.0
Beef noodle soup	42.0
Beef noodle soup, home recipe	42.0
Beef noodle soup, Puerto Rican style (Sopa de carne y fideos)	42.0
Beef rice soup	64.0
Beef stroganoff soup, chunky style	42.0
Beef vegetable soup with noodles, stew type, chunky style	40.0
Beef vegetable soup with potato, stew type	44.0
Beef vegetable soup with rice, stew type, chunky style	51.0
Beef vegetable soup, Mexican style (Sopa / caldo de Res)	38.0
Beef with vegetables (including carrots, broccoli, and/or dark-green leafy (no potatoes)), (mushroom) soup (mixture)	38.0
Beef, broth, bouillon, or consomme	50.0

Food Name	Glycemic Index
Beef, noodles, and vegetables (excluding carrots, broccoli, and dark-green leafy), (mushroom) soup (mixture)	34.7
Beef, rice, and vegetables (excluding carrots, broccoli, and dark-green leafy), (mushroom) soup (mixture)	49.1
Beef, rice, and vegetables (including carrots, broccoli, and/or dark-green leafy), (mushroom) soup (mixture)	47.4
Black bean soup	64.0
Broccoli cheese soup, prepared with milk	27.0
Broccoli soup	27.0
Carrot soup, cream of, prepared with milk	37.0
Cauliflower soup, cream of, prepared with milk	27.0
Celery soup, cream of, NS as to made with milk or water	27.0
Celery soup, cream of, prepared with milk	27.0
Celery soup, cream of, prepared with water	27.0
Cheddar cheese soup	27.0
Chicken and mushroom soup, cream of, prepared with milk	27.0
Chicken broth, with tomato, home recipe	38.0
Chicken gumbo soup	38.0
Chicken noodle soup	42.0
Chicken noodle soup, canned, low sodium, ready-to-serve	42.0
Chicken noodle soup, canned, reduced sodium, ready-to-serve	42.0
Chicken noodle soup, chunky style	40.0
Chicken noodle soup, cream of	34.5
Chicken noodle soup, home recipe	42.0
Chicken or turkey rice soup, home recipe	64.0
Chicken or turkey soup, cream of, canned, made with milk, reduced sodium	27.0
Chicken or turkey soup, cream of, canned, made with water, reduced sodium	27.0
Chicken or turkey soup, cream of, canned, undiluted	27.0
Chicken or turkey soup, cream of, NS as to prepared with milk or water	27.0
Chicken or turkey soup, cream of, prepared with milk	27.0

Food Name	Glycemic Index
Chicken or turkey soup, cream of, prepared with water	27.0
Chicken or turkey vegetable soup, home recipe	38.0
Chicken or turkey vegetable soup, stew type	38.0
Chicken rice soup	64.0
Chicken rice soup, canned, reduced sodium, prepared with water or ready-to-serve	64.0
Chicken soup	42.0
Chicken soup with noodles and potatoes, Puerto Rican style	57.0
Chicken soup with vegetables (broccoli, carrots, celery, potatoes and onions), Oriental style	38.0
Chicken vegetable soup with noodles, stew type, chunky style	40.0
Chicken vegetable soup with potato and cheese, chunky style	44.0
Chicken vegetable soup with rice, Mexican style (Sopa / Caldo de Pollo)	51.0
Chicken vegetable soup with rice, stew type, chunky style	51.0
Chicken, broth, bouillon, or consomme	50.0
Chili beef soup	51.0
Chili beef soup, chunky style	51.0
Chow fun noodles with meat and vegetables	50.5
Chow fun rice noodles, cooked, fat added in cooking	50.5
Chow fun rice noodles, cooked, fat not added in cooking	50.5
Chow fun rice noodles, cooked, NS as to fat added in cooking	50.5
Chunky pea and ham soup	66.0
Clam chowder, Manhattan	38.0
Clam chowder, New England, canned, reduced sodium, ready-to-serve	27.0
Clam chowder, New England, NS as to prepared with water or milk	27.0
Clam chowder, New England, prepared with milk	27.0
Clam chowder, New England, prepared with water	27.0
Clam chowder, NS as to Manhattan or New England style	29.7
Corn soup, cream of, prepared with milk	40.5
Corn soup, cream of, prepared with water	40.5

Food Name	Glycemic Index
Couscous, plain, cooked, fat added in cooking	65.0
Couscous, plain, cooked, fat not added in cooking	65.0
Couscous, plain, cooked, NS as to fat added in cooking	65.0
Crab soup, cream of, prepared with milk	27.0
Crab soup, tomato-base	38.0
Cucumber soup, cream of, prepared with milk	27.0
Dark-green leafy vegetable soup with meat, Oriental style	38.0
Dark-green leafy vegetable soup, meatless, Oriental style	38.0
Duck egg, cooked	50.0
Egg omelet or scrambled egg with chicken	50.0
Egg omelet or scrambled egg, fat added in cooking	50.0
Egg omelet or scrambled egg, fat not added in cooking	50.0
Egg omelet or scrambled egg, NS as to fat added in cooking	50.0
Egg omelet or scrambled egg, with beef	50.0
Egg omelet or scrambled egg, with cheese	50.0
Egg omelet or scrambled egg, with cheese and ham or bacon	50.0
Egg omelet or scrambled egg, with cheese, ham or bacon, and tomatoes	50.0
Egg omelet or scrambled egg, with chili, cheese, tomatoes, and beans	50.0
Egg omelet or scrambled egg, with chorizo	50.0
Egg omelet or scrambled egg, with dark-green vegetables	50.0
Egg omelet or scrambled egg, with fish	50.0
Egg omelet or scrambled egg, with ham or bacon	50.0
Egg omelet or scrambled egg, with mushrooms	50.0
Egg omelet or scrambled egg, with onions, peppers, tomatoes, and mushrooms	50.0
Egg omelet or scrambled egg, with peppers, onion, and ham	50.0
Egg omelet or scrambled egg, with potatoes and/or onions (Tortilla Espanola, traditional style Spanish omelet)	50.0
Egg omelet or scrambled egg, with sausage	50.0
Egg omelet or scrambled egg, with sausage and cheese	50.0

Food Name	Glycemic Index
Egg omelet or scrambled egg, with sausage and mushrooms	50.0
Egg omelet or scrambled egg, with vegetables other than dark-green vegetables	50.0
Egg roll, meatless	50.0
Egg roll, with beef and/or pork	50.0
Egg roll, with chicken or turkey	50.0
Egg roll, with shrimp	50.0
Egg salad	50.0
Egg substitute, NS as to powdered, frozen, or liquid	50.0
Egg, deviled	50.0
Egg, white only, cooked	50.0
Egg, whole, baked, fat added in cooking	50.0
Egg, whole, baked, fat not added in cooking	50.0
Egg, whole, baked, NS as to fat added in cooking	50.0
Egg, whole, boiled	50.0
Egg, whole, cooked, NS as to cooking method	50.0
Egg, whole, fried	50.0
Egg, whole, pickled	50.0
Egg, whole, poached	50.0
Egg, whole, raw	50.0
Fish chowder	27.0
Flavored pasta	42.0
Garbanzo or chickpea soup	64.0
Gnocchi, cheese	68.0
Ham, rice, and potato soup, Puerto Rican style	51.0
Huevos rancheros	50.0
Instant soup, noodle	42.0
Instant soup, noodle with egg, shrimp or chicken	42.0
Instant soup, rice	64.0

Food Name	Glycemic Index
Lasagna with meat and/or poultry	46.0
Lasagna, meatless	46.0
Leek soup, cream of, prepared with milk	27.0
Lentil soup	44.0
Lima bean soup	60.0
Long rice noodles (made from mung beans) cooked, NS as to fat added in cooking	33.0
Long rice noodles (made from mung beans), cooked, fat added in cooking	33.0
Long rice noodles (made from mung beans), cooked, fat not added in cooking	33.0
Macaroni and potato soup	62.5
Macaroni or noodles with beans or lentils and tomato sauce	36.3
Macaroni or noodles with cheese	64.0
Macaroni or noodles with cheese and tomato	40.0
Macaroni or noodles with cheese, canned	64.0
Macaroni or noodles with cheese, from boxed mix with already prepared cheese sauce	64.0
Macaroni or noodles with cheese, made from dry mix	64.0
Macaroni, cooked, fat added in cooking	47.0
Macaroni, cooked, fat not added in cooking	47.0
Macaroni, cooked, NS as to fat added in cooking	47.0
Macaroni, cooked, spinach, fat not added in cooking	47.0
Macaroni, cooked, spinach, NS as to fat added in cooking	47.0
Macaroni, cooked, vegetable, fat added in cooking	47.0
Macaroni, cooked, vegetable, fat not added in cooking	47.0
Macaroni, cooked, vegetable, NS as to fat added in cooking	47.0
Macaroni, creamed	50.5
Macaroni, creamed, with vegetables	41.6
Macaroni, whole wheat, cooked, fat not added in cooking	37.0
Meat and corn hominy soup, Mexican style (Pozole)	40.0

Food Name	Glycemic Index
Meatball soup, Mexican style (Sopa de Albondigas)	38.0
Minestrone soup, canned, reduced sodium, ready-to-serve	39.0
Minestrone soup, home recipe	39.0
Mushroom soup, cream of, canned, NS as to made with milk or water, reduced sodium	27.0
Mushroom soup, cream of, canned, prepared with milk, reduced sodium	27.0
Mushroom soup, cream of, canned, prepared with water, reduced sodium	27.0
Mushroom soup, cream of, canned, undiluted, reduced sodium	27.0
Mushroom soup, cream of, NS as to made with milk or water	27.0
Mushroom soup, cream of, prepared with milk	27.0
Mushroom soup, cream of, prepared with water	27.0
Mushroom soup, cream of, prepared with water, low sodium	27.0
Noodle and potato soup, Puerto Rican style	42.0
Noodle pudding	65.0
Noodle soup with vegetables, Oriental style	40.0
Noodle soup, NFS	42.0
Noodle soup, with fish ball, shrimp, and dark green leafy vegetable	42.0
Noodles, cooked, fat added in cooking	42.0
Noodles, cooked, fat not added in cooking	42.0
Noodles, cooked, NS as to fat added in cooking	42.0
Noodles, cooked, spinach, fat added in cooking	42.0
Noodles, cooked, spinach, fat not added in cooking	42.0
Noodles, cooked, spinach, NS as to fat added in cooking	42.0
Noodles, cooked, whole wheat, fat not added in cooking	37.0
Noodles, cooked, whole wheat, NS as to fat added in cooking	37.0
Oxtail soup	38.0
Pasta with carbonara sauce	42.0
Pasta with cheese and meat sauce	52.0
Pasta with cheese and tomato sauce, meatless	40.0

Food Name	Glycemic Index
Pasta with meat sauce	52.0
Pasta with tomato sauce and cheese, canned	40.0
Pasta with tomato sauce and meat or meatballs, canned	52.0
Pasta with tomato sauce, meatless	40.0
Pasta, cooked, corn-based, fat not added in cooking	78.0
Pasta, cooked, corn-based, NS as to fat added in cooking	78.0
Pea soup, canned, prepared with water, low sodium	66.0
Pea soup, instant type	66.0
Pea soup, NFS	66.0
Pea soup, prepared with milK	46.5
Pea soup, prepared with water	66.0
Pepperpot (tripe) soup	38.0
Pork and rice soup, stew type, chunky style	51.0
Pork vegetable soup with noodles, stew type, chunky style	40.0
Pork with vegetable (excluding carrots, broccoli and/or dark-green leafy) soup, Oriental Style	38.0
Pork, vegetable soup with potatoes, stew type	38.0
Potato and cheese soup	53.9
Potato chowder	53.3
Potato soup, cream of, prepared with milk	49.5
Potato soup, NS as to made with milk or water	49.5
Potato soup, prepared with water	49.5
Quail egg, canned	50.0
Ravioli, cheese-filled, no sauce	50.0
Ravioli, cheese-filled, with meat sauce	38.5
Ravioli, meat-filled, no sauce	39.0
Ravioli, meat-filled, with tomato sauce or meat sauce	38.5
Ravioli, meat-filled, with tomato sauce or meat sauce, canned	59.1
Ravioli, NS as to filling, no sauce	39.0

Food Name	Glycemic Index
Ravioli, NS as to filling, with tomato sauce	38.5
Rice and potato soup, Puerto Rican style	64.0
Rice soup, NFS	64.0
Salmon soup, cream style	27.0
Scotch broth (lamb, vegetables, and barley)	31.5
Scrambled egg, made from cholesterol-free frozen mixture	50.0
Scrambled egg, made from cholesterol-free frozen mixture with cheese	50.0
Scrambled egg, made from cholesterol-free frozen mixture with vegetables	50.0
Scrambled egg, made from frozen mixture	50.0
Scrambled egg, made from packaged liquid mixture	50.0
Scrambled egg, made from powdered mixture	50.0
Shrimp soup, cream of, prepared with milk	27.0
Shrimp-egg patty (Torta de Cameron seco)	50.0
Soup, mostly noodles	42.0
Soup, NFS	38.0
Soybean soup, made with milk	43.5
Soybean soup, miso broth	29.2
Spaghetti with clam sauce, NS as to red or white	40.0
Spaghetti with red clam sauce	40.0
Spaghetti with tomato sauce and chicken or turkey	52.0
Spaghetti with tomato sauce and frankfurters or hot dogs	52.0
Spaghetti with tomato sauce and meatballs or spaghetti with meat sauce or spaghetti with meat sauce and meatballs	52.0
Spaghetti with tomato sauce and meatballs, whole wheat noodles or spaghetti with meat sauce, whole wheat noodles or spaghetti with meat sauce and meatballs, whole wheat noodles	52.0
Spaghetti with tomato sauce, meatless	40.0
Spaghetti with tomato sauce, meatless, made with spinach noodles	40.0
Spaghetti with white clam sauce	42.0
Spaghetti, cooked, fat added in cooking	42.0

Food Name	Glycemic Index
Spaghetti, cooked, fat not added in cooking	42.0
Spaghetti, cooked, NS as to fat added in cooking	42.0
Split pea and ham soup	60.0
Split pea and ham soup, canned, reduced sodium, prepared with water or ready-to-serve	60.0
Split pea soup	60.0
Split pea soup, canned, reduced sodium, prepared with water or ready-to-serve	60.0
Tomato beef noodle soup, prepared with water	40.0
Tomato beef soup, prepared with water	38.0
Tomato noodle soup, prepared with water	40.0
Tomato rice soup, prepared with water	51.0
Tomato soup, canned, low sodium, ready-to-serve	38.0
Tomato soup, canned, undiluted	38.0
Tomato soup, cream of, prepared with milk	35.7
Tomato soup, instant type, prepared with water	38.0
Tomato soup, NFS	38.0
Tomato soup, prepared with water	38.0
Tomato vegetable soup with noodles, prepared with water	40.0
Tomato vegetable soup, prepared with water	38.0
Tortellini, cheese-filled, meatless, with tomato sauce	50.0
Tortellini, cheese-filled, meatless, with vinaigrette dressing	50.0
Tortellini, cheese-filled, with cream sauce	50.0
Turkey noodle soup	42.0
Turkey noodle soup, home recipe	42.0
Vegetable bean soup, prepared with water or ready-to-serve	39.0
Vegetable beef soup with noodles or pasta, home recipe	40.0
Vegetable beef soup with rice, home recipe	51.0
Vegetable beef soup with rice, prepared with water or ready-to-serve	51.0
Vegetable beef soup, canned, undiluted	38.0

Food Name	Glycemic Index
Vegetable beef soup, chunky style	38.0
Vegetable beef soup, home recipe	38.0
Vegetable beef soup, prepared with water	38.0
Vegetable chicken noodle soup, prepared with water or ready-to-serve	40.0
Vegetable chicken or turkey soup, prepared with water or ready-to-serve	38.0
Vegetable chicken rice soup, prepared with water or ready-to-serve	51.0
Vegetable chicken soup, canned, prepared with water, low sodium	38.0
Vegetable noodle soup, canned, reduced sodium, prepared with water or ready-to-serve	40.0
Vegetable noodle soup, home recipe	40.0
Vegetable noodle soup, prepared with water	40.0
Vegetable rice soup, prepared with water	51.0
Vegetable soup with chicken broth, Mexican style (Sopa Ranchera)	38.0
Vegetable soup, canned, low sodium, prepared with water or ready-to-serve	38.0
Vegetable soup, canned, undiluted	38.0
Vegetable soup, chunky style	38.0
Vegetable soup, cream of, made from dry mix, low sodium, prepared with water	32.5
Vegetable soup, cream of, prepared with milk	32.5
Vegetable soup, home recipe	38.0
Vegetable soup, made from dry mix	38.0
Vegetable soup, prepared with water or ready-to-serve	38.0
Vegetable soup, with pasta, chunky style	40.0
Vegetarian vegetable soup, prepared with water	38.0
Vichyssoise soup	49.5
Zucchini soup, cream of, prepared with milk	27.0

Fish & Fish Products

Food Name	Glycemic Index
Anchovy, canned	0.0
Anchovy, cooked, NS as to cooking method	0.0
Carp, baked or broiled	50.0
Carp, floured or breaded, fried	95.0
Carp, steamed or poached	0.0
Catfish, baked or broiled	50.0
Catfish, battered, fried	95.0
Catfish, breaded or battered, baked	95.0
Catfish, floured or breaded, fried	95.0
Catfish, steamed or poached	0.0
Clams, baked or broiled	50.0
Clams, battered, fried	95.0
Clams, canned	50.0
Clams, floured or breaded, fried	95.0
Clams, raw	50.0
Clams, steamed or boiled	50.0
Cod, baked or broiled	50.0
Cod, battered, fried	95.0
Cod, breaded or battered, baked	95.0
Cod, floured or breaded, fried	95.0
Cod, steamed or poached	0.0
Conch, baked or broiled	50.0
Crab, baked or broiled	50.0
Crab, cooked, NS as to cooking method	0.0
Crab, hard shell, steamed	0.0
Crab, soft shell, floured or breaded, fried	95.0
Crayfish, floured or breaded, fried	95.0

Food Name	Glycemic Index
Croaker, baked or broiled	50.0
Croaker, floured or breaded, fried	95.0
Croaker, steamed or poached	0.0
Eel, cooked, NS as to cooking method	95.0
Fish stick, patty, or fillet, NS as to type, baked or broiled	95.0
Fish stick, patty, or fillet, NS as to type, battered, fried	95.0
Fish stick, patty, or fillet, NS as to type, breaded or battered, baked	95.0
Fish stick, patty, or fillet, NS as to type, cooked, NS as to cooking method	95.0
Fish stick, patty, or fillet, NS as to type, floured or breaded, fried	95.0
Fish, NS as to type, baked or broiled	50.0
Fish, NS as to type, battered, fried	95.0
Fish, NS as to type, breaded or battered, baked	95.0
Fish, NS as to type, canned	0.0
Fish, NS as to type, cooked, NS as to cooking method	0.0
Fish, NS as to type, floured or breaded, fried	95.0
Fish, NS as to type, smoked	0.0
Fish, NS as to type, steamed	0.0
Flounder, baked or broiled	50.0
Flounder, battered, fried	95.0
Flounder, breaded or battered, baked	95.0
Flounder, cooked, NS as to cooking method	50.0
Flounder, floured or breaded, fried	95.0
Flounder, steamed or poached	0.0
Haddock, baked or broiled	50.0
Haddock, battered, fried	95.0
Haddock, breaded or battered, baked	95.0
Haddock, cooked, NS as to cooking method	50.0
Haddock, floured or breaded, fried	95.0

Food Name	Glycemic Index
Haddock, steamed or poached	0.0
Herring, baked or broiled	50.0
Herring, pickled	50.0
Herring, raw	0.0
Herring, smoked, kippered	0.0
Lobster, baked or broiled	50.0
Lobster, cooked, NS as to cooking method	50.0
Lobster, steamed or boiled	50.0
Lobster, without shell, steamed or boiled	50.0
Mackerel, baked or broiled	50.0
Mackerel, canned	0.0
Mackerel, cooked, NS as to cooking method	50.0
Mackerel, floured or breaded, fried	95.0
Mullet, baked or broiled	50.0
Mullet, floured or breaded, fried	95.0
Mussels, cooked, NS as to cooking method	95.0
Mussels, steamed or poached	50.0
Ocean perch, baked or broiled	50.0
Ocean perch, battered, fried	95.0
Ocean perch, breaded or battered, baked	95.0
Ocean perch, floured or breaded, fried	95.0
Ocean perch, raw	0.0
Octopus, cooked, NS as to cooking method	95.0
Octopus, dried, boiled	50.0
Oysters, baked or broiled	50.0
Oysters, battered, fried	95.0
Oysters, canned	50.0
Oysters, cooked, NS as to cooking method	95.0

Food Name	Glycemic Index
Oysters, floured or breaded, fried	95.0
Oysters, raw	50.0
Oysters, smoked	50.0
Perch, baked or broiled	50.0
Perch, battered, fried	95.0
Perch, breaded or battered, baked	95.0
Perch, cooked, NS as to cooking method	95.0
Perch, floured or breaded, fried	95.0
Perch, steamed or poached	0.0
Pike, baked or broiled	50.0
Pompano, baked or broiled	50.0
Pompano, floured or breaded, fried	95.0
Pompano, raw	0.0
Porgy, baked or broiled	50.0
Porgy, battered, fried	95.0
Porgy, breaded or battered, baked	95.0
Porgy, cooked, NS as to cooking method	95.0
Porgy, floured or breaded, fried	95.0
Porgy, raw	0.0
Porgy, steamed or poached	0.0
Roe, shad, cooked	50.0
Roe, sturgeon	50.0
Salmon, baked or broiled	50.0
Salmon, battered, fried	95.0
Salmon, canned	0.0
Salmon, cooked, NS as to cooking method	0.0
Salmon, floured or breaded, fried	95.0
Salmon, smoked	0.0

Food Name	Glycemic Index
Salmon, steamed or poached	0.0
Sardines with mustard sauce (mixture)	0.0
Sardines, canned in oil	0.0
Sardines, cooked	0.0
Sardines, skinless, boneless, packed in water	0.0
Scallops, baked or broiled	50.0
Scallops, battered, fried	95.0
Scallops, cooked, NS as to cooking method	95.0
Scallops, floured or breaded, fried	95.0
Scallops, steamed or boiled	50.0
Sea bass, baked or broiled	50.0
Sea bass, floured or breaded, fried	95.0
Sea bass, steamed or poached	0.0
Shark, steamed or poached	0.0
Shrimp, baked or broiled	50.0
Shrimp, canned	50.0
Shrimp, cooked, NS as to cooking method	50.0
Shrimp, floured, breaded, or battered, fried	95.0
Shrimp, steamed or boiled	50.0
Smelt, battered, fried	95.0
Smelt, floured or breaded, fried	95.0
Snails, cooked, NS as to cooking method	50.0
Squid, baked, broiled	50.0
Squid, breaded, fried	95.0
Squid, canned	50.0
Squid, pickled	50.0
Squid, steamed or boiled	50.0
Swordfish, baked or broiled	50.0

Food Name	Glycemic Index
Swordfish, cooked, NS as to cooking method	50.0
Swordfish, floured or breaded, fried	95.0
Swordfish, steamed or poached	0.0
Trout, baked or broiled	50.0
Trout, battered, fried	95.0
Trout, breaded or battered, baked	95.0
Trout, floured or breaded, fried	95.0
Trout, smoked	0.0
Trout, steamed or poached	0.0
Tuna, canned, NS as to oil or water pack	0.0
Tuna, canned, oil pack	0.0
Tuna, canned, water pack	0.0
Tuna, fresh, baked or broiled	50.0
Tuna, fresh, floured or breaded, fried	95.0
Tuna, fresh, raw	0.0
Tuna, fresh, steamed or poached	0.0
Whiting, baked or broiled	50.0
Whiting, battered, fried	95.0
Whiting, floured or breaded, fried	95.0

Fruit and Fruit Products

Food Name	Glycemic Index
Apple chips	29.0
Apple, baked, NS as to added sweetener	38.0
Apple, baked, unsweetened	38.0
Apple, baked, with sugar	38.0
Apple, candied	34.2
Apple, cooked or canned, with syrup	38.0
Apple, dried, cooked, NS as to sweetened or unsweetened; sweetened, NS as to type of sweetener	29.0
Apple, dried, cooked, with sugar	29.0
Apple, dried, uncooked	29.0
Apple, fried	38.0
Apple, raw	38.0
Applesauce, stewed apples, NS as to sweetened or unsweetened; sweetened, NS as to type of sweetener	38.0
Applesauce, stewed apples, sweetened with low calorie sweetener	38.0
Applesauce, stewed apples, unsweetened	38.0
Applesauce, stewed apples, with sugar	38.0
Apricot, dried, uncooked	31.0
Avocado, raw	50.0
Banana, raw	52.0
Banana, red, ripe (guineo morado)	52.0
Banana, ripe, boiled	52.0
Banana, ripe, fried	52.0
Berries, raw, NFS	40.0
Blueberries, raw	40.0
Cantaloupe (muskmelon), raw	65.0
Cherries, frozen	22.0
Cherries, sour, red, cooked, unsweetened	22.0

Food Name	Glycemic Index
Cherries, sweet, cooked or canned, drained solids	22.0
Cherries, sweet, cooked or canned, in heavy syrup	22.0
Cherries, sweet, cooked or canned, in light syrup	22.0
Cherries, sweet, cooked or canned, juice pack	22.0
Cherries, sweet, cooked or canned, NS as to sweetened or unsweetened; sweetened, NS as to type of sweetener	22.0
Cherries, sweet, raw (Queen Anne, Bing)	22.0
Currants, dried	64.0
Currants, raw	64.0
Date	103.0
Fig, dried, cooked, with sugar	61.0
Fig, dried, uncooked	61.0
Fig, raw	61.0
Figs, cooked or canned, in light syrup	61.0
Fried green plantain, Puerto Rican style (Tostones)	39.0
Fruit cocktail or mix (excluding citrus fruits), raw	55.0
Fruit cocktail or mix (including citrus fruits), raw	55.0
Fruit cocktail or mix, frozen	55.0
Fruit cocktail, cooked or canned, drained solids	55.0
Fruit cocktail, cooked or canned, in heavy syrup	55.0
Fruit cocktail, cooked or canned, in light syrup	55.0
Fruit cocktail, cooked or canned, juice pack	55.0
Fruit cocktail, cooked or canned, NS as to sweetened or unsweetened; sweetened, NS as to type of sweetener	55.0
Fruit cocktail, cooked or canned, unsweetened, water pack	55.0
Fruit juice bar with cream, frozen	42.0
Fruit juice bar, frozen, flavor other than orange	59.0
Fruit juice bar, frozen, orange flavor	59.0
Fruit juice bar, frozen, sweetened with low calorie sweetener, flavors other than orange	59.0

Food Name	Glycemic Index
Fruit mixture, dried (mixture includes three or more of the following: apples, apricots, dates, papaya, peaches, pears, pineapples, prunes, raisins)	38.3
Fruit, dried, NFS (assume uncooked)	38.3
Grapefruit, canned or frozen, in light syrup	25.0
Grapefruit, canned or frozen, NS as to sweetened or unsweetened; sweetened, NS as to type of sweetener	25.0
Grapefruit, canned or frozen, unsweetened, water pack	25.0
Grapefruit, raw	25.0
Grapes, American type, slip skin, raw	46.0
Grapes, European type, adherent skin, raw	46.0
Grapes, raw, NS as to type	46.0
Green banana, cooked (in salt water)	38.0
Green banana, fried	30.0
Green plantains, boiled	39.0
Guacamole with tomatoes	50.0
Guacamole with tomatoes and chili peppers	50.0
Guacamole, NFS	50.0
Honeydew melon, raw	65.0
Honeydew, frozen (balls)	65.0
Ice, fruit	59.0
Kiwi fruit, raw	53.0
Nectarine, raw	42.0
Orange, mandarin, canned or frozen, drained	42.0
Orange, mandarin, canned or frozen, in light syrup	42.0
Orange, mandarin, canned or frozen, NS as to sweetened or unsweetened; sweetened, NS as to type of sweetener	42.0
Orange, raw	42.0
Papaya, cooked or canned, in sugar or syrup	59.0
Papaya, green, cooked	59.0
Papaya, raw	59.0

Food Name	Glycemic Index
Peach, cooked or canned, drained solids	42.0
Peach, cooked or canned, in heavy syrup	58.0
Peach, cooked or canned, in light or medium syrup	52.0
Peach, cooked or canned, juice pack	38.0
Peach, cooked or canned, NS as to sweetened or unsweetened; sweetened, NS as to type of sweetener	58.0
Peach, cooked or canned, unsweetened, water pack	38.0
Peach, frozen, NS as to added sweetener	58.0
Peach, frozen, unsweetened	42.0
Peach, frozen, with sugar	58.0
Peach, raw	42.0
Peaches, baby food, junior	38.0
Pear, cooked or canned, drained solids	38.0
Pear, cooked or canned, in heavy syrup	43.5
Pear, cooked or canned, in light syrup	25.0
Pear, cooked or canned, juice pack	43.5
Pear, cooked or canned, NS as to sweetened or unsweetened; sweetened, NS as to type of sweetener	43.5
Pear, Japanese, raw	38.0
Pear, raw	38.0
Pineapple, cooked or canned, drained solids	59.0
Pineapple, cooked or canned, in heavy syrup	59.0
Pineapple, cooked or canned, in light syrup	59.0
Pineapple, cooked or canned, juice pack	59.0
Pineapple, cooked or canned, NS as to sweetened or unsweetened; sweetened, NS as to type of sweetener	59.0
Pineapple, cooked or canned, unsweetened, waterpack	59.0
Pineapple, raw	59.0
Plantain, boiled, NS as to green or ripe	39.0
Plantain, fried, NS as to green or ripe	39.0
Plum, cooked or canned, in heavy syrup	39.0

Food Name	Glycemic Index
Plum, cooked or canned, in light syrup	39.0
Plum, raw	39.0
Plums, baby food, strained	39.0
Prune, dried, cooked, NS as to sweetened or unsweetened; sweetened, NS as to type of sweetener	29.0
Prune, dried, cooked, unsweetened	29.0
Prune, dried, cooked, with sugar	29.0
Prune, dried, uncooked	29.0
Prunes with tapioca, baby food, strained	29.0
Raisins	64.0
Raisins, cooked	64.0
Sorbet, fruit, citrus flavor	59.0
Sorbet, fruit, noncitrus flavor	59.0
Strawberries, cooked or canned, in syrup	54.8
Strawberries, cooked or canned, NS as to sweetened or unsweetened; sweetened, NS as to type of sweetener	54.8
Strawberries, frozen, NS as to added sweetener	54.8
Strawberries, frozen, unsweetened	40.0
Strawberries, frozen, with sugar	54.8
Strawberries, raw	40.0
Strawberries, raw, with sugar	54.8
Tangelo, raw	42.0
Tangerine, raw	42.0
Watermelon, raw	72.0

Honey, Syrups & Gravy

Food Name	Glycemic Index
Milk gravy, quick gravy	50.0
Topping, chocolate, thick, fudge type	19.0
Topping, butterscotch or caramel	19.0
Syrup, pancake, reduced calorie	19.0
Sugar, white, granulated or lump	68.0
Sugar, white, granulated or lump	68.0
Sugar, white, confectioner's, powdered	68.0
Sugar, white, confectioner's, powdered	68.0
Sugar, raw	68.0
Sugar, raw	68.0
Sugar, NFS	68.0
Sugar, NFS	68.0
Sugar, cinnamon	68.0
Sugar, brown	68.0
Sugar, brown	68.0
Sugar substitute, saccharin-based, liquid	50.0
Sugar substitute, low-calorie, powdered, NFS	50.0
Sugar substitiute, saccharin-based, dry powder and tablets	50.0
Sugar replacement, saccharin-based, dry powder	50.0
Sugar (white) and water syrup	68.0
Sugar (white) and water syrup	68.0
Sausage gravy	50.0
Saccharin, sugar substitute	50.0
Maple and corn and/or cane pancake syrup blends (formerly Corn and maple syrup (2% maple))	19.0
Honey	55.0
Honey	55.0

Food Name	Glycemic Index
Milk gravy, quick gravy	50.0
Gravy, redeye	50.0
Gravy, poultry	50.0
Gravy, mushroom	50.0
Gravy, meat, with fruit	50.0
Gravy, meat or poultry, with wine	50.0
Gravy, giblet	50.0
Gravy, beef or meat	50.0
Gravy or sauce, poultry-based from Puerto Rican-style chicken fricasse	50.0
Gravy or sauce, Chinese (soy sauce, stock or bouillon, cornstarch)	50.0
Gelatin dessert with fruit	59.9
Gelatin dessert	68.0
Fruit syrup	51.0
Fructose sweetener, sugar substitute, dry powder	19.0
Fructose sweetener, sugar substitute, dry powder	19.0
Flour and water gravy	50.0
Corn syrup, light or dark	19.0
Chocolate syrup, thin type	19.0

Legumes and Nuts

Food Name	Glycemic Index
Baked beans, low sodium	48.0
Baked beans, NFS	48.0
Baked beans, with pork and sweet sauce	48.0
Baked beans, with tomato sauce	48.0
Beans, dry, cooked with ground beef	48.0
Beans, dry, cooked with pork	48.0
Beans, dry, cooked, NS as to type and as to fat added in cooking	29.0
Beans, dry, cooked, NS as to type, fat added in cooking	29.0
Beans, dry, cooked, NS as to type, fat not added in cooking	29.0
Beans, green string, with onions, cooked, fat not added in cooking	32.0
Beans, lima, immature, canned, low sodium, NS as to fat added in cooking	32.0
Beans, lima, immature, cooked, from canned, fat added in cooking	32.0
Beans, lima, immature, cooked, from canned, fat not added in cooking	32.0
Beans, lima, immature, cooked, from canned, NS as to fat added in cooking	32.0
Beans, lima, immature, cooked, from fresh, fat added in cooking	32.0
Beans, lima, immature, cooked, from fresh, fat not added in cooking	32.0
Beans, lima, immature, cooked, from frozen, fat added in cooking	32.0
Beans, lima, immature, cooked, from frozen, fat not added in cooking	32.0
Beans, lima, immature, cooked, from frozen, NS as to fat added in cooking	32.0
Beans, lima, immature, cooked, NS as to form, fat added in cooking	32.0
Beans, lima, immature, cooked, NS as to form, fat not added in cooking	32.0
Beans, lima, immature, cooked, NS as to form, NS as to fat added in cooking	32.0

Food Name	Glycemic Index
Baked beans, low sodium	48.0
Beans, lima, immature, from frozen, creamed or with cheese sauce	31.1
Beans, string, cooked, from canned, NS as to color, fat not added in cooking	32.0
Beans, string, cooked, from fresh, NS as to color, fat not added in cooking	32.0
Beans, string, cooked, from frozen, NS as to color, fat not added in cooking	32.0
Beans, string, cooked, NS as to form, NS as to color, fat not added in cooking	32.0
Beans, string, green, canned, low sodium, fat not added in cooking	32.0
Beans, string, green, cooked, from canned, fat not added in cooking	32.0
Beans, string, green, cooked, from fresh, fat not added in cooking	32.0
Beans, string, green, cooked, from frozen, fat not added in cooking	32.0
Beans, string, green, cooked, NS as to form, fat not added in cooking	32.0
Beans, string, green, raw	32.0
Beans, string, yellow, cooked, from canned, fat not added in cooking	32.0
Beans, string, yellow, cooked, from fresh, fat not added in cooking	32.0
Beans, string, yellow, cooked, from frozen, fat not added in cooking	32.0
Beans, string, yellow, cooked, NS as to form, fat not added in cooking	32.0
Black, brown, or Bayo beans, dry, cooked, fat added in cooking	20.0
Black, brown, or Bayo beans, dry, cooked, fat not added in cooking	20.0
Black, brown, or Bayo beans, dry, cooked, NS as to fat added in cooking	20.0
Boston baked beans	48.0
Chickpeas stewed with pig's feet, Puerto Rican style (Garbanzos guisados con patitos de cerdo)	28.0
Chickpeas, dry, cooked, fat added in cooking	28.0

Food Name	Glycemic Index
Baked beans, low sodium	48.0
Chickpeas, dry, cooked, fat not added in cooking	28.0
Chickpeas, dry, cooked, NS as to fat added in cooking	28.0
Chili beans, barbecue beans, ranch style beans or Mexican- style beans	48.0
Cowpeas, dry, cooked with pork	42.0
Cowpeas, dry, cooked, fat added in cooking	42.0
Cowpeas, dry, cooked, fat not added in cooking	42.0
Cowpeas, dry, cooked, NS as to fat added in cooking	42.0
Green or yellow split peas, dry, cooked, fat added in cooking	32.0
Green or yellow split peas, dry, cooked, NS as to fat added in cooking	32.0
Lentils, dry, cooked, fat added in cooking	28.3
Lentils, dry, cooked, fat not added in cooking	28.3
Lentils, dry, cooked, NS as to fat added in cooking	28.3
Lima beans, dry, cooked, fat added in cooking	31.0
Lima beans, dry, cooked, fat not added in cooking	31.0
Lima beans, dry, cooked, NS as to fat added in cooking	31.0
Mung beans, fat added in cooking	36.5
Mung beans, fat not added in cooking	36.5
Peas, cowpeas, field peas, or blackeye peas (not dried), cooked, from fresh, NS as to fat added in cooking	42.0
Pinto, calico, or red Mexican beans, dry, cooked, fat added in cooking	39.0
Pinto, calico, or red Mexican beans, dry, cooked, fat not added in cooking	39.0
Pinto, calico, or red Mexican beans, dry, cooked, NS as to fat added in cooking	39.0
Pork and beans	48.0

Food Name	Glycemic Index
Baked beans, low sodium	48.0
Red kidney beans, dry, cooked, fat added in cooking	28.0
Red kidney beans, dry, cooked, fat not added in cooking	28.0
Red kidney beans, dry, cooked, NS as to fat added in cooking	28.0
Refried beans	42.0
Soybean curd	16.0
Soybean curd, breaded, fried	16.0
Soybean curd, deep fried	16.0
Soybean meal	16.0
Soybeans, cooked, fat not added in cooking	16.0
Soyburger, meatless, no bun	16.0
Stewed dry lima beans, Puerto Rican style	31.0
Stewed dry red beans, Puerto Rican style (Habichuelas coloradas guisadas)	28.0
White beans, dry, cooked, fat added in cooking	13.0
White beans, dry, cooked, fat not added in cooking	13.0
White beans, dry, cooked, NS as to fat added in cooking	13.0

Meat Sandwiches and Ham

Food Name	Glycemic Index
Capicola	50.0
Ham and pork, luncheon meat, chopped, minced, pressed, spiced, canned	50.0
Ham loaf, luncheon meat	50.0
Ham, breaded or floured, fried, lean and fat eaten	95.0
Ham, breaded or floured, fried, lean only eaten	95.0
Ham, breaded or floured, fried, NS as to fat eaten	95.0
Ham, deviled or potted	50.0
Ham, fried, lean and fat eaten	50.0
Ham, fried, NS as to fat eaten	50.0
Ham, luncheon meat, chopped, minced, pressed, spiced, lowfat, not canned	50.0
Ham, luncheon meat, chopped, minced, pressed, spiced, not canned	50.0
Ham, pork and chicken, luncheon meat, chopped, minced, pressed, spiced, canned	50.0
Ham, pork, and chicken, luncheon meat, chopped, minced, pressed, spiced, canned, reduced sodium	50.0
Ham, prosciutto	50.0
Ham, sliced, extra lean, prepackaged or deli, luncheon meat	50.0
Ham, sliced, low salt, prepackaged or deli, luncheon meat	50.0
Ham, sliced, prepackaged or deli, luncheon meat	50.0
Ham, smoked or cured, canned, lean and fat eaten	50.0
Ham, smoked or cured, cooked, lean and fat eaten	50.0
Ham, smoked or cured, cooked, NS as to fat eaten	50.0
Ham, smoked or cured, ground patty	50.0
Ham, smoked or cured, low sodium, cooked, lean and fat eaten	50.0
Ham, smoked or cured, low sodium, cooked, NS as to fat eaten	50.0

Mixed Meals and Convenience Foods

Food Name	Glycemic Index
Chicken and beef sausage, smoked	0.0
Turkey breakfast sausage, bulk	0.0
Beef sausage, NFS	28.0
Beef sausage, brown and serve, links, cooked	28.0
Beef sausage, smoked, stick	28.0
Beef sausage, smoked	28.0
Beef sausage, fresh, bulk, patty or link, cooked	28.0
Blood sausage	28.0
Bratwurst, cooked	28.0
Chorizos	28.0
Polish sausage	28.0
Italian sausage	28.0
Sausage (not cold cut), NFS	28.0
Pork sausage, fresh, bulk, patty or link, cooked	28.0
Pork sausage, brown and serve, cooked	28.0
Pork sausage, country style, fresh, cooked	28.0
Pork and beef sausage	28.0
Pork and beef sausage, brown and serve, cooked	28.0
Smoked link sausage, pork	28.0
Smoked link sausage, pork and beef	28.0
Smoked sausage, pork	28.0
Vienna sausage, canned	28.0
Knockwurst	28.0
Mettwurst	28.0
Scrapple, cooked	28.0
Souse	28.0

Food Name	Glycemic Index
Turkey sausage, smoked	28.0
Turkey and pork sausage, fresh, bulk, patty or link, cooked	28.0
Turkey, pork, and beef sausage, reduced fat, smoked	28.0
Turkey, pork, and beef sausage, lowfat, smoked	28.0
Vienna sausage, chicken, canned	28.0
Frankfurter, wiener, or hot dog, NFS	28.0
Frankfurter or hot dog, beef	28.0
Frankfurter or hot dog, beef and pork	28.0
Frankfurter or hot dog, meat and poultry	28.0
Frankfurter or hot dog, low salt	28.0
Frankfurter or hot dog, beef and pork, lowfat	28.0
Frankfurter or hot dog, meat and poultry, fat free	28.0
Frankfurter or hot dog, chicken	28.0
Frankfurter or hot dog, turkey	28.0
Frankfurter or hot dog, beef, lowfat	28.0
Frankfurter or hot dog, meat & poultry, lowfat	28.0
Pork roll, cured, fried	28.0
Deer bologna	28.0
Cold cut, NFS	28.0
Bologna, pork and beef	28.0
Bologna, NFS	28.0
Bologna, Lebanon	28.0
Bologna, beef	28.0
Bologna ring, smoked	28.0
Bologna, pork	28.0
Bologna, beef, lower sodium	28.0
Bologna, chicken, beef, and pork	28.0
Mortadella	28.0

Food Name	Glycemic Index
Pepperoni	28.0
Salami, NFS	28.0
Salami, soft, cooked	28.0
Salami, dry or hard	28.0
Salami, beef	28.0
Thuringer	28.0
Luncheon meat, NFS	28.0
Luncheon loaf (olive, pickle, or pimiento)	28.0
Sandwich loaf, luncheon meat	28.0
Bologna, beef, lowfat	28.0
Bologna, beef and pork, lowfat	28.0
Bologna, turkey	28.0
Pizza with meat, NS as to type of crust	30.0
Pizza with meat, thin crust	30.0
Pizza with meat and vegetables, NS as to type of crust	30.0
Pizza with meat and vegetables, thin crust	30.0
Pizza with meat and fruit, thin crust	30.0
Pizza with meat and vegetables, lowfat, thin crust	30.0
Pizza with meat, thick crust	36.0
Pizza with meat and vegetables, thick crust	36.0
Pizza with meat and fruit, thick crust	36.0
Beef pot pie	45.0
Pizza, cheese, with vegetables, NS as to type of crust	49.0
Pizza, cheese, with vegetables, thin crust	49.0
Pizza, cheese, with vegetables, thick crust	49.0
Beef, bacon, cooked	50.0
Beef, bacon, formed, lean meat added, cooked	50.0
Bacon, NS as to type of meat, cooked	50.0

Food Name	Glycemic Index
Pork bacon, NS as to fresh, smoked or cured, cooked	50.0
Pork bacon, smoked or cured, cooked	50.0
Bacon or side pork, fresh, cooked	50.0
Pork bacon, smoked or cured, lower sodium	50.0
Pork bacon, formed, lean meat added, cooked	50.0
Canadian bacon, cooked	50.0
Pork bacon, smoked or cured, cooked, lean only eaten	50.0
Turkey bacon, cooked	50.0
Pizza, cheese, NS as to type of crust	60.0
Pizza, cheese, thin crust	60.0
Pizza, cheese, thick crust	60.0
Pizza, cheese, with fruit, thick crust	60.0
Italian pie, meatless	60.0
Pizza, no cheese, thick crust	80.0

Recipes

Food Name	Glycemic Index
Beef and noodles with tomato-based sauce (mixture)	39.5
Beef and vegetables (including carrots, broccoli, and/or dark-green leafy (no potatoes)), soy-based sauce (mixture)	48.7
Beef sloppy joe (no bun)	42.3
Beef stew with potatoes and vegetables (including carrots, broccoli, and/ or dark-green leafy), gravy	63.6
Beef stew with potatoes and vegetables (including carrots, broccoli, and/ or dark-green leafy), tomato-based sauce	62.6
Beef stew with potatoes, tomato-based sauce (mixture)	69.7
Beef stroganoff with noodles	45.6
Beef with barbecue sauce (mixture)	38.0
Beef with gravy (mixture)	70.6
Beef with tomato-based sauce (mixture)	36.7
Burrito with beans and cheese, meatless	34.0
Burrito with beef and beans	34.0
Burrito with beef and cheese, no beans	29.9
Burrito with beef, beans, and cheese	34.0
Burrito with beef, beans, cheese, and sour cream	32.9
Burrito with eggs, sausage, cheese and vegetables	30.8
Chicken fillet, (broiled), sandwich, on whole wheat roll, with lettuce, tomato and spread	69.1
Chicken fillet, broiled, sandwich with cheese, on bun, with lettuce, tomato and spread	58.9
Chicken or turkey and noodles with cream or white sauce (mixture)	46.3
Chicken or turkey and noodles, no sauce (mixture)	40.0
Chicken or turkey and vegetables (including carrots, broccoli, and/or dark-green leafy (no potatoes)), no sauce (mixture)	42.5
Chicken or turkey and vegetables (including carrots, broccoli, and/or dark-green leafy (no potatoes)), soy-based sauce (mixture)	55.1
Chicken or turkey cacciatore	61.0
Chicken or turkey cordon bleu	81.5
Chicken or turkey garden salad (chicken and/or turkey, tomato and/or carrots, other vegetables), no dressing	32.2

Food Name	Glycemic Index
Chicken or turkey parmigiana	79.0
Chicken or turkey pot pie	85.2
Chicken or turkey salad	40.8
Chicken or turkey teriyaki (chicken or turkey with soy-based sauce)	57.2
Chicken or turkey with barbecue sauce (mixture)	38.0
Chicken or turkey with dumplings (mixture)	90.7
Chicken patty sandwich, with lettuce and spread	67.3
Chiles rellenos, cheese-filled (stuffed chili peppers)	34.5
Chili con carne with beans	34.0
Chili con carne with beans and cheese	33.9
Chili con carne with beans and macaroni	40.5
Chili con carne with beans and rice	54.6
Chili con carne with beans, made with pork	34.0
Chili con carne with chicken or turkey and beans	33.9
Chili con carne with venison/deer and beans	34.0
Chili con carne without beans	37.2
Chili con carne, NS as to beans	34.0
Chili con carne, NS as to beans, with cheese	33.9
Cream, heavy, whipped, sweetened	55.4
Cream, whipped, pressurized container	55.4
Fajita with chicken and vegetables	30.5
Fruit salad (excluding citrus fruits) with cream	48.4
Fruit salad (excluding citrus fruits) with cream substitute	45.8
Fruit salad (excluding citrus fruits) with salad dressing or mayonnaise	48.8
Fruit salad (including citrus fruits) with salad dressing or mayonnaise	41.4
Fruit, chocolate covered	54.3
Macaroni salad	45.0
Macaroni, creamed, with cheese	43.4

Food Name	Glycemic Index
Meat loaf made with beef	60.6
Meat loaf made with beef, with tomato-based sauce	55.8
Meat loaf made with chicken or turkey	60.1
Pasta salad (macaroni or noodles, vegetables, dressing)	45.6
Pepper steak	46.1
Potato salad	65.9
Potato salad with egg	65.8
Potato salad, German style	68.2
Pudding, bread	61.6
Pudding, with fruit and vanilla wafers	59.1
Roast beef sandwich	70.0
Roast beef sandwich with cheese	69.2
Salisbury steak with gravy (mixture)	63.8
Soft taco with beef, cheese, and lettuce	30.0
Sweet and sour chicken or turkey	53.3
Taco or tostada salad with beef and cheese, corn chips	56.1
Taco or tostada with beans, cheese, meat, lettuce, tomato and salsa	55.0
Taco or tostada with beef, cheese and lettuce	67.5
Taco or tostada with beef, cheese, lettuce, tomato and salsa	57.7
Tamale with meat and/or poultry	61.7
Whipped cream substitute, nondairy, lowfat, low sugar, made from powdered mix	55.4
Whipped cream substitute, nondairy, made from powdered mix	55.4
Whipped topping, nondairy, frozen	55.4
Whipped topping, nondairy, frozen, lowfat	55.4
Whipped topping, nondairy, NS as to canned, frozen, or made from powdered mix	55.4
Whipped topping, nondairy, pressurized can	55.4

Snack Foods and Confectionery

Food Name	Glycemic Index
Bagel chip	72.0
Biscuit dough, fried	66.0
Biscuit, baking powder or buttermilk type, commercially baked	92.0
Biscuit, baking powder or buttermilk type, made from home recipe	92.0
Biscuit, baking powder or buttermilk type, made from mix	92.0
Biscuit, baking powder or buttermilk type, made from refrigerated dough	92.0
Biscuit, baking powder or buttermilk type, made from refrigerated dough, lowfat	92.0
Biscuit, baking powder or buttermilk type, NS as to made from mix, refrigerated dough, or home recipe	92.0
Bread stick, hard, whole wheat, NS as to 100%	83.0
Bread sticks, hard	70.0
Cashew butter	22.0
Cashew nuts, dry roasted	22.0
Cashew nuts, NFS	22.0
Cashew nuts, roasted (assume salted)	22.0
Cashew nuts, roasted, without salt	22.0
Chocolate, milk, plain	43.0
Chocolate, milk, with almonds	43.0
Chocolate, milk, with cereal	43.0
Chocolate, milk, with fruit and nuts	43.0
Chocolate, milk, with nuts, not almond or peanuts	43.0
Chocolate, milk, with peanuts	43.0
Chocolate, semi-sweet morsel	43.0
Chocolate, sweet or dark	43.0
Chocolate, white	44.0
Chocolate, white, with almonds	44.0
Chocolate, white, with cereal	44.0

Food Name	Glycemic Index
Coconut candy, chocolate covered	43.0
Cookie, almond	64.0
Cookie, batter or dough, raw, not chocolate	64.0
Cookie, brownie, diet, NS as to icing	51.0
Cookie, brownie, fat free, cholesterol free, with icing	51.0
Cookie, brownie, fat free, without icing	51.0
Cookie, brownie, lowfat, with icing	51.0
Cookie, brownie, lowfat, without icing	51.0
Cookie, brownie, NS as to icing	51.0
Cookie, brownie, with cream cheese filling, without icing	51.0
Cookie, brownie, with icing	51.0
Cookie, brownie, with peanut butter fudge icing	51.0
Cookie, brownie, without icing	51.0
Cookie, butter or sugar cookie	55.0
Cookie, butter or sugar cookie, with fruit and / or nuts	55.0
Cookie, butter or sugar, with chocolate icing or filling	49.0
Cookie, butterscotch chip	64.0
Cookie, butterscotch, brownie	53.0
Cookie, chocolate and vanilla sandwich	49.0
Cookie, chocolate chip	49.0
Cookie, chocolate chip sandwich	49.0
Cookie, chocolate chip, made from home recipe or purchased at a bakery	49.0
Cookie, chocolate chip, reduced fat	42.0
Cookie, chocolate chip, with raisins	49.0
Cookie, chocolate fudge, with / without nuts	49.0
Cookie, chocolate sandwich, reduced fat	42.0
Cookie, chocolate-covered, chocolate sandwich	49.0
Cookie, chocolate, chocolate sandwich or chocolate-coated or striped	49.0

Food Name	Glycemic Index
Cookie, chocolate, sandwich, with extra filling	49.0
Cookie, chocolate, with chocolate filling or coating, fat free	42.0
Cookie, date bar	51.0
Cookie, dietetic, NFS	58.0
Cookie, dietetic, oatmeal with raisins	58.0
Cookie, dietetic, sugar or plain	58.0
Cookie, fig bar	51.0
Cookie, fig bar, fat free	51.0
Cookie, fortune	77.0
Cookie, fruit-filled bar	51.0
Cookie, fruit-filled bar, fat free	51.0
Cookie, gingersnaps	77.0
Cookie, graham cracker sandwich with chocolate and marshmallow filling	74.0
Cookie, NS as to type	56.5
Cookie, oatmeal	54.0
Cookie, oatmeal sandwich, with creme filling	54.0
Cookie, oatmeal, fat free, with raisins	54.0
Cookie, oatmeal, reduced fat, with raisins	54.0
Cookie, oatmeal, with chocolate chips	54.0
Cookie, oatmeal, with fruit filling	54.0
Cookie, oatmeal, with raisins	54.0
Cookie, peanut butter	64.0
Cookie, rich, all chocolate, with chocolate filling or chocolate chips	49.0
Cookie, rich, chocolate chip, with chocolate filling	49.0
Cookie, shortbread	64.0
Cookie, shortbread, reduced fat	64.0
Cookie, shortbread, with chocolate filling	56.5
Cookie, tea, Japanese	55.0

Food Name	Glycemic Index
Cookie, vanilla sandwich	77.0
Cookie, vanilla sandwich, reduced fat	77.0
Cookie, vanilla wafer	77.0
Cookie, vanilla wafer, reduced fat	77.0
Cookie, vanilla waffle creme	77.0
Cookie, vanilla with caramel, coconut, and chocolate coating	63.0
Cracker, 100% whole wheat	67.0
Cracker, 100% whole wheat, low sodium	67.0
Cracker, 100% whole wheat, reduced fat	67.0
Cracker, animal	65.0
Cracker, cheese	55.0
Cracker, cheese, low sodium	55.0
Cracker, cheese, reduced fat	55.0
Cracker, graham, sugar-honey coated, cinnamon crisps	74.0
Cracker, sandwich-type, peanut butter filled	59.0
Cracker, snack	55.0
Cracker, snack, fat free	55.0
Cracker, snack, low sodium	55.0
Cracker, snack, lowfat, low sodium	55.0
Cracker, snack, reduced fat	55.0
Crackers, graham	74.0
Crackers, graham, chocolate covered	74.0
Crackers, graham, fat free	74.0
Crackers, graham, higher fat	74.0
Crackers, graham, lowfat	74.0
Crackers, matzo	71.0
Crackers, matzo, low sodium	71.0
Crackers, milk	55.0

Food Name	Glycemic Index
Crackers, NS as to sweet or nonsweet	74.0
Crackers, oyster	71.0
Crackers, saltine	74.0
Crackers, saltine, fat free, low sodium	74.0
Crackers, saltine, low sodium	74.0
Crackers, saltine, whole wheat	67.0
Crackers, toast thins (rye, pumpernickel, white flour)	70.0
Crackers, toast thins (rye, wheat, white flour), low sodium	70.0
Crackers, water biscuits	71.0
Crackers, wheat	67.0
Crackers, wheat, reduced fat	67.0
Crispbread, rye, no added fat	64.0
Crispbread, wheat or rye, extra crispy	64.0
Crispbread, wheat, no added fat	55.0
Fondant, chocolate covered	43.0
Fruit butter, all flavors	51.0
Fruit leather	99.0
Granola bar with nuts, chocolate-coated	62.0
Granola bar, chocolate-coated	62.0
Granola bar, coated with non-chocolate coating	51.0
Granola bar, high fiber, coated with non-chocolate yogurt coating	51.0
Granola bar, nonfat	61.0
Granola bar, oats, fruit and nuts, lowfat	61.0
Granola bar, oats, sugar, raisins, coconut	61.0
Granola bar, peanuts, oats, sugar, wheat germ	61.0
Granola bar, with coconut, chocolate-coated	62.0
Granola bar, with rice cereal	63.0
Gumdrops	78.0

Food Name	Glycemic Index
Hard candy	70.0
Jam, preserves, all flavors	51.0
Jams, preserves, marmalades, dietetic, all flavors, sweetened with artificial sweetener	55.0
Jams, preserves, marmalades, low sugar (all flavors)	55.0
Jams, preserves, marmalades, sweetened with fruit juice concentrates, all flavors	51.0
Jelly, all flavors	51.0
Jelly, dietetic, all flavors, sweetened with artificial sweetener	55.0
Jelly, reduced sugar, all flavors	55.0
Licorice	78.0
M & M's Almond Chocolate Candies	33.0
M & M's Peanut Butter Chocolate Candies	33.0
M & M's Peanut Chocolate Candies	33.0
M & M's Plain Chocolate Candies	43.0
Marmalade, all flavors	48.0
MARS Bar	65.0
Melba toast	70.0
MILKY WAY Bar	43.0
Mixed nuts, dry roasted	18.0
Mixed nuts, honey-roasted, with peanuts	18.0
Mixed nuts, in shell	18.0
Mixed nuts, NFS	18.0
Mixed nuts, roasted, with peanuts	18.0
Mixed nuts, roasted, without peanuts	22.0
Nougat, chocolate covered	65.0
Nougat, plain	32.0
Nougat, with caramel, chocolate covered	65.0
Peanut bar	23.0
Peanut butter	14.0

Food Name	Glycemic Index
Peanut butter, low sodium	14.0
Peanut butter, reduced fat	14.0
Peanut butter, reduced sodium	14.0
Peanuts, boiled	14.0
Peanuts, dry roasted, salted	14.0
Peanuts, dry roasted, without salt	14.0
Peanuts, honey-roasted	14.0
Peanuts, in shell, NFS (shell not eaten)	14.0
Peanuts, NFS	14.0
Peanuts, roasted, salted	14.0
Peanuts, roasted, without salt	14.0
Pecans	20.0
Planters Peanut Bar	23.0
Popcorn, air-popped (no butter or no oil added)	72.0
Popcorn, air-popped, buttered	72.0
Popcorn, flavored	72.0
Popcorn, popped in oil, buttered	72.0
Popcorn, popped in oil, lowfat	72.0
Popcorn, popped in oil, lowfat, low sodium	72.0
Popcorn, popped in oil, unbuttered	72.0
Popcorn, popped in oil, unsalted	72.0
Popcorn, with cheese	72.0
Pretzel, hard, unsalted	83.0
Pretzel, oatbran, hard	83.0
Pretzels, hard	83.0
Pretzels, NFS	83.0
Pretzels, soft	83.0
Puffed rice cake	78.0

Food Name	Glycemic Index
Puffed rice cake without salt	78.0
Reese's Peanut Butter Cup	43.0
Rice cake, cracker-type	78.0
Salty snack mixture, mostly corn or cornmeal based, with pretzels, without nuts	63.0
Salty snacks, corn based puffs and twists, cheese puffs and twists, lowfat	63.0
Salty snacks, corn or cornmeal base, corn chips, corn-cheese chips	63.0
Salty snacks, corn or cornmeal base, corn chips, corn-cheese chips, unsalted	63.0
Salty snacks, corn or cornmeal base, corn puffs and twists; corn-cheese puffs and twists	63.0
Salty snacks, corn or cornmeal base, nuts or nuggets, toasted	63.0
Salty snacks, corn or cornmeal base, tortilla chips	63.0
Salty snacks, corn or cornmeal base, tortilla chips, light (baked with less oil)	63.0
Salty snacks, corn or cornmeal base, tortilla chips, lowfat, baked without fat	63.0
Salty snacks, corn or cornmeal base, tortilla chips, lowfat, baked without fat, unsalted	63.0
Salty snacks, corn or cornmeal base, tortilla chips, unsalted	63.0
Salty snacks, multigrain, chips	63.0
Scone	92.0
Scone, with fruit	92.0
Skittles	70.0
SNICKERS Bar	55.0
Snickers Peanut Butter Bar	55.0
Special Dark	43.0
Sunflower seeds, hulled, unroasted	20.0
TWIX Chocolate Fudge Cookie Bars	44.0
TWIX Cookie Bars	44.0
TWIX Peanut Butter Cookie Bars	44.0
Walnuts	20.0
White potato skins, chips	54.0

Food Name	Glycemic Index
White potato, chips	54.0
White potato, chips, fat free	54.0
White potato, chips, reduced fat	54.0
White potato, chips, restructured	54.0
White potato, chips, restructured, baked	54.0
White potato, chips, restructured, reduced fat and reduced sodium	54.0
White potato, chips, unsalted	54.0
White potato, chips, unsalted, reduced fat	54.0
White potato, sticks	54.0

Vegetables

Food Name	Glycemic Index
Alfalfa sprouts, raw	32.0
Algae, dried	32.0
Apple, pickled	38.0
Artichoke salad in oil	32.0
Artichoke, globe (French), cooked, from canned, NS as to fat added in cooking	32.0
Artichoke, globe (French), cooked, from fresh, fat added in cooking	32.0
Artichoke, globe (French), cooked, from fresh, fat not added in cooking	32.0
Artichoke, globe (French), cooked, from fresh, NS as to fat added in cooking	32.0
Artichoke, globe (French), cooked, from frozen, NS as to fat added in cooking	32.0
Artichoke, globe (French), cooked, NS as to form, fat not added in cooking	32.0
Artichoke, globe (French), cooked, NS as to form, NS as to fat added in cooking	32.0
Artichoke, Jerusalem, raw	32.0
Asparagus, cooked, from canned, fat added in cooking	32.0
Asparagus, cooked, from canned, fat not added in cooking	32.0
Asparagus, cooked, from canned, NS as to fat added in cooking	32.0
Asparagus, cooked, from fresh, fat added in cooking	32.0
Asparagus, cooked, from fresh, fat not added in cooking	32.0
Asparagus, cooked, from fresh, NS as to fat added in cooking	32.0
Asparagus, cooked, from frozen, fat added in cooking	32.0
Asparagus, cooked, from frozen, fat not added in cooking	32.0
Asparagus, cooked, NS as to form, fat added in cooking	32.0
Asparagus, cooked, NS as to form, fat not added in cooking	32.0
Asparagus, cooked, NS as to form, NS as to fat added in cooking	32.0
Asparagus, from canned, creamed or with cheese sauce	28.3
Asparagus, from fresh, creamed or with cheese sauce	29.2
Asparagus, raw	32.0

Food Name	Glycemic Index
Bamboo shoots, cooked, fat added in cooking	32.0
Bamboo shoots, cooked, fat not added in cooking	32.0
Bean sprouts, cooked, from canned, fat added in cooking	32.0
Bean sprouts, cooked, from canned, fat not added in cooking	32.0
Bean sprouts, cooked, from fresh, fat added in cooking	32.0
Bean sprouts, cooked, from fresh, fat not added in cooking	32.0
Bean sprouts, cooked, from fresh, NS as to fat added in cooking	32.0
Bean sprouts, cooked, NS as to form, fat added in cooking	32.0
Bean sprouts, cooked, NS as to form, NS as to fat added in cooking	32.0
Bean sprouts, raw (soybean or mung)	32.0
Beans, green string, with tomatoes, cooked, fat not added in cooking	35.0
Beans, green, and potatoes, cooked, fat not added in cooking	63.3
Beans, green, with pinto beans, cooked, fat not added in cooking	38.0
Beet greens, raw	32.0
Beets with Harvard sauce	66.2
Beets, cooked, from canned, fat added in cooking	64.0
Beets, cooked, from canned, fat not added in cooking	64.0
Beets, cooked, from canned, NS as to fat added in cooking	64.0
Beets, cooked, from fresh, fat not added in cooking	64.0
Beets, cooked, from fresh, NS as to fat added in cooking	64.0
Beets, cooked, NS as to form, fat added in cooking	64.0
Beets, cooked, NS as to form, fat not added in cooking	64.0
Beets, cooked, NS as to form, NS as to fat added in cooking	64.0
Beets, pickled	65.5
Beets, raw	64.0
Bitter melon, cooked, fat not added in cooking	32.0
Breadfruit, cooked, fat not added in cooking	68.0
Broccoflower, cooked, fat not added in cooking	32.0

Food Name	Glycemic Index
Broccoli, cooked, from fresh, fat not added in cooking	32.0
Broccoli, cooked, from frozen, fat not added in cooking	32.0
Broccoli, cooked, NS as to form, fat not added in cooking	32.0
Broccoli, raw	32.0
Brussels sprouts, cooked, from fresh, fat not added in cooking	32.0
Brussels sprouts, cooked, from frozen, fat not added in cooking	32.0
Brussels sprouts, cooked, NS as to form, fat not added in cooking	32.0
Brussels sprouts, raw	32.0
Cabbage salad or coleslaw, with dressing	44.1
Cabbage, Chinese, cooked, fat added in cooking	32.0
Cabbage, Chinese, cooked, fat not added in cooking	32.0
Cabbage, Chinese, cooked, NS as to fat added in cooking	32.0
Cabbage, Chinese, raw	32.0
Cabbage, Chinese, salad, with dressing	32.0
Cabbage, fresh, pickled, Japanese style	32.0
Cabbage, green, cooked, fat added in cooking	32.0
Cabbage, green, cooked, fat not added in cooking	32.0
Cabbage, green, cooked, NS as to fat added in cooking	32.0
Cabbage, green, raw	32.0
Cabbage, Kim Chee style	32.0
Cabbage, red, cooked, fat added in cooking	32.0
Cabbage, red, cooked, fat not added in cooking	32.0
Cabbage, red, cooked, NS as to fat added in cooking	32.0
Cabbage, red, pickled	32.0
Cabbage, red, raw	32.0
Cactus, cooked, fat added in cooking	7.0
Cactus, cooked, fat not added in cooking	7.0
Cactus, cooked, NS as to fat added in cooking	7.0

Food Name	Glycemic Index
Cactus, raw	7.0
Calabaza (Spanish pumpkin), cooked	75.0
Carrots, canned, low sodium, fat not added in cooking	47.0
Carrots, cooked, from canned, fat not added in cooking	47.0
Carrots, cooked, from fresh, fat not added in cooking	47.0
Carrots, cooked, from frozen, fat not added in cooking	47.0
Carrots, cooked, NS as to form, fat not added in cooking	47.0
Carrots, raw	16.0
Casabe, cassava bread	56.0
Cassava (yuca blanca), cooked, fat not added in cooking	46.0
Cassava (yuca blanca), cooked, NS as to fat added in cooking	46.0
Cauliflower, cooked, from fresh, fat not added in cooking	32.0
Cauliflower, cooked, from frozen, fat not added in cooking	32.0
Cauliflower, cooked, NS as to form, fat not added in cooking	32.0
Cauliflower, pickled	32.0
Cauliflower, raw	32.0
Celery juice	32.0
Celery, cooked, fat added in cooking	32.0
Celery, cooked, fat not added in cooking	32.0
Celery, cooked, NS as to fat added in cooking	32.0
Celery, raw	32.0
Chard, cooked, fat not added in cooking	32.0
Chives, raw	32.0
Christophine, cooked, fat not added in cooking	32.0
Cilantro, raw	32.0
Cocktail sauce	38.0
Collards, cooked, from canned, fat not added in cooking	32.0
Collards, cooked, from fresh, fat not added in cooking	32.0

Food Name	Glycemic Index
Collards, cooked, from frozen, fat not added in cooking	32.0
Corn relish	54.0
Corn with peppers, red or green, cooked, fat not added in cooking	53.5
Cucumber pickles, dill	32.0
Cucumber pickles, dill, reduced salt	32.0
Cucumber pickles, fresh	32.0
Cucumber pickles, relish	32.0
Cucumber pickles, sour	32.0
Cucumber pickles, sweet	32.0
Cucumber salad made with cucumber, oil, and vinegar	32.0
Cucumber salad with creamy dressing	32.0
Cucumber, cooked, fat added in cooking	32.0
Cucumber, cooked, fat not added in cooking	32.0
Cucumber, cooked, NS as to fat added in cooking	32.0
Cucumber, raw	32.0
Dandelion greens, cooked, fat not added in cooking	32.0
Dandelion greens, raw	32.0
Dasheen, boiled	32.0
Dumpling, potato- or cheese-filled	52.0
Eggplant in tomato sauce, cooked, fat not added in cooking	35.0
Eggplant, cooked, fat added in cooking	32.0
Eggplant, cooked, fat not added in cooking	32.0
Eggplant, cooked, NS as to fat added in cooking	32.0
Eggplant, pickled	32.0
Endive, chicory, escarole, or romaine lettuce, raw	32.0
Escarole, cooked, fat not added in cooking	32.0
Garlic, cooked	32.0
Garlic, raw	32.0

Food Name	Glycemic Index
Green tomato-chile sauce, cooked (Salsa verde, NFS)	38.0
Greens, cooked, from canned, fat not added in cooking	32.0
Greens, cooked, from fresh, fat not added in cooking	32.0
Jicama, raw	32.0
Kale, cooked, from fresh, fat not added in cooking	32.0
Leek, raw	32.0
Lettuce, arugula, raw	32.0
Lettuce, Boston, raw	32.0
Lettuce, cooked, fat not added in cooking	32.0
Lettuce, raw	32.0
Lotus root, cooked, fat not added in cooking	32.0
Mixed salad greens, raw	32.0
Mixed vegetables (corn, lima beans, peas, green beans, and carrots), canned, low sodium, fat not added in cooking	42.6
Mixed vegetables (corn, lima beans, peas, green beans, and carrots), cooked, from canned, fat not added in cooking	42.6
Mixed vegetables (corn, lima beans, peas, green beans, and carrots), cooked, from frozen, fat not added in cooking	42.6
Mixed vegetables (corn, lima beans, peas, green beans, and carrots), cooked, NS as to form, fat not added in cooking	42.6
Mushroom, Oriental, cooked, from dried	32.0
Mushrooms, cooked, from canned, fat added in cooking	32.0
Mushrooms, cooked, from canned, fat not added in cooking	32.0
Mushrooms, cooked, from canned, NS as to fat added in cooking	32.0
Mushrooms, cooked, from fresh, fat added in cooking	32.0
Mushrooms, cooked, from fresh, fat not added in cooking	32.0
Mushrooms, cooked, from fresh, NS as to fat added in cooking	32.0
Mushrooms, cooked, from frozen, fat added in cooking	32.0
Mushrooms, cooked, from frozen, NS as to fat added in cooking	32.0
Mushrooms, cooked, NS as to form, fat added in cooking	32.0
Mushrooms, cooked, NS as to form, fat not added in cooking	32.0

Food Name	Glycemic Index
Mushrooms, cooked, NS as to form, NS as to fat added in cooking	32.0
Mushrooms, pickled	32.0
Mushrooms, raw	32.0
Mustard greens, cooked, from canned, fat not added in cooking	32.0
Mustard greens, cooked, from fresh, fat not added in cooking	32.0
Mustard greens, cooked, from frozen, fat not added in cooking	32.0
Mustard greens, cooked, NS as to form, fat not added in cooking	32.0
Mustard pickles	32.0
Okra, cooked, from canned, fat added in cooking	32.0
Okra, cooked, from canned, fat not added in cooking	32.0
Okra, cooked, from fresh, fat added in cooking	32.0
Okra, cooked, from fresh, fat not added in cooking	32.0
Okra, cooked, from fresh, NS as to fat added in cooking	32.0
Okra, cooked, from frozen, fat added in cooking	32.0
Okra, cooked, from frozen, fat not added in cooking	32.0
Okra, cooked, from frozen, NS as to fat added in cooking	32.0
Okra, cooked, NS as to form, fat added in cooking	32.0
Okra, cooked, NS as to form, fat not added in cooking	32.0
Okra, cooked, NS as to form, NS as to fat added in cooking	32.0
Okra, pickled	32.0
Olives, black	50.0
Olives, green	50.0
Olives, green, stuffed	50.0
Olives, NFS	50.0
Onion, young green, cooked, NS as to form, NS as to fat added in cooking	32.0
Onions, mature, cooked, from fresh, fat not added in cooking	32.0
Onions, mature, cooked, from frozen, fat not added in cooking	32.0
Onions, mature, cooked, NS as to form, fat not added in cooking	32.0

Food Name	Glycemic Index
Onions, mature, raw	32.0
Onions, pearl, cooked, from canned	32.0
Onions, pearl, cooked, from fresh	32.0
Onions, pearl, cooked, NS as to form	32.0
Onions, young green, cooked, from fresh, fat not added in cooking	32.0
Onions, young green, cooked, NS as to form, fat not added in cooking	32.0
Onions, young green, raw	32.0
Palm hearts, cooked (assume fat not added in cooking)	32.0
Parsley, cooked (assume fat not added in cooking)	32.0
Parsley, raw	32.0
Parsnips, cooked, fat added in cooking	97.0
Parsnips, cooked, fat not added in cooking	97.0
Peas and carrots, canned, low sodium, fat not added in cooking	47.5
Peas and carrots, cooked, from canned, fat not added in cooking	47.5
Peas and carrots, cooked, from fresh, fat not added in cooking	47.5
Peas and carrots, cooked, from frozen, fat not added in cooking	47.5
Peas and carrots, cooked, NS as to form, fat not added in cooking	47.5
Peas and corn, cooked, fat not added in cooking	51.0
Peas and onions, cooked, fat not added in cooking	40.0
Peas and potatoes, cooked, fat not added in cooking	63.2
Peas with mushrooms, cooked, fat not added in cooking	46.8
Peas, cowpeas, field peas, or blackeye peas (not dried), cooked, from canned, fat not added in cooking	42.0
Peas, cowpeas, field peas, or blackeye peas (not dried), cooked, from fresh, fat not added in cooking	42.0
Peas, cowpeas, field peas, or blackeye peas (not dried), cooked, from frozen, fat not added in cooking	42.0
Peas, cowpeas, field peas, or blackeye peas (not dried), cooked, NS as to form, fat not added in cooking	42.0
Peas, green, canned, low sodium, fat not added in cooking	48.0
Peas, green, cooked, from canned, fat not added in cooking	48.0

Food Name	Glycemic Index
Peas, green, cooked, from fresh, fat not added in cooking	48.0
Peas, green, cooked, from frozen, fat not added in cooking	48.0
Peas, green, cooked, NS as to form, fat not added in cooking	48.0
Peas, green, raw	48.0
Pepper, banana, raw	32.0
Pepper, hot chili, raw	32.0
Pepper, hot, pickled	32.0
Pepper, poblano, raw	32.0
Pepper, raw, NFS	32.0
Pepper, Serrano, raw	32.0
Pepper, sweet, green, raw	32.0
Pepper, sweet, red, raw	32.0
Peppers, green, cooked, fat not added in cooking	32.0
Peppers, hot, cooked, from canned, fat added in cooking	32.0
Peppers, hot, cooked, from canned, fat not added in cooking	32.0
Peppers, hot, cooked, from canned, NS as to fat added in cooking	32.0
Peppers, hot, cooked, from fresh, fat added in cooking	32.0
Peppers, hot, cooked, from fresh, fat not added in cooking	32.0
Peppers, hot, cooked, from fresh, NS as to fat added in cooking	32.0
Peppers, hot, cooked, from frozen, fat not added in cooking	32.0
Peppers, hot, cooked, NS as to form, fat added in cooking	32.0
Peppers, hot, cooked, NS as to form, fat not added in cooking	32.0
Peppers, hot, cooked, NS as to form, NS as to fat added in cooking	32.0
Peppers, pickled	32.0
Peppers, red, cooked, fat not added in cooking	32.0
Pickles, NS as to vegetable	32.0
Pigeon peas, cooked, NS as to form, fat not added in cooking	22.0
Pimiento	32.0

Food Name	Glycemic Index
Pumpkin, cooked, from canned, fat not added in cooking	75.0
Pumpkin, cooked, from fresh, fat added in cooking	75.0
Pumpkin, cooked, from fresh, fat not added in cooking	75.0
Pumpkin, cooked, NS as to form, fat not added in cooking	75.0
Radicchio, raw	32.0
Radish, Japanese (daikon), cooked, fat not added in cooking	32.0
Radish, raw	32.0
Radishes, pickled, Hawaiian style	32.0
Raw vegetable, NFS	32.1
Recaito (Puerto Rican little coriander)	32.0
Rutabaga, cooked, fat added in cooking	72.0
Rutabaga, cooked, fat not added in cooking	72.0
Salsa, NFS	38.0
Salsa, red, cooked, homemade	38.0
Salsa, red, cooked, not homemade	38.0
Salsa, red, uncooked	38.0
Sauerkraut, canned, low sodium	32.0
Sauerkraut, cooked, fat added in cooking	32.0
Sauerkraut, cooked, fat not added in cooking	32.0
Sauerkraut, cooked, NS as to fat added in cooking	32.0
Seaweed, dried	32.0
Seaweed, prepared with soy sauce	32.0
Seaweed, raw	32.0
Snowpea (pea pod), cooked, from fresh, fat not added in cooking	32.0
Snowpea (pea pod), cooked, from frozen, fat not added in cooking	32.0
Snowpea (pea pod), cooked, NS as to form, fat not added in cooking	32.0
Snowpeas (pea pod), raw	32.0
Spinach, cooked, from canned, fat not added in cooking	32.0

Food Name	Glycemic Index
Spinach, cooked, from fresh, fat not added in cooking	32.0
Spinach, cooked, from frozen, fat not added in cooking	32.0
Spinach, cooked, NS as to form, fat not added in cooking	32.0
Spinach, raw	32.0
Sprouts, NFS	32.0
Squash, spaghetti, cooked, fat not added in cooking	32.0
Squash, spaghetti, cooked, NS as to fat added in cooking	32.0
Squash, summer, and onions, cooked, fat added in cooking	32.0
Squash, summer, and onions, cooked, fat not added in cooking	32.0
Squash, summer, cooked, from canned, fat added in cooking	32.0
Squash, summer, cooked, from canned, fat not added in cooking	32.0
Squash, summer, cooked, from canned, NS as to fat added in cooking	32.0
Squash, summer, cooked, from fresh, fat added in cooking	32.0
Squash, summer, cooked, from fresh, fat not added in cooking	32.0
Squash, summer, cooked, from fresh, NS as to fat added in cooking	32.0
Squash, summer, cooked, from frozen, fat added in cooking	32.0
Squash, summer, cooked, from frozen, fat not added in cooking	32.0
Squash, summer, cooked, NS as to form, fat added in cooking	32.0
Squash, summer, cooked, NS as to form, fat not added in cooking	32.0
Squash, summer, cooked, NS as to form, NS as to fat added in cooking	32.0
Squash, summer, from fresh, creamed	28.6
Squash, summer, green, raw	32.0
Squash, summer, yellow, raw	32.0
Squash, winter type, baked, fat added in cooking, no sugar added in cooking	75.0
Squash, winter type, baked, fat and sugar added in cooking	71.3
Squash, winter type, baked, no fat added in cooking, sugar added in cooking	71.3
Squash, winter type, baked, no fat or sugar added in cooking	75.0
Squash, winter type, baked, NS as to fat or sugar added in cooking	71.3

Food Name	Glycemic Index
Squash, winter type, mashed, fat added in cooking, no sugar added in cooking	75.0
Squash, winter type, mashed, fat and sugar added in cooking	71.3
Squash, winter type, mashed, no fat or sugar added in cooking	75.0
Squash, winter type, mashed, NS as to fat or sugar added in cooking	75.0
Sweetpotato leaves, squash leaves, pumpkin leaves, chrysanthemum leaves, bean leaves, or swamp cabbage, cooked, fat not added in cooking	32.0
Sweetpotato with fruit	53.2
Sweetpotato, baked, peel eaten, fat not added in cooking	61.0
Sweetpotato, baked, peel not eaten, fat not added in cooking	61.0
Sweetpotato, boiled, with peel, fat not added in cooking	61.0
Sweetpotato, boiled, without peel, fat not added in cooking	61.0
Sweetpotato, canned in syrup	61.0
Sweetpotato, canned without syrup	61.0
Sweetpotato, canned, NS as to syrup	61.0
Tannier, cooked	32.0
Taro leaves, cooked, fat not added in cooking	32.0
Taro, baked	55.0
Tomato and corn, cooked, fat not added in cooking	50.3
Tomato and okra, cooked, fat not added in cooking	35.0
Tomato and onion, cooked, fat not added in cooking	35.0
Tomato and onion, cooked, NS as to fat added in cooking	35.0
Tomato catsup	38.0
Tomato catsup, low sodium	38.0
Tomato chili sauce (catsup-type)	38.0
Tomato paste	38.0
Tomato relish	32.0
Tomato, green, pickled	32.0
Tomatoes, green, raw	38.0
Tomatoes, raw	38.0

Food Name	Glycemic Index
Turnip greens with roots, cooked, from frozen, fat not added in cooking	32.0
Turnip greens, cooked, from canned, fat not added in cooking	32.0
Turnip greens, cooked, from fresh, fat not added in cooking	32.0
Turnip greens, cooked, from frozen, fat not added in cooking	32.0
Turnip greens, cooked, NS as to form, fat not added in cooking	32.0
Turnip, cooked, from fresh, fat added in cooking	72.0
Turnip, cooked, from fresh, fat not added in cooking	72.0
Turnip, cooked, from fresh, NS as to fat added in cooking	72.0
Turnip, cooked, NS as to form, fat added in cooking	72.0
Turnip, cooked, NS as to form, fat not added in cooking	72.0
Turnip, raw	72.0
Turnips, from fresh, creamed	39.9
Vegetable combination (excluding carrots, broccoli, and dark-green leafy), cooked, with soy-based sauce	49.1
Vegetable combination (green beans, broccoli, onions, mushrooms), cooked, fat not added in cooking	32.0
Vegetable combination (including carrots, broccoli, and/or dark-green leafy), cooked, with soy-based sauce	48.2
Vegetable combinations (broccoli, carrots, corn, cauliflower, etc.), cooked, fat not added in cooking	48.6
Vegetable combinations, Oriental style, (broccoli, green pepper, water chestnuts, etc), cooked, fat not added in cooking	32.0
Vegetable relish	32.0
Vegetables, NS as to type, cooked, fat not added in cooking	42.6
Vegetables, NS as to type, cooked, NS as to fat added in cooking	42.6
Vegetables, pickled	32.0
Vegetables, stew type (including potatoes, carrots, onions, celery) cooked, fat not added in cooking	62.1
Water chestnut	32.0
Watercress, raw	32.0
White potato skins, with adhering flesh, baked	72.5
White potato, baked, peel eaten, fat not added in cooking	72.5
White potato, baked, peel not eaten	72.5

Food Name	Glycemic Index
White potato, boiled, with peel, fat not added in cooking	66.2
White potato, boiled, without peel, canned, low sodium, fat not added in cooking	63.0
White potato, boiled, without peel, fat not added in cooking	66.2
White potato, french fries, breaded or battered	75.0
White potato, french fries, from fresh, deep fried	75.0
White potato, french fries, from frozen, deep fried	75.0
White potato, french fries, from frozen, oven baked	75.0
White potato, french fries, NS as to from fresh or frozen	75.0
White potato, from complete dry mix, mashed, made with water	85.0
White potato, from dry, mashed, made with milk, no fat	85.0
White potato, from fresh, mashed, made with milk	79.3
White potato, from fresh, mashed, not made with milk or fat	79.3
White potato, hash brown, from dry mix	75.0
White potato, hash brown, from fresh	75.0
White potato, hash brown, from frozen	75.0
White potato, hash brown, NS as to from fresh, frozen, or dry mix	75.0
White potato, hash brown, with cheese	75.0
White potato, home fries	75.0
White potato, NFS	66.2
White potato, roasted, fat not added in cooking	72.5
Winter melon, cooked	32.0
Yam, Puerto Rican (Name), cooked	37.0
Zucchini with tomato sauce, cooked, fat not added in cooking	35.0

PART III: Net carb, Fat, Protein, and Calories Counting Tables

You can use our "Keto Carb Counter" search engine if you want to have the macros for given foods, in the following address: https://www.easyketodiet.net/glycemic-index-counter/

BACKED PRODUCTS

Food Name ---> per 100 g	Protein (g)	Fat (g)	Calorie	Net Carb (g)
Bagels, plain, enriched, with calcium propionate (includes onion, poppy, sesame)	10.56	1.32	264	50.78
Bagels, plain (includes onion, poppy, sesame), toasted	11.14	1.43	287	55.59
Bagels, egg	10.6	2.1	278	50.7
Bagels, cinnamon-raisin	9.8	1.7	274	52.9
Bagels, cinnamon-raisin, toasted	10.6	1.8	294	56.8
Bagels, oat bran	10.7	1.2	255	49.7
Biscuits, plain or buttermilk, frozen, baked	6.2	11.03	338	52.57
Biscuits, plain or buttermilk, dry mix	8	15.4	428	61.3
Biscuits, plain or buttermilk, dry mix, prepared	7.3	12.1	335	46.6
Biscuits, plain or buttermilk, refrigerated dough, lower fat	6.7	7.83	270	41.7
Biscuits, plain or buttermilk, refrigerated dough, lower fat, baked	7.8	9.1	319	49.3
Biscuits, plain or buttermilk, refrigerated dough, higher fat	6.66	10.58	307	45.62
Biscuits, plain or buttermilk, refrigerated dough, higher fat, baked	6.79	11.22	324	46.25
Biscuits, plain or buttermilk, prepared from recipe	7	16.3	353	43.1
Biscuits, mixed grain, refrigerated dough	6.1	5.6	263	47.4
Bread, banana, prepared from recipe, made with margarine	4.3	10.5	326	53.5
Bread, boston brown, canned	5.2	1.5	195	38.6
Bread, cornbread, dry mix, enriched (includes corn muffin mix)	7	12.2	418	63
Bread, cornbread, dry mix, prepared with 2% milk, 80% margarine, and eggs	6.59	9.58	330	52.16
Bread, cornbread, prepared from recipe, made with low fat (2%) milk	6.7	7.1	266	43.5
Bread, cracked-wheat	8.7	3.9	260	44
Bread, egg	9.5	6	287	45.5
Bread, egg, toasted	10.5	6.6	315	50.1
Bread, french or vienna (includes sourdough)	10.75	2.42	272	49.68
Bread, french or vienna, toasted (includes sourdough)	13	2.14	319	58.83
Bread, irish soda, prepared from recipe	6.6	5	290	53.4
Bread, italian	8.8	3.5	271	46.9

Food Name ---> per 100 g	Protein (g)	Fat (g)	Calorie	Net Carb (g)
Bread, multi-grain, toasted (includes whole-grain)	14.52	4.6	288	39.01
Bread, oat bran	10.4	4.4	236	35.3
Bread, oat bran, toasted	11.4	4.8	259	38.8
Bread, oatmeal	8.4	4.4	269	44.5
Bread, oatmeal, toasted	9.2	4.8	292	48.4
Bread, pita, white, enriched	9.1	1.2	275	53.5
Bread, pita, whole-wheat	9.8	1.71	262	49.79
Bread, protein (includes gluten)	12.1	2.2	245	40.8
Bread, pumpernickel	8.7	3.1	250	41
Bread, pumpernickel, toasted	9.5	3.4	275	45.1
Bread, raisin, enriched	7.9	4.4	274	48
Bread, raisin, enriched, toasted	8.6	4.8	297	52.2
Bread, reduced-calorie, oat bran	8	3.2	201	29.3
Bread, reduced-calorie, oat bran, toasted	9.5	3.8	239	34.9
Bread, reduced-calorie, oatmeal	7.6	3.5	210	43.3
Bread, reduced-calorie, rye	9.1	2.9	203	28.5
Bread, reduced-calorie, wheat	13.32	2.92	217	31.37
Bread, reduced-calorie, white	8.7	2.5	207	34.6
Bread, rice bran	8.9	4.6	243	38.6
Bread, rye	8.5	3.3	259	42.5
Bread, rye, toasted	9.4	3.6	284	46.7
Bread, wheat	10.72	3.24	267	44.68
Bread, wheat, toasted	12.96	4.27	313	51.07
Bread, wheat bran	8.8	3.4	248	43.8
Bread, white, commercially prepared (includes soft bread crumbs)	8.85	3.33	266	46.72
Bread, white, commercially prepared, toasted	9	4	290	51.6
Bread, white, prepared from recipe, made with nonfat dry milk	7.7	2.6	274	51.6
Bread, white, prepared from recipe, made with low fat (2%) milk	7.9	5.7	285	47.6
Bread, whole-wheat, commercially prepared	12.45	3.5	252	36.71
Bread, whole-wheat, commercially prepared, toasted	16.27	4.07	306	43.66
Bread, whole-wheat, prepared from recipe	8.4	5.4	278	45.4

Food Name ---> per 100 g	Protein (g)	Fat (g)	Calorie	Net Carb (g)
Bread, whole-wheat, prepared from recipe, toasted	9.2	5.9	305	49.7
Bread crumbs, dry, grated, plain	13.35	5.3	395	67.48
Bread sticks, plain	12	9.5	412	65.4
Bread stuffing, bread, dry mix	11	3.4	386	73
Bread stuffing, bread, dry mix, prepared	2.73	12.05	195	18.04
Bread stuffing, cornbread, dry mix	10	4.2	389	62.4
Bread stuffing, cornbread, dry mix, prepared	2.9	8.8	179	19
Cake, angelfood, commercially prepared	5.9	0.8	258	56.3
Cake, angelfood, dry mix	6.4	0.27	366	85.63
Cake, angelfood, dry mix, prepared	6.1	0.3	257	58.5
Cake, boston cream pie, commercially prepared	2.4	8.5	252	41.5
Cake, pudding-type, carrot, dry mix	5.1	9.8	415	79.2
Cake, cherry fudge with chocolate frosting	2.4	12.5	264	37.5
Cake, chocolate, commercially prepared with chocolate frosting, in-store bakery	3.48	20.05	389	50.64
Cake, pudding-type, chocolate, dry mix	4.6	8.14	391	77.86
Cake, chocolate, prepared from recipe without frosting	5.3	15.1	371	51.8
Cake, white, prepared from recipe with coconut frosting	4.4	10.3	356	62.2
Coffeecake, cheese	7	15.2	339	43.3
Coffeecake, cinnamon with crumb topping, commercially prepared, enriched	6.8	23.3	418	44.7
Coffeecake, creme-filled with chocolate frosting	5	10.8	331	51.8
Coffeecake, fruit	5.2	10.2	311	49
Coffeecake, cinnamon with crumb topping, dry mix	4.8	12	436	75.9
Coffeecake, cinnamon with crumb topping, dry mix, prepared	5.5	9.6	318	51.6
Cake, fruitcake, commercially prepared	2.9	9.1	324	57.9
Cake, pudding-type, german chocolate, dry mix	4.17	3.24	350	79.15
Cake, gingerbread, dry mix	4.4	13.8	437	72.9
Cake, gingerbread, prepared from recipe	3.9	16.4	356	49.2
Cake, pudding-type, marble, dry mix	3.4	11.7	416	76.6
Cake, pineapple upside-down, prepared from recipe	3.5	12.1	319	49.7

Food Name ---> per 100 g	Protein (g)	Fat (g)	Calorie	Net Carb (g)
Cake, pound, commercially prepared, butter (includes fresh and frozen)	5	13.96	353	53.04
Cake, pound, commercially prepared, other than all butter, enriched	5.2	17.9	389	51.5
Cake, shortcake, biscuit-type, prepared from recipe	6.1	14.2	346	48.5
Cake, snack cakes, creme-filled, chocolate with frosting	3.63	15.93	399	57.11
Cake, snack cakes, creme-filled, sponge	3.47	11.54	374	63.03
Cake, white, dry mix, special dietary (includes lemon-flavored)	3	8.4	397	79.6
Cake, sponge, commercially prepared	5.4	2.7	290	60.5
Cake, sponge, prepared from recipe	7.3	4.3	297	57.7
Cake, pudding-type, white, enriched, dry mix	3.9	9.5	423	80.2
Cake, white, prepared from recipe without frosting	5.4	12.4	357	56.4
Cake, yellow, commercially prepared, with chocolate frosting, in-store bakery	3.16	17.75	379	53.86
Cake, yellow, commercially prepared, with vanilla frosting	2.99	17.91	391	55.9
Cake, pudding-type, yellow, dry mix	4	9.8	423	79.3
Cake, yellow, enriched, dry mix	3.7	3.5	374	80.72
Cake, yellow, prepared from recipe without frosting	5.3	14.6	361	52.3
Cheesecake commercially prepared	5.5	22.5	321	25.1
Cheesecake prepared from mix, no-bake type	5.5	12.7	274	33.6
Cookies, brownies, commercially prepared	4.8	16.3	405	61.8
Cookies, brownies, dry mix, regular	4	14.9	434	76.6
Cookies, brownies, prepared from recipe	6.2	29.1	466	50.2
Cookies, butter, commercially prepared, enriched	6.1	18.8	467	68.1
Cookies, fudge, cake-type (includes trolley cakes)	5	3.7	349	75.5
Cookies, chocolate wafers	6.6	14.2	433	69.3
Cookies, chocolate chip, commercially prepared, regular, lower fat	5.97	17.91	451	64.49
Cookies, chocolate chip, commercially prepared, regular, higher fat, enriched	5.1	24.72	492	63.36
Cookies, chocolate chip, commercially prepared, soft-type	3.63	19.77	444	63.95
Cookies, chocolate chip, dry mix	4.6	25.2	497	66.1
Cookies, chocolate chip, refrigerated dough	3.98	21.33	451	59.52
Cookies, chocolate chip, refrigerated dough, baked	4.9	22.6	492	66.5

Food Name ---> per 100 g	Protein (g)	Fat (g)	Calorie	Net Carb (g)
Cookies, chocolate chip, prepared from recipe, made with margarine	5.7	28.3	488	55.6
Cookies, chocolate sandwich, with creme filling, regular	5.21	19.14	464	68.1
Cookies, chocolate sandwich, with creme filling, regular, chocolate-coated	3.6	26.4	481	61.2
Cookies, chocolate sandwich, with extra creme filling	4.33	24.52	497	65.5
Cookies, fig bars	3.7	7.3	348	66.3
Cookies, fortune	4.2	2.7	378	82.4
Cookies, gingersnaps	5.6	9.8	416	74.7
Cookies, graham crackers, plain or honey (includes cinnamon)	6.69	10.6	430	74.26
Cookies, graham crackers, chocolate-coated	4	25.8	500	64.58
Cookies, ladyfingers, with lemon juice and rind	10.6	9.1	365	58.7
Cookies, marshmallow, chocolate-coated (includes marshmallow pies)	4	16.9	421	65.7
Cookies, molasses	5.6	12.8	430	72.8
Cookies, oatmeal, commercially prepared, regular	6.2	18.1	450	65.9
Cookies, oatmeal, commercially prepared, soft-type	6.1	14.7	409	63
Cookies, oatmeal, dry mix	6.5	19.2	462	67.3
Cookies, oatmeal, refrigerated dough	5.4	18.9	424	56.6
Cookies, oatmeal, refrigerated dough, baked	6	21	471	62.9
Cookies, oatmeal, prepared from recipe, with raisins	6.5	16.2	435	68.4
Cookies, peanut butter, commercially prepared, regular	8.92	23.82	473	56.05
Cookies, peanut butter, commercially prepared, soft-type	5.3	24.4	457	56
Cookies, peanut butter, refrigerated dough	8.2	25	458	51
Cookies, peanut butter, refrigerated dough, baked	9.1	27.5	503	56.1
Cookies, peanut butter, prepared from recipe	9	23.8	475	58.9
Cookies, peanut butter sandwich, regular	8.8	21.1	478	63.7
Cookies, raisin, soft-type	4.1	13.6	401	66.8
Cookies, shortbread, commercially prepared, plain	5.37	26.22	514	62.48
Cookies, shortbread, commercially prepared, pecan	4.9	32.5	542	56.5
Cookies, brownies, dry mix, sugar free	2.9	12.5	426	76.2
Cookies, chocolate chip, commercially prepared, special dietary	3.9	16.8	450	71.8

Food Name ---> per 100 g	Protein (g)	Fat (g)	Calorie	Net Carb (g)
Cookies, chocolate sandwich, with creme filling, special dietary	4.5	22.1	461	63.9
Cookies, oatmeal, commercially prepared, special dietary	4.8	18	449	67
Cookies, peanut butter sandwich, special dietary	10	34	535	50.8
Cookies, sugar wafer, with creme filling, sugar free	3.57	28.57	531	51.96
Cookies, sugar, commercially prepared, regular (includes vanilla)	5.35	19.55	464	66.04
Cookies, sugar, refrigerated dough	4	19.48	436	60.32
Cookies, sugar, refrigerated dough, baked	4.7	23.1	489	64.7
Cookies, sugar, prepared from recipe, made with margarine	5.9	23.4	472	58.8
Cookies, sugar wafers with creme filling, regular	3.84	23.24	502	69.04
Cookies, vanilla sandwich with creme filling	4.5	20	483	70.6
Puff pastry, frozen, ready-to-bake, baked	7.4	38.5	558	44.2
Cookies, vanilla wafers, lower fat	5	15.2	441	71.7
Cookies, vanilla wafers, higher fat	4.9	16.41	455	71
Crackers, cheese, regular	10.93	22.74	489	57.12
Crackers, cheese, sandwich-type with peanut butter filling	12.41	25.12	496	53.34
Crackers, crispbread, rye	7.9	1.3	366	65.7
Crackers, matzo, plain	10	1.4	395	80.7
Crackers, matzo, egg	12.3	2.1	391	75.8
Crackers, matzo, whole-wheat	13.1	1.5	351	67.1
Crackers, melba toast, plain	12.1	3.2	390	70.3
Crackers, melba toast, rye (includes pumpernickel)	11.6	3.4	389	69.3
Crackers, melba toast, wheat	12.9	2.3	374	69
Crackers, milk	7.6	13.77	446	68.33
Crackers, rusk toast	13.5	7.2	407	72.3
Crackers, rye, sandwich-type with cheese filling	9.2	22.3	481	57.2
Crackers, rye, wafers, plain	9.6	0.9	334	57.5
Crackers, rye, wafers, seasoned	9	9.2	381	52.9
Crackers, saltines (includes oyster, soda, soup)	9.46	8.64	418	71.25
Crackers, standard snack-type, regular	6.64	26.43	510	59
Crackers, standard snack-type, sandwich, with cheese filling	9.3	21.1	477	59.8
Crackers, standard snack-type, sandwich, with peanut butter filling	11.47	24.54	494	56.08

Food Name ---> per 100 g	Protein (g)	Fat (g)	Calorie	Net Carb (g)
Crackers, wheat, regular	7.3	16.4	455	63.83
Crackers, wheat, sandwich, with cheese filling	9.8	25	497	55.1
Crackers, wheat, sandwich, with peanut butter filling	13.5	26.7	495	49.4
Crackers, whole-wheat	10.58	14.13	427	59.25
Cracker meal	9.3	1.7	383	78.3
Cream puff shell, prepared from recipe	9	25.9	360	22
Croissants, butter	8.2	21	406	43.2
Croissants, apple	7.4	8.7	254	34.6
Croissants, cheese	9.2	20.9	414	44.4
Croutons, plain	11.9	6.6	407	68.4
Croutons, seasoned	10.8	18.3	465	58.5
Danish pastry, cinnamon, enriched	7	22.4	403	43.3
Danish pastry, cheese	8	21.9	374	36.2
Danish pastry, fruit, enriched (includes apple, cinnamon, raisin, lemon, raspberry, strawberry)	5.4	18.5	371	45.9
Danish pastry, nut (includes almond, raisin nut, cinnamon nut)	7.1	25.2	430	43.7
Doughnuts, cake-type, plain (includes unsugared, old-fashioned)	5.31	24.93	434	45.36
Doughnuts, cake-type, plain, chocolate-coated or frosted	4.93	25.25	452	49.43
Doughnuts, cake-type, plain, sugared or glazed	5.2	22.9	426	49.3
Doughnuts, cake-type, chocolate, sugared or glazed	4.5	19.9	417	55.2
Doughnuts, french crullers, glazed	3.1	18.3	412	58.3
Doughnuts, yeast-leavened, with creme filling	6.4	24.5	361	29.2
Doughnuts, yeast-leavened, glazed, enriched (includes honey buns)	6.14	22.7	421	45.83
Doughnuts, yeast-leavened, with jelly filling	5.9	18.7	340	38.1
English muffins, plain, enriched, with ca prop (includes sourdough)	8.87	1.69	227	40.67
English muffins, plain, toasted, enriched, with calcium propionate (includes sourdough)	10.32	2.02	270	49.85
English muffins, mixed-grain (includes granola)	9.1	1.8	235	43.5
English muffins, mixed-grain, toasted (includes granola)	9.9	1.9	255	47.3
English muffins, raisin-cinnamon (includes apple-cinnamon)	7.91	1.8	240	45.5

Food Name ---> per 100 g	Protein (g)	Fat (g)	Calorie	Net Carb (g)
English muffins, raisin-cinnamon, toasted (includes apple-cinnamon)	8.87	2.21	276	52.04
English muffins, wheat	8.7	2	223	40.2
English muffins, wheat, toasted	9.4	2.1	243	43.7
English muffins, whole-wheat	8.8	2.1	203	33.7
English muffins, whole-wheat, toasted	9.6	2.3	221	36.8
French toast, frozen, ready-to-heat	7.4	6.1	213	31
French toast, prepared from recipe, made with low fat (2%) milk	7.7	10.8	229	25
Hush puppies, prepared from recipe	7.7	13.5	337	43.2
Ice cream cones, cake or wafer-type	8.1	6.9	417	76
Ice cream cones, sugar, rolled-type	7.9	3.8	402	82.4
Muffins, plain, prepared from recipe, made with low fat (2%) milk	6.9	11.4	296	38.7
Muffins, blueberry, commercially prepared (Includes mini-muffins)	4.49	16.07	375	51.9
Muffins, blueberry, dry mix	3.48	3.25	293	59.6
Muffins, blueberry, toaster-type	4.6	9.5	313	51.5
Muffins, blueberry, prepared from recipe, made with low fat (2%) milk	6.5	10.8	285	40.7
Muffins, corn, commercially prepared	5.9	8.4	305	47.6
Muffins, corn, dry mix, prepared	7.4	10.2	321	46.7
Muffins, corn, toaster-type	5.3	11.3	346	56.3
Muffins, corn, prepared from recipe, made with low fat (2%) milk	7.1	12.3	316	44.2
Muffins, oat bran	7	7.4	270	43.7
Muffins, wheat bran, dry mix	7.1	12	396	73
Pancakes plain, frozen, ready-to-heat (includes buttermilk)	5.23	6.83	233	36.75
Pancakes, plain, dry mix, complete (includes buttermilk)	9.77	3.1	368	70.75
Pancakes, plain, dry mix, complete, prepared	5.2	2.5	194	35.4
Pancakes, plain, dry mix, incomplete (includes buttermilk)	10	1.7	355	68.2
Pancakes, plain, dry mix, incomplete, prepared	7.8	7.7	218	27
Pancakes, plain, prepared from recipe	6.4	9.7	227	28.3
Pancakes, blueberry, prepared from recipe	6.1	9.2	222	29
Pancakes, buckwheat, dry mix, incomplete	10.9	2.7	340	62.8

Food Name ---> per 100 g	Protein (g)	Fat (g)	Calorie	Net Carb (g)
Pancakes, special dietary, dry mix	8.9	1.4	349	73.9
Pancakes, whole-wheat, dry mix, incomplete	12.8	1.5	344	71
Pancakes, whole-wheat, dry mix, incomplete, prepared	8.5	6.5	208	26.6
Pie, apple, commercially prepared, enriched flour	1.9	11	237	32.4
Pie, apple, prepared from recipe	2.4	12.5	265	37.1
Pie, banana cream, prepared from mix, no-bake type	3.4	12.9	251	31
Pie, banana cream, prepared from recipe	4.4	13.6	269	32.2
Pie, blueberry, commercially prepared	1.8	10	232	33.9
Pie, blueberry, prepared from recipe	2.7	11.9	245	33.5
Pie, cherry, commercially prepared	2	11	260	39
Pie, cherry, prepared from recipe	2.8	12.2	270	38.5
Pie, chocolate creme, commercially prepared	4.15	22.41	353	37.64
Pie, chocolate mousse, prepared from mix, no-bake type	3.5	15.4	260	29.6
Pie, coconut creme, commercially prepared	2.1	16.6	298	36
Pie, coconut cream, prepared from mix, no-bake type	2.8	17.6	276	28
Pie, coconut custard, commercially prepared	5.9	13.2	260	28.4
Pie, egg custard, commercially prepared	5.5	11.6	210	19.2
Pie, fried pies, fruit	3	16.1	316	40
Pie, lemon meringue, commercially prepared	1.5	8.7	268	46
Pie, lemon meringue, prepared from recipe	3.8	12.9	285	39.1
Pie, mince, prepared from recipe	2.6	10.8	289	45.4
Pie, peach	1.9	10	224	32.1
Pie, pecan, commercially prepared	4.5	16.69	407	57.51
Pie, pecan, prepared from recipe	4.9	22.2	412	52.2
Pie, pumpkin, commercially prepared	3.9	9.75	243	33.03
Pie, pumpkin, prepared from recipe	4.5	9.3	204	26.4
Pie, vanilla cream, prepared from recipe	4.8	14.4	278	32
Pie crust, standard-type, dry mix	6.9	31.4	518	52.1
Pie crust, standard-type, dry mix, prepared, baked	6.7	30.4	501	48.6
Pie crust, standard-type, frozen, ready-to-bake, enriched	6.16	26.07	457	46.12
Pie crust, standard-type, frozen, ready-to-bake, enriched, baked	6.5	28.59	508	52.94

Food Name ---> per 100 g	Protein (g)	Fat (g)	Calorie	Net Carb (g)
Pie crust, standard-type, prepared from recipe, baked	6.4	34.6	527	45.8
Puff pastry, frozen, ready-to-bake	7.3	38.1	551	43.6
Phyllo dough	7.1	6	299	50.7
Popovers, dry mix, enriched	10.4	4.3	371	71
Rolls, dinner, plain, commercially prepared (includes brown-and-serve)	10.86	6.47	310	50.04
Rolls, dinner, egg	9.5	6.4	307	48.3
Rolls, dinner, oat bran	9.5	4.6	236	36.1
Rolls, dinner, rye	10.3	3.4	286	48.2
Rolls, dinner, wheat	8.6	6.3	273	42.2
Rolls, dinner, whole-wheat	8.7	4.7	266	43.6
Rolls, french	8.6	4.3	277	47
Rolls, hamburger or hotdog, plain	9.77	3.91	279	48.32
Rolls, hamburger or hotdog, mixed-grain	9.6	6	263	40.8
Rolls, hamburger or hotdog, reduced-calorie	8.3	2	196	35.9
Rolls, hard (includes kaiser)	9.9	4.3	293	50.4
Strudel, apple	3.3	11.2	274	38.9
Sweet rolls, cheese	7.1	18.3	360	42.5
Sweet rolls, cinnamon, commercially prepared with raisins	6.2	16.4	372	48.5
Sweet rolls, cinnamon, refrigerated dough with frosting	5	12.2	333	51.6
Sweet rolls, cinnamon, refrigerated dough with frosting, baked	5.4	13.2	362	56.1
Taco shells, baked	6.41	21.79	476	56.79
Toaster pastries, brown-sugar-cinnamon	4.06	7.98	370	70.34
Toaster pastries, fruit (includes apple, blueberry, cherry, strawberry)	4.2	9.95	388	69.32
Tortillas, ready-to-bake or -fry, corn	5.7	2.85	218	38.34
Tortillas, ready-to-bake or -fry, flour, refrigerated	8.2	7.99	306	45.88
Waffles, plain, frozen, ready-to-heat	6.47	9.7	285	40.78
Waffles, plain, prepared from recipe	7.9	14.1	291	32.9
Wonton wrappers (includes egg roll wrappers)	9.8	1.5	291	56.1
Leavening agents, baking powder, double-acting, sodium aluminum sulfate	0	0	53	27.5

Food Name ---> per 100 g	Protein (g)	Fat (g)	Calorie	Net Carb (g)
Leavening agents, baking powder, double-acting, straight phosphate	0.1	0	51	23.9
Leavening agents, baking powder, low-sodium	0.1	0.4	97	44.7
Leavening agents, baking soda	0	0	0	0
Leavening agents, cream of tartar	0	0	258	61.3
Leavening agents, yeast, baker's, compressed	8.4	1.9	105	10
Leavening agents, yeast, baker's, active dry	40.44	7.61	325	14.32
Bread crumbs, dry, grated, seasoned	14.13	5.48	383	63.59
Cookies, oatmeal, prepared from recipe, without raisins	6.8	17.9	447	66.4
Cookies, chocolate chip, prepared from recipe, made with butter	5.7	28.4	488	58.2
Bread, protein, (includes gluten), toasted	13.2	2.4	270	44.8
Bread, rice bran, toasted	9.7	5	264	42
Bread, wheat germ, toasted	10.7	3.3	293	52
Muffins, blueberry, toaster-type, toasted	4.9	10.1	333	54.8
Muffins, wheat bran, toaster-type with raisins, toasted	5.5	9.4	313	47.3
Pancakes, buttermilk, prepared from recipe	6.8	9.3	227	28.7
Rolls, dinner, plain, prepared from recipe, made with low fat (2%) milk	8.5	7.3	316	51.5
Pie crust, cookie-type, prepared from recipe, graham cracker, chilled	4.1	24.4	484	62.4
Crackers, matzo, egg and onion	10	3.9	391	72.1
Pie crust, cookie-type, prepared from recipe, vanilla wafer, chilled	3.7	36.2	531	50.1
Pie crust, standard-type, prepared from recipe, unbaked	5.7	30.8	469	38.9
Waffles, plain, frozen, ready -to-heat, toasted	7.19	9.61	312	46.89
Bagels, plain, enriched, without calcium propionate (includes onion, poppy, sesame)	10.5	1.6	275	51.1
Bagels, plain, unenriched, with calcium propionate (includes onion, poppy, sesame)	10.5	1.6	275	51.1
Bagels, plain, unenriched, without calcium propionate(includes onion, poppy, sesame)	10.5	1.6	275	51.1
Bread, cornbread, dry mix, unenriched (includes corn muffin mix)	7	12.2	418	63
Bread, pita, white, unenriched	9.1	1.2	275	53.5
Bread, raisin, unenriched	7.9	4.4	274	48

Food Name ---> per 100 g	Protein (g)	Fat (g)	Calorie	Net Carb (g)
Bread, white, commercially prepared, low sodium, no salt	8.2	3.6	267	47.3
Coffeecake, cinnamon with crumb topping, commercially prepared, unenriched	6.8	23.3	418	44.7
Cake, pound, commercially prepared, other than all butter, unenriched	5.2	17.9	389	51.5
Cake, pudding-type, white, unenriched, dry mix	3.9	9.5	423	80.3
Cake, yellow, unenriched, dry mix	4.4	11.6	432	77
Cookies, butter, commercially prepared, unenriched	6.1	18.8	467	68.1
Cookies, chocolate chip, commercially prepared, regular, higher fat, unenriched	5.4	22.6	481	64.3
Cookies, ladyfingers, without lemon juice and rind	10.6	9.1	363	58.7
Crackers, melba toast, plain, without salt	12.1	3.2	390	70.3
Crackers, saltines, low salt (includes oyster, soda, soup)	9.5	8.85	421	71.44
Crackers, saltines, unsalted tops (includes oyster, soda, soup)	9.2	11.8	434	68.5
Crackers, standard snack-type, regular, low salt	7.4	25.3	502	59.4
Crackers, wheat, low salt	8.6	20.6	473	60.4
Crackers, whole-wheat, low salt	8.8	17.2	443	58.1
Danish pastry, cinnamon, unenriched	7	22.4	403	43.4
Danish pastry, fruit, unenriched (includes apple, cinnamon, raisin, strawberry)	5.4	18.5	371	45.9
Bread, white, commercially prepared, toasted, low sodium no salt	9	4	293	54.4
Danish pastry, lemon, unenriched	5.4	18.5	371	45.9
Crackers, cheese, low sodium	10.1	25.3	503	55.8
Danish pastry, raspberry, unenriched	5.4	18.5	371	45.9
Doughnuts, yeast-leavened, glazed, unenriched (includes honey buns)	6.4	22.8	403	43.1
English muffins, plain, enriched, without calcium propionate(includes sourdough)	7.7	1.8	235	43.3
English muffins, plain, unenriched, with calcium propionate (includes sourdough)	7.7	1.8	235	43.3
English muffins, plain, unenriched, without calcium propionate (includes sourdough)	7.7	1.8	235	43.3
Pie, apple, commercially prepared, unenriched flour	1.9	11	237	32.4
Pie, fried pies, cherry	3	16.1	316	40

Food Name ---> per 100 g	Protein (g)	Fat (g)	Calorie	Net Carb (g)
Pie, fried pies, lemon	3	16.1	316	40
Pie crust, standard-type, frozen, ready-to-bake, unenriched	3.9	29.2	457	43.2
Popovers, dry mix, unenriched	10.4	4.3	371	71
Taco shells, baked, without added salt	7.2	22.6	468	54.9
Tortillas, ready-to-bake or -fry, corn, without added salt	5.7	2.5	222	41.4
Tortillas, ready-to-bake or -fry, flour, without added calcium	8.7	7.1	325	52.3
Cake, pound, commercially prepared, fat-free	5.4	1.2	283	59.9
Cake, yellow, light, dry mix	4.7	5.5	404	82.8
Crackers, saltines, fat-free, low-sodium	10.5	1.6	393	79.6
Breakfast tart, low fat	3.99	5.99	372	75.3
Toaster Pastries, KELLOGG, KELLOGG'S POP TARTS, Blueberry	4.6	13.3	412	67.31
Toaster Pastries, KELLOGG, KELLOGG'S POP TARTS, Frosted blueberry	4.6	10	391	70.67
Toaster Pastries, KELLOGG, KELLOGG'S POP TARTS, Brown sugar cinnamon	5.4	18.4	438	62.9
Toaster Pastries, KELLOGG, KELLOGG'S POP TARTS, Frosted brown sugar cinnamon	4.6	13.8	417	67.6
Toaster Pastries, KELLOGG, KELLOGG'S POP TARTS, Frosted cherry	4.2	10.2	397	71
Toaster Pastries, KELLOGG, KELLOGG'S POP TARTS, Frosted chocolate fudge	4.9	9.3	384	68.3
Toaster Pastries, KELLOGG, KELLOGG'S POP TARTS, Frosted raspberry	4.2	10.6	399	70.62
Toaster Pastries, KELLOGG, KELLOGG'S POP TARTS, S'mores	6.2	10.5	392	68.2
Toaster Pastries, KELLOGG, KELLOGG'S POP TARTS, Strawberry	4.7	10.5	398	70
Toaster Pastries, KELLOGG, KELLOGG'S POP TARTS, Frosted strawberry	4.1	9.8	390	70.4
Toaster Pastries, KELLOGG, KELLOGG'S POP TARTS, Frosted wild berry	4	9.5	390	71.1
Toaster Pastries, KELLOGG, KELLOGG'S LOW FAT POP TARTS, Frosted brown sugar cinnamon	4.7	5.9	366	68.2
Toaster Pastries, KELLOGG, KELLOGG'S LOW FAT POP TARTS, Frosted strawberry	4.2	5.4	363	68.8
KELLOGG, KELLOGG'S EGGO, Buttermilk Pancake	5.3	8	245	37.6

Food Name ---> per 100 g	Protein (g)	Fat (g)	Calorie	Net Carb (g)
KELLOGG, KELLOG'S NUTRI-GRAIN CEREAL BARS, Mixed Berry	4.3	7.6	370	70.9
KELLOGG'S, EGGO, Waffles, Homestyle, Low Fat	6.3	3.5	229	43.6
KELLOGG'S, EGGO, NUTRI-GRAIN, Waffles, Low Fat	6.5	3.5	201	35
KELLOGG'S EGGO Lowfat Blueberry Nutri-Grain Waffles	5.95	2.83	208	39.21
ARCHWAY Home Style Cookies, Sugar Free Oatmeal	5.54	20.92	442	65.3
ARCHWAY Home Style Cookies, Chocolate Chip Ice Box	4.28	24.4	497	63.02
ARCHWAY Home Style Cookies, Coconut Macaroon	3.02	22.55	460	56.13
ARCHWAY Home Style Cookies, Date Filled Oatmeal	4.67	12.05	400	66.06
ARCHWAY Home Style Cookies, Dutch Cocoa	4.5	14.99	431	66.84
ARCHWAY Home Style Cookies, Frosty Lemon	4.41	17.11	430	64.08
ARCHWAY Home Style Cookies, Iced Molasses	3.5	14.43	420	68.12
ARCHWAY Home Style Cookies, Iced Oatmeal	4.89	16.53	435	64.76
ARCHWAY Home Style Cookies, Molasses	4.25	12.06	403	68.21
ARCHWAY Home Style Cookies, Oatmeal	5.48	14.08	421	65.27
ARCHWAY Home Style Cookies, Oatmeal Raisin	5.17	12.08	406	66.57
ARCHWAY Home Style Cookies, Old Fashioned Molasses	4.27	11.83	406	69.45
ARCHWAY Home Style Cookies, Old Fashioned Windmill Cookies	5.17	17.55	468	70.43
ARCHWAY Home Style Cookies, Peanut Butter	9	24.28	480	55.68
ARCHWAY Home Style Cookies, Raspberry Filled	4.35	13.26	400	63.72
ARCHWAY Home Style Cookies, Strawberry Filled	4.35	13.26	400	63.72
ARCHWAY Home Style Cookies, Reduced Fat Ginger Snaps	4.67	11.14	424	75.13
Artificial Blueberry Muffin Mix, dry	4.7	8.7	407	77.45
KRAFT, STOVE TOP Stuffing Mix Chicken Flavor	12.6	4.1	381	70.6
GEORGE WESTON BAKERIES, Brownberry Sage and Onion Stuffing Mix, dry	13.3	5.1	390	67.3
KEEBLER, KEEBLER Chocolate Graham SELECTS	7.1	16.6	465	71.8
KEEBLER, Vanilla Wafers	4	17.4	462	71.7
CONTINENTAL MILLS, KRUSTEAZ Almond Poppyseed Muffin Mix, Artificially Flavored, dry	5.6	10.3	418	73.9
MCKEE BAKING, LITTLE DEBBIE NUTTY BARS, Wafers with Peanut Butter, Chocolate Covered	8	32.8	548	55.2

Food Name ---> per 100 g	Protein (g)	Fat (g)	Calorie	Net Carb (g)
MARTHA WHITE FOODS, Martha White's Chewy Fudge Brownie Mix, dry	4.42	6.16	407	80.68
MARTHA WHITE FOODS, Martha White's Buttermilk Biscuit Mix, dry	7.81	13.23	388	57.91
MISSION FOODS, MISSION Flour Tortillas, Soft Taco, 8 inch	8.7	6	287	49.6
NABISCO, NABISCO GRAHAMS Crackers	6.99	10	424	72.8
NABISCO, NABISCO OREO CRUNCHIES, Cookie Crumb Topping	4.78	21.5	476	67.03
NABISCO, NABISCO RITZ Crackers	7.23	23.21	492	61.21
PILLSBURY, Buttermilk Biscuits, Artificial Flavor, refrigerated dough	6.4	2.79	236	45.47
PILLSBURY, Chocolate Chip Cookies, refrigerated dough	3.82	21.26	450	59.05
PILLSBURY, Crusty French Loaf, refrigerated dough	8.59	2.88	243	43.75
PILLSBURY, Traditional Fudge Brownie Mix, dry	4.8	12.1	441	78.3
PILLSBURY GRANDS, Buttermilk Biscuits, refrigerated dough	6.16	11.34	293	40.91
PILLSBURY Golden Layer Buttermilk Biscuits, Artificial Flavor, refrigerated dough	5.88	13.24	307	39.98
PILLSBURY, Cinnamon Rolls with Icing, refrigerated dough	4.34	11.27	330	52.02
KRAFT FOODS, SHAKE 'N' BAKE ORIGINAL RECIPE, Coating for Pork, dry	6.1	3.7	377	79.8
GEORGE WESTON BAKERIES, Thomas English Muffins	8	1.8	232	46
HEINZ, WEIGHT WATCHER, Chocolate Eclair, frozen	4.4	6.9	241	38.2
INTERSTATE BRANDS CORP, WONDER Hamburger Rolls	8.07	4.15	273	48.24
GENERAL MILLS, BETTY CROCKER SUPERMOIST Yellow Cake Mix, dry	3.8	8.1	413	81.3
NABISCO, NABISCO SNACKWELL'S Fat Free Devil's Food Cookie Cakes	5	1.09	305	72.65
Crackers, cheese, sandwich-type with cheese filling	8.92	24.41	490	56.86
USDA Commodity, Bakery, Flour Mix	8.47	12.9	400	55.43
USDA Commodity, Bakery, Flour Mix Low-fat	9.07	4.7	361	67.09
Waffles, buttermilk, frozen, ready-to-heat	6.58	9.22	273	38.85
Waffle, buttermilk, frozen, ready-to-heat, toasted	7.42	9.49	309	45.79
Waffle, buttermilk, frozen, ready-to-heat, microwaved	6.92	9.4	289	41.76
Waffle, plain, frozen, ready-to-heat, microwave	6.71	9.91	298	43.01

Food Name ---> per 100 g	Protein (g)	Fat (g)	Calorie	Net Carb (g)
Pancakes, plain, frozen, ready-to-heat, microwave (includes buttermilk)	5.88	4.73	239	40.83
Toaster Pastries, fruit, frosted (include apples, blueberry, cherry, strawberry)	4.01	9.02	385	70.03
Toaster pastries, fruit, toasted (include apple, blueberry, cherry, strawberry)	4.7	11.03	409	71.7
Muffin, blueberry, commercially prepared, low-fat	4.23	4.22	255	45.85
Pie Crust, Cookie-type, Graham Cracker, Ready Crust	5.1	24.83	501	62.4
Pie Crust, Cookie-type, Chocolate, Ready Crust	6.08	22.42	484	61.78
Pie, Dutch Apple, Commercially Prepared	2.17	11.5	290	42.94
Pie crust, deep dish, frozen, unbaked, made with enriched flour	5.52	28.74	468	45.39
Pie crust, refrigerated, regular, baked	3.41	28.69	506	57.12
Pie crust, deep dish, frozen, baked, made with enriched flour	6.1	31.84	521	50.17
Pie crust, refrigerated, regular, unbaked	2.97	25.46	445	49.31
Crackers, whole-wheat, reduced fat	11.34	7.59	416	64.62
Crackers, wheat, reduced fat	9.34	13.37	444	68.12
Waffles, chocolate chip, frozen, ready-to-heat	5.8	10.1	297	44.18
Tostada shells, corn	6.15	23.38	474	58.63
Bread, salvadoran sweet cheese (quesadilla salvadorena)	7.12	17.12	374	47.14
Bread, pound cake type, pan de torta salvadoran	7.06	17.45	390	49.59
Bread, pan dulce, sweet yeast bread	9.42	11.58	367	54.08
Keikitos (muffins), Latino bakery item	6.81	25.24	467	51.96
Cake, pound, BIMBO Bakeries USA, Panque Casero, home baked style	6.62	21.7	418	47.94
Pan Dulce, LA RICURA, Salpora de Arroz con Azucar, cookie-like, contains wheat flour and rice flour	8.81	16.11	445	65.08
Pastry, Pastelitos de Guava (guava pastries)	5.48	18.5	379	45.56
Crackers, snack, GOYA CRACKERS	14.25	13.35	433	60.55
Crackers, cream, GAMESA SABROSAS	7.01	20.37	484	62.15
Crackers, cream, LA MODERNA RIKIS CREAM CRACKERS	7.19	19.5	464	62.48
Garlic bread, frozen	8.36	16.61	350	39.22
Cinnamon buns, frosted (includes honey buns)	4.45	26.61	452	47.4
Crackers, cheese, reduced fat	10	11.67	418	64.89

Food Name ---> per 100 g	Protein (g)	Fat (g)	Calorie	Net Carb (g)
Crackers, saltines, whole wheat (includes multi-grain)	7.14	10.71	398	61.55
Bread, white wheat	10.66	2.15	238	34.71
Bagels, wheat	10.2	1.53	250	44.79
Cream puff, eclair, custard or cream filled, iced	4.41	18.52	334	36.53
Tortillas, ready-to-bake or -fry, flour, shelf stable	8.01	7.58	297	46.87
Bread, potato	12.5	3.13	266	40.77
Bread, cheese	10.42	20.83	408	42.73
Focaccia, Italian flatbread, plain	8.77	7.89	249	34.02
KASHI, TLC, Honey Sesame Crackers	8.7	10.4	398	66.4
KASHI, TLC, Original 7-Grain Crackers	13.9	11.9	385	54.2
KASHI, TLC, Country Cheddar Crackers	9.8	15.5	445	65.5
KASHI, TLC, Toasted Asiago Crackers	12.7	13.8	420	56.8
KASHI, Blueberry Waffle	5.7	7.1	192	25.6
KASHI, H2H Woven Wheat Cracker, Original	10.6	11.6	396	61.2
KASHI, Original Waffle	6	7.4	197	26.1
KASHI, TLC, Fire Roasted Vegetable Crackers	12	12.2	389	55.9
KASHI, H2H Woven Wheat Cracker, Roasted Garlic	10.5	11.7	440	61
AUSTIN, Cheddar Cheese on Wheat Crackers, sandwich-type	7.9	24.5	495	59.6
AUSTIN, Cheddar Cheese on Cheese Crackers, sandwich-type	7.5	24.9	494	58.7
AUSTIN, Chocolatey Peanut Butter Crackers, sandwich-type	7.7	20.8	479	64.2
AUSTIN, Grilled Cheese on Wafer Crackers, sandwich-type	7.9	23.8	493	60.7
AUSTIN, Cheddar Cheese on Cheese Crackers, sandwich-type, reduced fat	7.8	17.5	461	66.6
AUSTIN, Peanut Butter on Cheese Crackers, sandwich-type, reduced fat	9.7	17.9	461	63.6
AUSTIN, Peanut Butter on Toasty Crackers, sandwich-type, reduced fat	9.5	18	463	64.5
AUSTIN, PB & J Crackers, sandwich-type	7.6	21.7	484	63.7
BARBARA DEE, Winter Mints Cookies	3.9	26	515	65.1
KELLOGG'S, BEANATURAL, Original 3-Bean Chips	22.9	25.3	487	32.3
BEAR NAKED, Double Chocolate Cookies	6.6	16.9	423	59.9
BEAR NAKED, Fruit & Nut Cookies	7.5	21.4	443	54.5

Food Name ---> per 100 g	Protein (g)	Fat (g)	Calorie	Net Carb (g)
KELLOGG'S, EGGO, Biscuit Scramblers, Bacon, Egg & Cheese	8.8	7.9	258	36.2
KELLOGG'S, EGGO, Biscuit Scramblers, Egg & Cheese	8.8	7.6	254	36
KELLOGG'S, EGGO, French Toaster Sticks, Cinnamon	4.8	6.9	250	41.6
KELLOGG'S, EGGO, French Toaster Sticks, Original	5.3	7	239	38.5
KELLOGG'S, EGGO, Mini Muffin Tops, Blueberry	5	10.2	293	44.8
Rolls, pumpernickel	10.8	2.8	276	46.47

Beverages

Food Name ---> per 100 g	Protein (g)	Fat (g)	Calories	Net Carb (g)
Alcoholic beverage, beer, regular, all	0.46	0	43	3.55
Alcoholic beverage, beer, regular, BUDWEISER	0.36	0	41	2.97
Alcoholic beverage, beer, light, BUDWEISER SELECT	0.2	0	28	0.87
Alcoholic beverage, beer, light	0.24	0	29	1.64
Alcoholic beverage, beer, light, BUD LIGHT	0.25	0	29	1.3
Alcoholic beverage, daiquiri, canned	0	0	125	15.7
Alcoholic beverage, daiquiri, prepared-from-recipe	0.06	0.06	186	6.84
Alcoholic beverage, beer, light, low carb	0.17	0	27	0.73
Alcoholic beverage, pina colada, canned	0.6	7.6	237	27.5
Beverages, almond milk, sweetened, vanilla flavor, ready-to-drink	0.42	1.04	38	6.19
Alcoholic beverage, pina colada, prepared-from-recipe	0.42	1.88	174	22.36
Alcoholic beverage, tequila sunrise, canned	0.3	0.1	110	11.3
Beverages, Energy drink, Citrus	0	0	45	11.27
Beverages, MONSTER energy drink, low carb	0	0	5	1.38
Beverages, Whiskey sour mix, powder	0.6	0.1	383	97.3
Alcoholic beverage, whiskey sour, prepared with water, whiskey and powder mix	0.1	0.02	164	15.85
Beverages, THE COCA-COLA COMPANY, NOS Zero, energy drink, sugar-free with guarana, fortified with vitamins B6 and B12	0	0	4	1.03
Alcoholic beverage, whiskey sour, canned	0	0	119	13.3
Beverages, Whiskey sour mix, bottled	0.1	0.1	87	21.4
Alcoholic beverage, whiskey sour, prepared from item 14028	0.06	0.06	153	12.82
Beverages, THE COCA-COLA COMPANY, NOS energy drink, Original, grape, loaded cherry, charged citrus, fortified with vitamins B6 and B12	0	0	44	11.25
Beverages, water, bottled, yumberry, pomegranate with anti-oxidants, zero calories	0	0	5	1.25

Food Name ---> per 100 g	Protein (g)	Fat (g)	Calories	Net Carb (g)
Beverages, ABBOTT, EAS whey protein powder	66.67	5.13	385	17.95
Alcoholic beverage, creme de menthe, 72 proof	0	0.3	371	41.6
Beverages, ABBOTT, EAS soy protein powder	47.62	3.57	405	43.94
Beverages, CYTOSPORT, Muscle Milk, ready-to-drink	5.87	2.01	49	1.86
Alcoholic beverage, distilled, all (gin, rum, vodka, whiskey) 80 proof	0	0	231	0
Beverages, OCEAN SPRAY, Cran-Energy, Cranberry Energy Juice Drink	0	0	15	3.75
Beverages, NESTLE, Boost plus, nutritional drink, ready-to-drink	5.38	5.38	138	16.09
Beverages, SLIMFAST, Meal replacement, High Protein Shake, Ready-To-Drink, 3-2-1 plan	6.59	2.88	58	0.45
Beverages, UNILEVER, SLIMFAST, meal replacement, regular, ready-to-drink, 3-2-1 Plan	3.32	1.93	57	6.14
Beverages, UNILEVER, SLIMFAST Shake Mix, powder, 3-2-1 Plan	8.13	13.34	448	55.82
Beverages, FUZE, orange mango, fortified with vitamins A, C, E, B6	0.68	0.06	38	9
Alcoholic beverage, distilled, gin, 90 proof	0	0	263	0
Alcoholic beverage, distilled, rum, 80 proof	0	0	231	0
Alcoholic beverage, distilled, vodka, 80 proof	0	0	231	0
Alcoholic beverage, distilled, whiskey, 86 proof	0	0	250	0.1
Beverages, almond milk, chocolate, ready-to-drink	0.63	1.25	50	8.98
Beverages, UNILEVER, SLIMFAST Shake Mix, high protein, whey powder, 3-2-1 Plan,	27.87	11.62	368	31.8
Beverages, Acai berry drink, fortified	0.83	0.83	62	11.63
Alcoholic beverage, wine, dessert, sweet	0.2	0	160	13.69
Beverages, Whey protein powder isolate	58.14	1.16	359	29.07
Beverages, KELLOGG'S, SPECIAL K Protein Shake	3.2	1.6	64	7.5
Beverages, Energy Drink with carbonated water and high fructose corn syrup	0.42	0	62	15
Beverages, Energy Drink, sugar free	0.42	0	4	0.42
Beverages, ABBOTT, ENSURE, Nutritional Shake, Ready-to-Drink	3.8	2.53	105	16.88
Beverages, chocolate powder, no sugar added	9.09	9.09	373	54.54
Beverages, Orange juice, light, No pulp	0.21	0	21	5.42
Beverages, The COCA-COLA company, Hi-C Flashin' Fruit Punch	0	0	45	12.5

Food Name ---> per 100 g	Protein (g)	Fat (g)	Calories	Net Carb (g)
Beverages, Protein powder whey based	78.13	1.56	352	3.15
Beverages, Protein powder soy based	55.56	5.56	388	22.19
Beverages, KELLOGG'S SPECIAL K20 protein powder	35.2	0.6	380	20.9
Beverages, ZEVIA, cola	0	0	0	1.13
Beverages, ZEVIA, cola, caffeine free	0	0	0	1.13
Beverages, GEROLSTEINER BRUNNEN GmbH & Co. KG,Gerolsteiner naturally sparkling mineral water,	0	0	0	0
Beverages, ICELANDIC, Glacial Natural spring water	0	0	0	0
Beverages, yellow green colored citrus soft drink with caffeine	0	0	49	12.83
Beverages, rich chocolate, powder	0	0	372	92.96
Beverages, GEROLSTEINER BRUNNEN GmbH & Co. KG (Gerolsteiner), naturally sparkling, mineral bottled water	0	0	0	0
Beverages, chocolate malt, powder, prepared with fat free milk	3.25	0.17	49	8.64
Alcoholic beverage, wine, table, all	0.07	0	83	2.72
Beverages, V8 SPLASH Smoothies, Peach Mango	1.22	0	37	7.76
Beverages, V8 SPLASH Smoothies, Strawberry Banana	1.22	0	37	8.16
Beverages, V8 SPLASH Smoothies, Tropical Colada	1.22	0	41	8.14
Beverages, Coconut water, ready-to-drink, unsweetened	0.22	0	18	4.24
Beverages, almond milk, unsweetened, shelf stable	0.59	1.1	15	0.58
Beverages, chocolate almond milk, unsweetened, shelf-stable, fortified with vitamin D2 and E	0.83	1.46	21	0.85
Beverages, The COCA-COLA company, Glaceau Vitamin Water, Revive Fruit Punch, fortified	0	0	0	0
Beverages, MINUTE MAID, Lemonada, Limeade	0	0	50	13.75
Alcoholic beverage, wine, table, red	0.07	0	85	2.61
Alcoholic Beverage, wine, table, red, Cabernet Sauvignon	0.07	0	83	2.6
Alcoholic Beverage, wine, table, red, Cabernet Franc	0.07	0	83	2.45
Alcoholic Beverage, wine, table, red, Pinot Noir	0.07	0	82	2.31
Alcoholic Beverage, wine, table, red, Syrah	0.07	0	83	2.58
Alcoholic Beverage, wine, table, red, Barbera	0.07	0	85	2.79
Alcoholic Beverage, wine, table, red, Zinfandel	0.07	0	88	2.86
Alcoholic Beverage, wine, table, red, Petite Sirah	0.07	0	85	2.68
Alcoholic Beverage, wine, table, red, Claret	0.07	0	83	3.01

Food Name ---> per 100 g	Protein (g)	Fat (g)	Calories	Net Carb (g)
Alcoholic beverage, wine, table, white	0.07	0	82	2.6
Alcoholic Beverage, wine, table, red, Lemberger	0.07	0	80	2.46
Alcoholic Beverage, wine, table, red, Sangiovese	0.07	0	86	2.62
Alcoholic Beverage, wine, table, red, Carignane	0.07	0	74	2.4
Alcoholic beverage, wine, table, white, Pinot Gris (Grigio)	0.07	0	83	2.06
Alcoholic beverage, wine, table, white, Chenin Blanc	0.07	0	80	3.31
Alcoholic beverage, wine, table, white, Fume Blanc	0.07	0	82	2.27
Beverages, Mixed vegetable and fruit juice drink, with added nutrients	0.04	0.01	29	7.47
Alcoholic beverage, wine, table, white, Muller Thurgau	0.07	0	76	3.48
Beverages, carbonated, club soda	0	0	0	0
Alcoholic beverage, wine, table, white, Gewurztraminer	0.07	0	81	2.6
Alcoholic beverage, wine, table, white, late harvest, Gewurztraminer	0.07	0	108	11.39
Alcoholic beverage, wine, table, white, Semillon	0.07	0	82	3.12
Carbonated beverage, cream soda	0	0	51	13.3
Alcoholic beverage, wine, table, white, Riesling	0.07	0	80	3.74
Alcoholic beverage, wine, table, white, Sauvignon Blanc	0.07	0	81	2.05
Alcoholic beverage, wine, table, white, late harvest	0.07	0	112	13.39
Beverages, carbonated, ginger ale	0	0	34	8.76
Beverages, NESTEA, tea, black, ready-to-drink, lemon	0	0	36	9.09
Alcoholic beverage, wine, table, white, Pinot Blanc	0.07	0	81	1.94
Alcoholic beverage, wine, table, white, Muscat	0.07	0	82	5.23
Beverages, carbonated, grape soda	0	0	43	11.2
Beverages, carbonated, low calorie, other than cola or pepper, without caffeine	0.1	0	0	0
Beverages, carbonated, lemon-lime soda, no caffeine	0.09	0	41	10.42
Beverages, carbonated, SPRITE, lemon-lime, without caffeine	0.05	0.02	40	10.14
Beverages, carbonated, low calorie, cola or pepper-type, with aspartame, without caffeine	0.12	0	1	0.12
Beverages, carbonated, cola, without caffeine	0	0	41	10.58
Beverages, carbonated, cola, regular	0	0.25	42	10.36

Food Name ---> per 100 g	Protein (g)	Fat (g)	Calories	Net Carb (g)
Beverages, carbonated, reduced sugar, cola, contains caffeine and sweeteners	0	0	20	5.16
Beverages, carbonated, orange	0	0	48	12.3
Beverages, carbonated, low calorie, other than cola or pepper, with aspartame, contains caffeine	0.1	0	0	0
Alcoholic Beverage, wine, table, red, Burgundy	0.07	0	86	3.69
Beverages, carbonated, pepper-type, contains caffeine	0	0.1	41	10.4
Beverages, Energy drink, RED BULL	0.46	0	43	10.23
Beverages, carbonated, tonic water	0	0	34	8.8
Beverages, Energy drink, RED BULL, sugar free, with added caffeine, niacin, pantothenic acid, vitamins B6 and B12	0.25	0.08	5	0.7
Beverages, carbonated, root beer	0	0	41	10.6
Alcoholic Beverage, wine, table, red, Gamay	0.07	0	78	2.38
Alcoholic Beverage, wine, table, red, Mouvedre	0.07	0	88	2.64
Alcoholic beverage, wine, table, white, Chardonnay	0.07	0	84	2.16
Beverages, Kiwi Strawberry Juice Drink	0	0	47	12.26
Beverages, Apple juice drink, light, fortified with vitamin C	0	0.1	22	5.1
Beverages, chocolate drink, milk and soy based, ready to drink, fortified	4.22	1.69	101	16
Beverages, chocolate malt powder, prepared with 1% milk, fortified	3.32	0.97	57	8.81
Beverages, carbonated, limeade, high caffeine	0	0.11	18	4.16
Beverages, carbonated, low calorie, cola or pepper-types, with sodium saccharin, contains caffeine	0	0	0	0.1
Beverages, POWERADE, Zero, Mixed Berry	0	0	0	0.14
Beverages, Carob-flavor beverage mix, powder	1.8	0.2	372	85.3
Beverages, Carob-flavor beverage mix, powder, prepared with whole milk	3.16	3.11	75	8.28
Beverages, coconut milk, sweetened, fortified with calcium, vitamins A, B12, D2	0.21	2.08	31	2.92
Beverages, coffee, ready to drink, vanilla, light, milk based, sweetened	2.14	1.07	36	4.27
Beverages, Lemonade fruit juice drink light, fortified with vitamin E and C	0	0	21	5

Food Name ---> per 100 g	Protein (g)	Fat (g)	Calories	Net Carb (g)
Beverages, chocolate-flavor beverage mix, powder, prepared with whole milk	3.23	3.24	85	11.51
Beverages, coffee, ready to drink, milk based, sweetened	1.98	1.38	71	12.6
Beverages, coffee, brewed, breakfast blend	0.3	0	2	0.23
Beverages, chocolate syrup	2.1	1.13	279	62.5
Beverages, chocolate syrup, prepared with whole milk	3.07	2.96	90	12.48
Beverages, coffee, ready to drink, iced, mocha, milk based	1.48	0.98	60	11.42
Beverages, tea, Oolong, brewed	0	0	1	0.15
Beverages, Clam and tomato juice, canned	0.6	0.2	48	10.55
Beverages, tea, green, ready to drink, ginseng and honey, sweetened	0	0.18	30	7.16
Beverages, The COCA-COLA company, Minute Maid, Lemonade	0	0	46	12.08
Beverages, tea, green, ready-to-drink, diet	0	0	0	0
Beverages, tea, green, ready-to-drink, citrus, diet, fortified with vitamin C	0	0	1	0.31
Beverages, Cocoa mix, powder	6.67	4	398	80.03
Beverages, Cocoa mix, powder, prepared with water	0.92	0.55	55	11.04
Beverages, Cocoa mix, NESTLE, Hot Cocoa Mix Rich Chocolate With Marshmallows	2.8	15	400	71.3
Beverages, Cocoa mix, no sugar added, powder	15.49	3	377	64.43
Cocoa mix, NESTLE, Rich Chocolate Hot Cocoa Mix	3	15	400	71
Beverages, tea, black, ready-to-drink, lemon, sweetened	0	0.22	45	10.8
Beverages, coffee, brewed, prepared with tap water, decaffeinated	0.1	0	0	0
Beverages, coffee, brewed, espresso, restaurant-prepared, decaffeinated	0.1	0.18	9	1.69
Beverages, coffee, instant, regular, half the caffeine	14.42	0.5	352	73.18
Beverages, coffee and cocoa, instant, decaffeinated, with whitener and low calorie sweetener	9	13.21	440	66.6
Beverages, tea, green, ready-to-drink, sweetened	0	0.22	27	6.2
Beverages, tea, ready-to-drink, lemon, diet	0	0	2	0.41
Beverages, coffee, brewed, prepared with tap water	0.12	0.02	1	0
Beverages, coffee, brewed, espresso, restaurant-prepared	0.12	0.18	9	1.67
Beverages, tea, black, ready-to-drink, lemon, diet	0	0	1	0.22

Food Name ---> per 100 g	Protein (g)	Fat (g)	Calories	Net Carb (g)
Beverages, coffee, instant, regular, powder	12.2	0.5	353	75.4
Beverages, coffee, instant, regular, prepared with water	0.1	0	2	0.34
Beverages, aloe vera juice drink, fortified with Vitamin C	0	0	15	3.75
Beverages, OCEAN SPRAY, Cran Grape	0.21	0	54	12.56
Beverages, coffee, instant, decaffeinated, powder	11.6	0.2	351	76
Beverages, coffee, instant, decaffeinated, prepared with water	0.12	0	2	0.43
Beverages, OCEAN SPRAY, Cranberry-Apple Juice Drink, bottled	0.29	0	56	13.08
Beverages, OCEAN SPRAY, Diet Cranberry Juice	0.07	0	4	0.2
Beverages, coffee, instant, with chicory	9.3	0.2	355	78.4
Beverages, coffee, instant, chicory	0.09	0	3	0.75
Beverages, coffee, instant, mocha, sweetened	5.29	15.87	460	72.14
Beverages, OCEAN SPRAY, Light Cranberry and Raspberry Flavored Juice	0.73	0	26	5.07
Beverages, OCEAN SPRAY, White Cranberry Strawberry Flavored Juice Drink	0.22	0.01	49	11.38
Beverages, KRAFT, coffee, instant, French Vanilla Cafe	2.5	19.2	481	73.2
Beverages, OCEAN SPRAY, Cran Raspberry Juice Drink	0.28	0	49	11.36
Beverages, OCEAN SPRAY, Cran Lemonade	0.07	0	45	10.52
Beverages, OCEAN SPRAY, Diet Cran Cherry	0.21	0	4	0.1
Beverages, coffee substitute, cereal grain beverage, powder	6.01	2.52	360	55.12
Beverages, coffee substitute, cereal grain beverage, prepared with water	0.1	0.04	6	0.9
Beverages, cranberry-apple juice drink, bottled	0	0.11	63	15.85
Alcoholic beverage, malt beer, hard lemonade	0	0	68	10.07
Beverages, cranberry-apricot juice drink, bottled	0.2	0	64	16.1
Beverages, cranberry-grape juice drink, bottled	0.2	0.1	56	13.9
Cranberry juice cocktail, bottled	0	0.1	54	13.52
Cranberry juice cocktail, bottled, low calorie, with calcium, saccharin and corn sweetener	0.02	0.01	19	4.6
Beverages, Eggnog-flavor mix, powder, prepared with whole milk	2.93	3.02	95	14.2
Beverages, tea, green, instant, decaffeinated, lemon, unsweetened, fortified with vitamin C	0	0	378	94.45
Beverages, tea, black, ready to drink	0	0	0	0

Food Name ---> per 100 g	Protein (g)	Fat (g)	Calories	Net Carb (g)
Alcoholic beverage, beer, light, higher alcohol	0.25	0	46	0.77
Beverages, AMBER, hard cider	0	0	56	5.92
Alcoholic beverages, beer, higher alcohol	0.9	0	58	0.27
Beverages, Malt liquor beverage	0.35	0	40	0
Alcoholic beverages, wine, rose	0.36	0	83	3.8
Beverages, OCEAN SPRAY, Cran Pomegranate	0.07	0.01	47	11.96
Beverages, OCEAN SPRAY, Cran Cherry	0.19	0	46	12.16
Beverages, OCEAN SPRAY, Light Cranberry	0.22	0.01	19	4.02
Beverages, OCEAN SPRAY, White Cranberry Peach	0.13	0.01	45	11.28
Beverages, OCEAN SPRAY, Light Cranberry, Concord Grape	0.36	0.02	23	5.08
Beverages, tea, green, brewed, decaffeinated	0	0	0	0
Beverages, tea, green, ready to drink, unsweetened	0	0	0	0
Beverages, citrus fruit juice drink, frozen concentrate	1.2	0.1	162	40
Beverages, citrus fruit juice drink, frozen concentrate, prepared with water	0.34	0.03	46	11.32
Beverages, fruit punch drink, without added nutrients, canned	0	0	48	11.97
Beverages, Fruit punch drink, with added nutrients, canned	0	0	47	11.74
Beverages, Fruit punch drink, frozen concentrate	0.2	0	162	41
Beverages, Fruit punch drink, frozen concentrate, prepared with water	0.06	0	46	11.56
Beverages, coffee, instant, vanilla, sweetened, decaffeinated, with non dairy creamer	0	13.33	465	86.28
Beverages, Tropical Punch, ready-to-drink	0	0	10	2.5
Beverages, grape drink, canned	0	0	61	15.72
Beverages, tea, green, brewed, regular	0.22	0	1	0
Beverages, tea, black, ready-to-drink, peach, diet	0	0	1	0.25
Beverages, tea, black, ready to drink, decaffeinated, diet	0	0	0	0.83
Beverages, tea, black, ready to drink, decaffeinated	0	0	38	8.75
Beverages, grape juice drink, canned	0	0	57	14.45
Beverages, Cranberry juice cocktail	0	0.34	52	12.25
Beverages, OCEAN SPRAY, Ruby Red cranberry	0.07	0.01	45	10.98
Beverages, MOTTS, Apple juice light, fortified with vitamin C	0	0.1	22	5.1

Food Name ---> per 100 g	Protein (g)	Fat (g)	Calories	Net Carb (g)
Beverages, Lemonade, powder	0	1.05	376	97.17
Lemonade, powder, prepared with water	0	0.04	14	3.59
Beverages, SNAPPLE, tea, black and green, ready to drink, peach, diet	0.1	0	2	0.1
Lemonade, frozen concentrate, white	0.22	0.7	196	49.59
Lemonade, frozen concentrate, white, prepared with water	0.07	0.04	40	10.42
Beverages, SNAPPLE, tea, black and green, ready to drink, lemon, diet	0.1	0	2	0.1
Beverages, lemonade-flavor drink, powder	0	1.01	380	97.9
Beverages, lemonade-flavor drink, powder, prepared with water	0	0.07	27	6.9
Limeade, frozen concentrate, prepared with water	0	0	52	13.79
Malt beverage, includes non-alcoholic beer	0.21	0.12	37	8.05
Beverages, OVALTINE, Classic Malt powder	0	0	372	93.33
Beverages, Malted drink mix, natural, with added nutrients, powder, prepared with whole milk	3.67	3.21	86	10.67
Beverages, Malted drink mix, natural, powder, dairy based.	14.29	9.52	428	71.11
Beverages, Malted drink mix, natural, powder, prepared with whole milk	3.86	3.62	88	10.13
Beverages, OVALTINE, chocolate malt powder	0	0	372	92.96
Beverages, Malted drink mix, chocolate, with added nutrients, powder, prepared with whole milk	3.29	3.26	87	10.79
Beverages, malted drink mix, chocolate, powder	5.1	4.76	411	82.14
Beverages, Malted drink mix, chocolate, powder, prepared with whole milk	3.37	3.29	85	10.7
Beverages, orange drink, canned, with added vitamin C	0	0.07	49	12.34
Beverages, orange and apricot juice drink, canned	0.3	0.1	51	12.6
Beverages, pineapple and grapefruit juice drink, canned	0.2	0.1	47	11.5
Beverages, pineapple and orange juice drink, canned	1.3	0	50	11.7
Shake, fast food, vanilla	3.37	6.52	148	18.69
Strawberry-flavor beverage mix, powder	0.1	0.2	389	99.1
Beverages, Strawberry-flavor beverage mix, powder, prepared with whole milk	3	3.1	88	12.3
Beverages, tea, black, brewed, prepared with tap water, decaffeinated	0	0	1	0.3

Food Name ---> per 100 g	Protein (g)	Fat (g)	Calories	Net Carb (g)
Beverages, tea, instant, decaffeinated, unsweetened	20.21	0	315	50.16
Beverages, tea, black, brewed, prepared with tap water	0	0	1	0.3
Beverages, tea, instant, decaffeinated, lemon, diet	3.3	0.6	338	85.4
Beverages, tea, instant, decaffeinated, lemon, sweetened	0.12	0.73	401	98.55
Beverages, tea, instant, unsweetened, powder	20.21	0	315	50.16
Beverages, tea, instant, unsweetened, prepared with water	0.06	0	1	0.17
Beverages, tea, instant, lemon, unsweetened	7.4	0.18	345	73.52
Beverages, tea, instant, lemon, sweetened, powder	0.12	0.73	401	97.85
Beverages, tea, instant, lemon, sweetened, prepared with water	0.01	0.06	35	8.51
Beverages, tea, instant, sweetened with sodium saccharin, lemon-flavored, powder	3.3	0.6	338	85.4
Beverages, tea, instant, lemon, diet	0.02	0	2	0.44
Beverages, tea, herb, other than chamomile, brewed	0	0	1	0.2
Beverages, water, bottled, PERRIER	0	0	0	0
Beverages, water, bottled, POLAND SPRING	0	0	0	0
Beverages, cocoa mix, with aspartame, powder, prepared with water	1.21	0.23	29	5.01
Beverages, carbonated, cola, fast-food cola	0.07	0.02	37	9.56
Beverages, fruit punch juice drink, frozen concentrate	0.3	0.7	175	42.9
Beverages, fruit punch juice drink, frozen concentrate, prepared with water	0.07	0.17	42	11.4
Beverages, orange-flavor drink, breakfast type, powder	0	0	386	98.54
Beverages, orange-flavor drink, breakfast type, powder, prepared with water	0	0	49	12.55
Beverages, Orange-flavor drink, breakfast type, low calorie, powder	3.6	0	217	82.1
Beverages, water, tap, drinking	0	0	0	0
Beverages, water, tap, well	0	0	0	0
Alcoholic beverage, liqueur, coffee, 53 proof	0.1	0.3	336	46.8
Alcoholic beverage, liqueur, coffee with cream, 34 proof	2.8	15.7	327	20.9
Beverages, carbonated, low calorie, cola or pepper-type, with aspartame, contains caffeine	0.11	0.03	2	0.29
Beverages, coffee substitute, cereal grain beverage, powder, prepared with whole milk	3.3	3.3	65	5.5

Food Name ---> per 100 g	Protein (g)	Fat (g)	Calories	Net Carb (g)
Beverages, Dairy drink mix, chocolate, reduced calorie, with low-calorie sweeteners, powder	25	2.6	329	42
Beverages, dairy drink mix, chocolate, reduced calorie, with aspartame, powder, prepared with water and ice	2.19	0.23	29	3.71
Beverages, Orange-flavor drink, breakfast type, with pulp, frozen concentrate. Not manufactured anymore.	0.1	0.5	172	42.7
Beverages, Orange-flavor drink, breakfast type, with pulp, frozen concentrate, prepared with water	0.03	0.14	49	12.21
Beverages, Orange drink, breakfast type, with juice and pulp, frozen concentrate	0.4	0	153	38.9
Beverages, Orange drink, breakfast type, with juice and pulp, frozen concentrate, prepared with water	0.12	0	45	11.32
Beverages, shake, fast food, strawberry	3.4	2.8	113	18.5
Beverages, water, tap, municipal	0	0	0	0
Cranberry juice cocktail, frozen concentrate	0.05	0	201	51.25
Cranberry juice cocktail, frozen concentrate, prepared with water	0.01	0	47	11.81
Beverages, water, bottled, non-carbonated, DANNON	0	0	0	0
Beverages, water, bottled, non-carbonated, PEPSI, AQUAFINA	0	0	0	0
Beverages, The COCA-COLA company, DASANI, water, bottled, non-carbonated	0	0	0	0
Beverages, orange breakfast drink, ready-to-drink, with added nutrients	0	0	53	13.1
Beverages, water, bottled, non-carbonated, CALISTOGA	0	0	0	0
Beverages, water, bottled, non-carbonated, CRYSTAL GEYSER	0	0	0	0
Water, bottled, non-carbonated, NAYA	0	0	0	0
Beverages, water, bottled, non-carbonated, DANNON Fluoride To Go	0	0	0	0.03
Beverages, drink mix, QUAKER OATS, GATORADE, orange flavor, powder	0	1.23	388	94.11
Beverages, PEPSICO QUAKER, Gatorade, G performance O 2, ready-to-drink.	0	0	26	6.43
Beverages, COCA-COLA, POWERADE, lemon-lime flavored, ready-to-drink	0	0.05	32	7.84
Beverages, Propel Zero, fruit-flavored, non-carbonated	0	0	5	1.14
Beverages, ARIZONA, tea, ready-to-drink, lemon	0	0	39	9.77
Beverages, LIPTON BRISK, tea, black, ready-to-drink, lemon	0	0	35	8.81

Food Name ---> per 100 g	Protein (g)	Fat (g)	Calories	Net Carb (g)
Whiskey sour mix, bottled, with added potassium and sodium	0.1	0.1	84	21.4
Alcoholic beverage, whiskey sour	0	0.03	149	13.17
Alcoholic beverage, distilled, all (gin, rum, vodka, whiskey) 94 proof	0	0	275	0
Alcoholic beverage, distilled, all (gin, rum, vodka, whiskey) 100 proof	0	0	295	0
Alcoholic beverage, liqueur, coffee, 63 proof	0.1	0.3	308	32.2
Alcoholic beverage, wine, dessert, dry	0.2	0	152	11.67
Carbonated beverage, low calorie, other than cola or pepper, with sodium saccharin, without caffeine	0	0	0	0.1
Beverages, Cocoa mix, low calorie, powder, with added calcium, phosphorus, aspartame, without added sodium or vitamin A	25.1	3	359	56.9
Beverages, fruit punch-flavor drink, powder, without added sodium, prepared with water	0	0.01	37	9.47
Lemonade, frozen concentrate, pink	0.22	0.69	192	48.56
Beverages, lemonade, frozen concentrate, pink, prepared with water	0.05	0.15	43	10.71
Beverages, tea, black, brewed, prepared with distilled water	0	0	1	0.3
Beverages, tea, herb, brewed, chamomile	0	0	1	0.2
Beverages, tea, instant, lemon, with added ascorbic acid	0.6	0.3	385	97.6
Alcoholic beverage, distilled, all (gin, rum, vodka, whiskey) 86 proof	0	0	250	0.1
Alcoholic beverage, distilled, all (gin, rum, vodka, whiskey) 90 proof	0	0	263	0
Carbonated beverage, chocolate-flavored soda	0	0	42	10.7
Beverages, Wine, non-alcoholic	0.5	0	6	1.1
Water, bottled, generic	0	0	0	0
Beverages, chocolate-flavor beverage mix for milk, powder, with added nutrients	4.55	2.27	400	85.78
Beverages, chocolate-flavor beverage mix for milk, powder, with added nutrients, prepared with whole milk	3.27	3.17	89	11.47
Beverages, water, bottled, non-carbonated, EVIAN	0	0	0	0
Beverages, Powerade Zero Ion4, calorie-free, assorted flavors	0	0	0	0
Beverages, WENDY'S, tea, ready-to-drink, unsweetened	0.22	0	1	0
Alcoholic Beverage, wine, table, red, Merlot	0.07	0	83	2.51

Food Name ---> per 100 g	Protein (g)	Fat (g)	Calories	Net Carb (g)
Water, non-carbonated, bottles, natural fruit flavors, sweetened with low calorie sweetener	0	0	1	0.13
Beverages, Water with added vitamins and minerals, bottles, sweetened, assorted fruit flavors	0	0	22	5.49
Beverages, V8 SPLASH Juice Drinks, Diet Berry Blend	0	0	4	1.23
Beverages, V8 SPLASH Juice Drinks, Diet Fruit Medley	0	0	4	1.26
Beverages, V8 SPLASH Juice Drinks, Diet Strawberry Kiwi	0	0	4	1.26
Beverages, V8 SPLASH Juice Drinks, Diet Tropical Blend	0	0	4	1.26
Beverages, V8 SPLASH Juice Drinks, Berry Blend	0	0	29	7.41
Beverages, V8 SPLASH Juice Drinks, Fruit Medley	0	0	33	7.82
Beverages, V8 SPLASH Juice Drinks, Guava Passion Fruit	0	0	33	7.82
Beverages, V8 SPLASH Juice Drinks, Mango Peach	0	0	33	8.23
Beverages, V8 SPLASH Juice Drinks, Orange Pineapple	0	0	29	7.41
Beverages, V8 SPLASH Juice Drinks, Orchard Blend	0	0	33	7.82
Beverages, V8 SPLASH Juice Drinks, Strawberry Banana	0	0	29	7.41
Beverages, V8 SPLASH Juice Drinks, Strawberry Kiwi	0	0	29	7.41
Beverages, V8 SPLASH Juice Drinks, Tropical Blend	0	0	29	7.41
Beverages, V8 V-FUSION Juices, Peach Mango	0.41	0	49	11.38
Beverages, V8 V-FUSION Juices, Strawberry Banana	0.41	0	49	11.79
Beverages, V8 V-FUSION Juices, Tropical	0.41	0	49	11.38
Beverages, V8 V- FUSION Juices, Acai Berry	0	0	45	10.98
Beverages, Energy drink, AMP	0.25	0.08	46	12.08
Beverages, Energy drink, FULL THROTTLE	0.25	0.08	46	12.08
Beverages, Energy Drink, Monster, fortified with vitamins C, B2, B3, B6, B12	0.47	0	47	11.28
Beverages, Energy drink, AMP, sugar free	0	0	2	1.03
Beverages, Energy drink, ROCKSTAR	0.34	0.22	58	12.7
Beverages, Energy drink, ROCKSTAR, sugar free	0.25	0.08	4	0.7
Beverages, Horchata, dry mix, unprepared, variety of brands, all with morro seeds	7.5	7.46	413	75.05
Beverages, Meal supplement drink, canned, peanut flavor	3.5	3.07	101	14.74
Beverages, Vegetable and fruit juice drink, reduced calorie, with low-calorie sweetener, added vitamin C	0	0	4	1.1

Food Name ---> per 100 g	Protein (g)	Fat (g)	Calories	Net Carb (g)
Beverages, milk beverage, reduced fat, flavored and sweetened, Ready-to-drink, added calcium, vitamin A and vitamin D	3.05	1.83	77	11.68
Beverages, vegetable and fruit juice blend, 100% juice, with added vitamins A, C, E	0.3	0.01	46	11.15
Beverages, fruit juice drink, reduced sugar, with vitamin E added	0	0.07	39	10
Water, with corn syrup and/or sugar and low calorie sweetener, fruit flavored	0	0	18	4.5
Beverages, Horchata, as served in restaurant	0.48	0.71	54	11.52
Beverages, rice milk, unsweetened	0.28	0.97	47	8.87
Beverages, Energy drink, VAULT, citrus flavor	0	0	49	12.99
Beverages, Energy drink, VAULT Zero, sugar-free, citrus flavor	0.25	0.08	1	0.7
Beverages, PEPSICO QUAKER, Gatorade G2, low calorie	0.05	0.01	8	1.94
Beverages, Fruit flavored drink, less than 3% juice, not fortified with vitamin C	0	0	64	16.03
Beverages, Fruit flavored drink containing less than 3% fruit juice, with high vitamin C	0	0	27	6.67
Beverages, Fruit flavored drink, reduced sugar, greater than 3% fruit juice, high vitamin C, added calcium	0	0.37	29	6.67
Beverages, fruit juice drink, greater than 3% fruit juice, high vitamin C and added thiamin	0.13	0	54	13.06
Beverages, tea, hibiscus, brewed	0	0	0	0
Beverages, fruit juice drink, greater than 3% juice, high vitamin C	0.13	0.11	46	11.25
Beverages, nutritional shake mix, high protein, powder	53.57	10.71	392	20.38
Beverages, fruit-flavored drink, dry powdered mix, low calorie, with aspartame	0.45	0.04	218	87.28
Beverages, Orange juice drink	0.2	0	54	13.21
Alcoholic beverage, wine, cooking	0.5	0	50	6.3
Alcoholic beverage, wine, light	0.07	0	49	1.17
Beverages, fruit-flavored drink, powder, with high vitamin C with other added vitamins, low calorie	0.25	0.16	227	88.8
Beverages, Chocolate-flavored drink, whey and milk based	0.64	0.4	49	10.08
Beverages, coffee, instant, with whitener, reduced calorie	1.96	29.1	509	59.44
Beverages, cranberry-apple juice drink, low calorie, with vitamin C added	0.1	0	19	4.6
Alcoholic beverage, rice (sake)	0.5	0	134	5

Food Name ---> per 100 g	Protein (g)	Fat (g)	Calories	Net Carb (g)
Beverages, ABBOTT, ENSURE PLUS, ready-to-drink	5.16	4.52	141	19.88
Beverages, Cocktail mix, non-alcoholic, concentrated, frozen	0.08	0.01	287	71.6

Baby Products

Food Name ---> per serving	Weight (g)	Measure	Calories	Net Carb (g)
Babyfood, apple yogurt dessert, strained	15	1 tbsp	14	2.82
Babyfood, apple-banana juice	31.2	1 fl oz	16	3.74
Babyfood, apples with ham, strained	15	1 tbsp	9	1.34
Babyfood, apples, dices, toddler	28.35	1 oz	14	2.78
Babyfood, Baby MUM MUM Rice Biscuits	8	4.0 biscuit	31	6.66
Babyfood, baked product, finger snacks cereal fortified	1.7	1 cookie	7	1.3
Babyfood, banana apple dessert, strained	15	1 tbsp	10	2.34
Babyfood, banana juice with low fat yogurt	31.5	1 fl oz	27	5.43
Babyfood, banana no tapioca, strained	15	1 tbsp	14	3
Babyfood, banana with mixed berries, strained	99	1 packet	91	20.1
Babyfood, beverage, GERBER, GRADUATES, FRUIT SPLASHERS	113	4.0 oz	33	8.31
Babyfood, carrots and beef, strained	15	1 tbsp	9	0.45
Babyfood, carrots, toddler	28.35	1 oz	6	0.78
Babyfood, cereal, barley, dry fortified	2.4	1 tbsp	9	1.47
Babyfood, cereal, barley, prepared with whole milk	28.35	1 oz	24	2.62
Babyfood, cereal, brown rice, dry, instant	3.7	1 tbsp	15	2.98
Babyfood, cereal, egg yolks and bacon, junior	28.35	1 oz	22	1.46
Babyfood, cereal, high protein, prepared with whole milk	28.35	1 oz	31	3.29
Babyfood, cereal, high protein, with apple and orange, dry	2.4	1 tbsp	9	1.18
Babyfood, cereal, high protein, with apple and orange, prepared with whole milk	28.35	1 oz	32	3.8
Babyfood, cereal, mixed, dry fortified	2.5	1 tbsp	10	1.76
Babyfood, cereal, mixed, prepared with whole milk	28.35	1 oz	27	3.29
Babyfood, cereal, mixed, with applesauce and bananas, junior, fortified	28.35	1 oz	24	5.03

Food Name ---> per serving	Weight (g)	Measure	Calories	Net Carb (g)
Babyfood, cereal, mixed, with applesauce and bananas, strained	28.35	1 oz	23	4.91
Babyfood, cereal, mixed, with bananas, dry	2.5	1 tbsp	10	1.73
Babyfood, cereal, mixed, with bananas, prepared with whole milk	28.35	1 oz	24	2.73
Babyfood, cereal, mixed, with honey, prepared with whole milk	28.35	1 oz	33	4.51
Babyfood, cereal, oatmeal, dry fortified	3.2	1 tbsp	13	2.15
Babyfood, cereal, oatmeal, prepared with whole milk	28.35	1 oz	33	4.04
Babyfood, cereal, oatmeal, with applesauce and bananas, junior, fortified	28.35	1 oz	22	4.24
Babyfood, cereal, oatmeal, with applesauce and bananas, strained	28.35	1 oz	21	4.13
Babyfood, cereal, oatmeal, with bananas, dry	15	1 serv	60	10.91
Babyfood, cereal, oatmeal, with bananas, prepared with whole milk	28.35	1 oz	24	2.73
Babyfood, cereal, oatmeal, with honey, dry	2.4	1 tbsp	9	1.66
Babyfood, cereal, oatmeal, with honey, prepared with whole milk	28.35	1 oz	33	4.34
Babyfood, cereal, rice with pears and apple, dry, instant fortified	15	1 serv	58	12.88
Babyfood, cereal, rice, dry fortified	2.5	1 tbsp	10	2.08
Babyfood, cereal, rice, prepared with whole milk	28.35	1 oz	24	2.92
Babyfood, cereal, rice, with applesauce and bananas, strained	16	1 tbsp	13	2.54
Babyfood, cereal, rice, with bananas, dry	2.5	1 tbsp	10	2
Babyfood, cereal, rice, with bananas, prepared with whole milk	28.35	1 oz	24	2.97
Babyfood, cereal, rice, with honey, prepared with whole milk	28.35	1 oz	33	4.85
Babyfood, cereal, whole wheat, with apples, dry fortified	15	0.5 oz	60	11.48
Babyfood, cereal, with egg yolks, junior	28.35	1 oz	15	1.71
Babyfood, cereal, with egg yolks, strained	28.35	1 oz	14	1.68
Babyfood, cereal, with eggs, strained	28.35	1 oz	16	2.27

Food Name ---> per serving	Weight (g)	Measure	Calories	Net Carb (g)
Babyfood, cherry cobbler, junior	28.35	1 oz	22	5.34
Babyfood, cookie, baby, fruit	8	1 cookie	35	5.6
Babyfood, cookies	28.35	1 oz	123	18.92
Babyfood, cookies, arrowroot	28.35	1 oz	120	21.28
Babyfood, corn and sweet potatoes, strained	28.35	1 oz	19	3.82
Babyfood, crackers, vegetable	0.7	1 cracker	3	0.47
Babyfood, dessert, banana pudding, strained	15	1 tbsp	10	2.02
Babyfood, dessert, banana yogurt, strained	15	1 tbsp	12	2.5
Babyfood, dessert, blueberry yogurt, strained	15	1 tbsp	12	2.46
Babyfood, dessert, cherry vanilla pudding, junior	28.35	1 oz	20	5.12
Babyfood, dessert, cherry vanilla pudding, strained	28.35	1 oz	19	4.95
Babyfood, dessert, custard pudding, vanilla, junior	229	1 cup	197	39.76
Babyfood, dessert, custard pudding, vanilla, strained	229	1 cup	195	36.64
Babyfood, dessert, dutch apple, junior	28.35	1 oz	22	5.04
Babyfood, dessert, dutch apple, strained	28.35	1 oz	21	5.2
Babyfood, dessert, fruit dessert, without ascorbic acid, junior	15	1 tbsp	9	2.48
Babyfood, dessert, fruit dessert, without ascorbic acid, strained	15	1 tbsp	9	2.3
Babyfood, dessert, fruit pudding, orange, strained	28.35	1 oz	23	4.82
Babyfood, dessert, fruit pudding, pineapple, strained	15	1 tbsp	12	2.94
Babyfood, dessert, peach cobbler, junior	15	1 tbsp	10	2.65
Babyfood, dessert, peach cobbler, strained	15	1 tbsp	10	2.57
Babyfood, dessert, peach melba, junior	28.35	1 oz	17	4.65
Babyfood, dessert, peach melba, strained	28.35	1 oz	17	4.68
Babyfood, dessert, peach yogurt	15	1 tbsp	12	2.54
Babyfood, dessert, tropical fruit, junior	28.35	1 oz	17	4.65
Babyfood, dinner, apples and chicken, strained	28.35	1 oz	18	2.58

Food Name ---> per serving	Weight (g)	Measure	Calories	Net Carb (g)
Babyfood, dinner, beef and rice, toddler	28.35	1 oz	23	2.49
Babyfood, dinner, beef lasagna, toddler	28.35	1 oz	22	2.83
Babyfood, dinner, beef noodle, junior	16	1 tbsp	9	0.97
Babyfood, dinner, beef noodle, strained	16	1 tbsp	10	1.11
Babyfood, dinner, beef with vegetables	113	4 oz	108	5.19
Babyfood, dinner, broccoli and chicken, junior	29	1 tbsp	18	1.44
Babyfood, dinner, chicken and rice	16	1 tbsp	8	1.27
Babyfood, dinner, chicken noodle, junior	16	1 tbsp	12	0.95
Babyfood, dinner, chicken noodle, strained	16	1 tbsp	12	0.95
Babyfood, dinner, chicken soup, strained	113	1 jar	56	6.94
Babyfood, dinner, chicken stew, toddler	16	1 tbsp	12	0.92
Babyfood, dinner, macaroni and cheese, junior	28.35	1 oz	17	2.22
Babyfood, dinner, macaroni and cheese, strained	28.35	1 oz	19	2.34
Babyfood, dinner, macaroni and tomato and beef, junior	16	1 tbsp	9	1.3
Babyfood, dinner, macaroni and tomato and beef, strained	16	1 tbsp	10	1.31
Babyfood, dinner, macaroni, beef and tomato sauce, toddler	16	1 tbsp	13	1.64
Babyfood, dinner, mixed vegetable, junior	99	1 serv	34	6.8
Babyfood, dinner, mixed vegetable, strained	28.35	1 oz	12	2.69
Babyfood, dinner, pasta with vegetables	113	1 jar, (4 oz)	68	7.79
Babyfood, dinner, spaghetti and tomato and meat, junior	16	1 tbsp	11	1.63
Babyfood, dinner, spaghetti and tomato and meat, toddler	28.35	1 oz	21	36
Babyfood, dinner, sweet potatoes and chicken, strained	16	1 tbsp	12	1.57
Babyfood, dinner, turkey and rice, junior	16	1 tbsp	9	1.33
Babyfood, dinner, turkey and rice, strained	16	1 tbsp	8	1.17
Babyfood, dinner, turkey, rice, and vegetables, toddler	28.35	1 oz	17	1.93
Babyfood, dinner, vegetables and beef, junior	256	1 cup	197	19.33

Food Name ---> per serving	Weight (g)	Measure	Calories	Net Carb (g)
Babyfood, dinner, vegetables and beef, strained	256	1 cup	197	19.33
Babyfood, dinner, vegetables and chicken, junior	256	1 cup	136	19.37
Babyfood, dinner, vegetables and dumplings and beef, junior	28.35	1 oz	14	2.27
Babyfood, dinner, vegetables and dumplings and beef, strained	28.35	1 oz	14	2.18
Babyfood, dinner, vegetables and lamb, junior	28.35	1 oz	14	1.71
Babyfood, dinner, vegetables and noodles and turkey, junior	28.35	1 oz	15	1.85
Babyfood, dinner, vegetables and noodles and turkey, strained	28.35	1 oz	12	1.63
Babyfood, dinner, vegetables and turkey, junior	256	1 cup	136	17.03
Babyfood, dinner, vegetables and turkey, strained	256	1 cup	123	15.71
Babyfood, dinner, vegetables chicken, strained	256	1 cup	151	16.16
Babyfood, dinner, vegetables, noodles and chicken, junior	28.35	1 oz	18	2.28
Babyfood, dinner, vegetables, noodles and chicken, strained	28.35	1 oz	18	1.94
Babyfood, fortified cereal bar, fruit filling	19	1 bar	65	12.74
Babyfood, fruit and vegetable, apple and sweet potato	113	1 jar, (4 oz)	72	15.69
Babyfood, fruit dessert, mango with tapioca	15	1 tbsp	10	2.65
Babyfood, fruit supreme dessert	15	1 tbsp	11	2.28
Babyfood, fruit, apple and blueberry, junior	28.35	1 oz	18	4.21
Babyfood, fruit, apple and blueberry, strained	28.35	1 oz	17	4.12
Babyfood, fruit, apple and raspberry, junior	28.35	1 oz	16	3.77
Babyfood, fruit, apple and raspberry, strained	28.35	1 oz	16	3.82
Babyfood, fruit, applesauce and apricots, junior	16	1 tbsp	8	1.68
Babyfood, fruit, applesauce and apricots, strained	16	1 tbsp	7	1.56
Babyfood, fruit, applesauce and cherries, junior	28.35	1 oz	14	3.7
Babyfood, fruit, applesauce and cherries, strained	28.35	1 oz	14	3.7

Food Name ---> per serving	Weight (g)	Measure	Calories	Net Carb (g)
Babyfood, fruit, applesauce and pineapple, junior	28.35	1 oz	11	2.58
Babyfood, fruit, applesauce and pineapple, strained	28.35	1 oz	10	2.46
Babyfood, fruit, applesauce with banana, junior	16	1 tbsp	11	2.29
Babyfood, fruit, applesauce, junior	16	1 tbsp	6	1.35
Babyfood, fruit, applesauce, strained	16	1 tbsp	7	1.43
Babyfood, fruit, apricot with tapioca, junior	15	1 tbsp	9	2.4
Babyfood, fruit, apricot with tapioca, strained	15	1 tbsp	9	2.24
Babyfood, fruit, banana and strawberry, junior	140	1 bottle	153	34.09
Babyfood, fruit, bananas and pineapple with tapioca, junior	15	1 tbsp	10	2.56
Babyfood, fruit, bananas and pineapple with tapioca, strained	15	1 tbsp	10	2.47
Babyfood, fruit, bananas with apples and pears, strained	15	1 tbsp	12	2.7
Babyfood, fruit, bananas with tapioca, junior	15	1 tbsp	10	2.47
Babyfood, fruit, bananas with tapioca, strained	15	1 tbsp	8	2.09
Babyfood, fruit, guava and papaya with tapioca, strained	28.35	1 oz	18	4.82
Babyfood, fruit, papaya and applesauce with tapioca, strained	28.35	1 oz	20	4.96
Babyfood, fruit, peaches, junior	17	1 tbsp	11	2.26
Babyfood, fruit, peaches, strained	17	1 tbsp	11	2.26
Babyfood, fruit, pears and pineapple, junior	16	1 tbsp	7	1.42
Babyfood, fruit, pears and pineapple, strained	16	1 tbsp	7	1.34
Babyfood, fruit, pears, junior	16	1 tbsp	7	1.46
Babyfood, fruit, pears, strained	16	1 tbsp	7	1.33
Babyfood, fruit, plums with tapioca, without ascorbic acid, junior	15	1 tbsp	11	2.88
Babyfood, fruit, plums with tapioca, without ascorbic acid, strained	15	1 tbsp	11	2.76
Babyfood, fruit, prunes with tapioca, without ascorbic acid, junior	28.35	1 oz	20	4.5

Food Name ---> per serving	Weight (g)	Measure	Calories	Net Carb (g)
Babyfood, fruit, prunes with tapioca, without ascorbic acid, strained	15	1 tbsp	10	2.37
Babyfood, fruit, tutti frutti, junior	15	1 tbsp	10	2.3
Babyfood, fruit, tutti frutti, strained	15	1 tbsp	10	2.22
Babyfood, GERBER, 2nd Foods, apple, carrot and squash, organic	99	1 serv	63	13.47
Babyfood, GERBER, 3rd Foods, apple, mango and kiwi	170	1 serv	82	18.5
Babyfood, GERBER, Banana with orange medley	113	1 jar	78	20.66
Babyfood, GERBER, GRADUATES Lil Biscuits Vanilla Wheat	28.35	1 oz	115	18.85
Babyfood, grape juice, no sugar, canned	118	4.0 fl oz	73	18.15
Babyfood, green beans and turkey, strained	14	1 tbsp	7	0.55
Babyfood, green beans, dices, toddler	28.35	1 oz	8	1.22
Babyfood, juice treats, fruit medley, toddler	28	1 packet	97	24.27
Babyfood, juice, apple	31.7	1 fl oz	15	3.71
Babyfood, juice, apple - cherry	31.2	1 fl oz	15	3.39
Babyfood, juice, apple and grape	31.2	1 fl oz	14	3.54
Babyfood, juice, apple and peach	31.2	1 fl oz	13	3.28
Babyfood, juice, apple and prune	31.2	1 fl oz	22	5.65
Babyfood, juice, apple-sweet potato	30.8	1 fl oz	87	3.31
Babyfood, juice, apple, with calcium	189	1 serv	14	20.18
Babyfood, juice, fruit punch, with calcium	31.2	1 fl oz	16	3.86
Babyfood, juice, mixed fruit	31.2	1 fl oz	15	3.65
Babyfood, juice, orange	31.2	1 fl oz	14	3.18
Babyfood, juice, orange and apple	31.2	1 fl oz	13	3.15
Babyfood, juice, orange and apple and banana	31.2	1 fl oz	15	3.59
Babyfood, juice, orange and apricot	31.2	1 fl oz	14	3.4
Babyfood, juice, orange and banana	31.2	1 fl oz	16	3.71
Babyfood, juice, orange and pineapple	31.2	1 fl oz	15	3.65
Babyfood, juice, orange-carrot	30.8	1 fl oz	13	2.95
Babyfood, juice, pear	31.2	1 fl oz	13	3.7

Food Name ---> per serving	Weight (g)	Measure	Calories	Net Carb (g)
Babyfood, juice, prune and orange	31.2	1 fl oz	22	5.24
Babyfood, macaroni and cheese, toddler	113	1 cont.	93	12.06
Babyfood, mashed cheddar potatoes and broccoli, toddlers	170	1 cont.	82	10.7
Babyfood, meat, beef with vegetables, toddler	179	1 jar	124	12.41
Babyfood, meat, beef, junior	28.35	1 oz	23	0.69
Babyfood, meat, beef, strained	14.7	1 tbsp	12	0.36
Babyfood, meat, chicken sticks, junior	10	1 stick	19	0.15
Babyfood, meat, chicken, junior	15	1 tbsp	22	0
Babyfood, meat, chicken, strained	15	1 tbsp	20	0.01
Babyfood, meat, ham, junior	28.35	1 oz	27	15
Babyfood, meat, ham, strained	15	1 tbsp	15	0.56
Babyfood, meat, lamb, junior	28.35	1 oz	32	0
Babyfood, meat, lamb, strained	22	1 tbsp	21	0.19
Babyfood, meat, meat sticks, junior	10	1 stick	18	0.11
Babyfood, meat, pork, strained	28.35	1 oz	35	0
Babyfood, meat, turkey sticks, junior	10	1 stick	19	0.14
Babyfood, meat, turkey, junior	19	1 tbsp	21	0.27
Babyfood, meat, turkey, strained	15	1 tbsp	17	0.21
Babyfood, meat, veal, strained	16	1 tbsp	13	0.24
Babyfood, mixed fruit juice with low fat yogurt	31.5	1 fl oz	23	4.52
Babyfood, mixed fruit yogurt, strained	15	1 tbsp	11	2.33
Babyfood, Multigrain whole grain cereal, dry fortified	16	3 tbsp	65	11.71
Babyfood, oatmeal cereal with fruit, dry, instant, toddler fortified	5.3	1 tbsp	21	3.53
Babyfood, peaches, dices, toddler	28.35	1 oz	14	3.15
Babyfood, pears, dices, toddler	28.35	1 oz	16	3.56
Babyfood, peas and brown rice	230	1 cup	147	20.63
Babyfood, peas, dices, toddler	28.35	1 oz	18	1.82
Babyfood, plums, bananas and rice, strained	28.35	1 oz	16	3.2
Babyfood, potatoes, toddler	163	1 cup	85	17.62

Food Name ---> per serving	Weight (g)	Measure	Calories	Net Carb (g)
Babyfood, pretzels	28.35	1 oz	113	22.6
Babyfood, prunes, without vitamin c, strained	15	1 tbsp	15	3.13
Babyfood, ravioli, cheese filled, with tomato sauce	16	1 tbsp	16	2.61
Babyfood, rice and apples, dry	2.5	1 tbsp	10	2.07
Babyfood, rice cereal, dry, EARTHS BEST ORGANIC WHOLE GRAIN, fortified only with iron	18	4.0 tbsp	69	13.95
Babyfood, snack, GERBER GRADUATE FRUIT STRIPS, Real Fruit Bars	9.9	1 bar	33	7.38
Babyfood, Snack, GERBER, GRADUATES, LIL CRUNCHIES, baked whole grain corn snack	7	18.0 piece	35	4.31
Babyfood, snack, GERBER, GRADUATES, YOGURT MELTS	7	1 serv	27	4.83
Babyfood, tropical fruit medley	88	1 serv	40	9.65
Babyfood, vegetable and brown rice, strained	230	1 cup	159	25.33
Babyfood, vegetable, butternut squash and corn	113	4 oz	56	8.16
Babyfood, vegetable, green beans and potatoes	113	4 oz	70	8.57
Babyfood, vegetables, beets, strained	224	1 cup	76	12.95
Babyfood, vegetables, carrots, junior	224	1 cup	72	12.33
Babyfood, vegetables, carrots, strained	224	1 cup	58	9.64
Babyfood, vegetables, corn, creamed, junior	240	1 cup	156	34
Babyfood, vegetables, corn, creamed, strained	113	1 jar	64	13.53
Babyfood, vegetables, garden vegetable, strained	28.35	1 oz	9	1.53
Babyfood, vegetables, green beans, junior	240	1 cup	58	9.32
Babyfood, vegetables, green beans, strained	240	1 cup	65	9.8
Babyfood, vegetables, mix vegetables junior	99	3.5 oz serv	36	6.62
Babyfood, vegetables, mix vegetables strained	28.35	1 oz	10	1.94
Babyfood, vegetables, peas, strained	16	1 tbsp	8	14
Babyfood, vegetables, spinach, creamed, strained	240	1 cup	89	9.38
Babyfood, vegetables, squash, junior	16	1 tbsp	4	0.82
Babyfood, vegetables, squash, strained	16	1 tbsp	4	0.82
Babyfood, vegetables, sweet potatoes strained	224	1 cup	128	26.17

Food Name ---> per serving	Weight (g)	Measure	Calories	Net Carb (g)
Babyfood, vegetables, sweet potatoes, junior	224	1 cup	134	27.96
Babyfood, water, bottled, GERBER, without added fluoride	113	1 serv	0	0
Babyfood, yogurt, whole milk, with fruit, multigrain cereal and added DHA fortified	31	1 oz	30	4
Babyfood, yogurt, whole milk, with fruit, multigrain cereal and added iron fortified	16	1 tbsp	15	1.98
Child formula, ABBOTT NUTRITION, PEDIASURE, ready-to-feed	31	1 fl oz	31	3.46
Child formula, ABBOTT NUTRITION, PEDIASURE, ready-to-feed, with iron and fiber	31	1 fl oz	31	3.3
Clif Z bar	36	1 bar	150	23.9
Fluid replacement, electrolyte solution (include PEDIALYTE)	31.2	1 fl oz	3	0.76
Infant formula, ABBOTT NUTRITION, ALIMENTUM ADVANCE, with iron, powder, not reconstituted, with DHA and ARA	8.7	1 scoop	45	4.52
Infant formula, ABBOTT NUTRITION, SIMILAC NEOSURE, ready-to-feed, with ARA and DHA	30.5	1 fl oz	21	2.12
Infant formula, ABBOTT NUTRITION, SIMILAC, ADVANCE, with iron, liquid concentrate, not reconstituted	31.4	1 fl oz	40	4.25
Infant formula, ABBOTT NUTRITION, SIMILAC, ADVANCE, with iron, powder, not reconstituted	8.5	1 scoop	44	4.65
Infant formula, ABBOTT NUTRITION, SIMILAC, ADVANCE, with iron, ready-to-feed	30.4	1 fl oz	20	2.06
Infant formula, ABBOTT NUTRITION, SIMILAC, ALIMENTUM, ADVANCE, ready-to-feed, with ARA and DHA	30.5	1 fl oz	20	2.06
Infant formula, ABBOTT NUTRITION, SIMILAC, ALIMENTUM, with iron, ready-to-feed	30.5	1 fl oz	20	2.06
Infant formula, ABBOTT NUTRITION, SIMILAC, Expert Care, Diarrhea, ready- to- feed with ARA and DHA	30.4	1 fl oz	20	1.83
Infant formula, ABBOTT NUTRITION, SIMILAC, For Spit Up, powder, with ARA and DHA	9.5	1 scoop	49	5.22

Food Name ---> per serving	Weight (g)	Measure	Calories	Net Carb (g)
Infant formula, ABBOTT NUTRITION, SIMILAC, For Spit Up, ready-to-feed, with ARA and DHA	30.4	1 fl oz	20	2.19
Infant formula, ABBOTT NUTRITION, SIMILAC, GO AND GROW, powder, with ARA and DHA	9.6	1 scoop	49	5.01
Infant formula, ABBOTT NUTRITION, SIMILAC, GO AND GROW, ready-to-feed, with ARA and DHA	153	5.0 fl oz	101	10.24
Infant formula, ABBOTT NUTRITION, SIMILAC, ISOMIL, ADVANCE with iron, liquid concentrate	31.4	1 fl oz	40	4.15
Infant formula, ABBOTT NUTRITION, SIMILAC, ISOMIL, ADVANCE with iron, powder, not reconstituted	8.7	1 scoop	45	4.66
Infant formula, ABBOTT NUTRITION, SIMILAC, ISOMIL, ADVANCE with iron, ready-to-feed	30.5	1 fl oz	20	2.04
Infant formula, ABBOTT NUTRITION, SIMILAC, ISOMIL, with iron, liquid concentrate	31.4	1 fl oz	40	4.15
Infant formula, ABBOTT NUTRITION, SIMILAC, ISOMIL, with iron, powder, not reconstituted	8.7	1 scoop	45	4.66
Infant formula, ABBOTT NUTRITION, SIMILAC, ISOMIL, with iron, ready-to-feed	30.5	1 fl oz	20	2.04
Infant formula, ABBOTT NUTRITION, SIMILAC, NEOSURE, powder, with ARA and DHA	30.5	1 fl oz	159	15.78
Infant formula, ABBOTT NUTRITION, SIMILAC, PM 60/40, powder not reconstituted	8.7	1 scoop	46	4.78
Infant formula, ABBOTT NUTRITION, SIMILAC, SENSITIVE (LACTOSE FREE) ready-to-feed, with ARA and DHA	30.5	1 fl oz	21	2.26
Infant formula, ABBOTT NUTRITION, SIMILAC, SENSITIVE, (LACTOSE FREE), liquid concentrate, with ARA and DHA	30.5	1 fl oz	39	4.16
Infant formula, ABBOTT NUTRITION, SIMILAC, SENSITIVE, (LACTOSE FREE), powder, with ARA and DHA	30.5	1 fl oz	159	16.98

Food Name ---> per serving	Weight (g)	Measure	Calories	Net Carb (g)
Infant formula, ABBOTT NUTRITION, SIMILAC, with iron, liquid concentrate, not reconstituted	31.4	1 fl oz	40	4.32
Infant formula, ABBOTT NUTRITION, SIMILAC, with iron, powder, not reconstituted	8.5	1 scoop	44	4.65
Infant Formula, GERBER GOOD START 2, GENTLE PLUS, powder	9.4	1 scoop	46	5.37
Infant Formula, GERBER GOOD START 2, GENTLE PLUS, ready-to-feed	30.4	1 fl oz	20	2.31
Infant formula, GERBER, GOOD START 2 SOY, with iron, powder	9.4	1 scoop	47	5.23
Infant formula, GERBER, GOOD START 2 Soy, with iron, ready-to-feed	30.4	1 fl oz	20	2.17
Infant formula, GERBER, GOOD START 2, PROTECT PLUS, powder	9.4	1 scoop	47	5.29
Infant formula, GERBER, GOOD START 2, PROTECT PLUS, ready-to-feed	30.4	1 fl oz	20	2.25
Infant formula, GERBER, GOOD START, PROTECT PLUS, powder	9.4	1 scoop	48	5.36
Infant formula, GERBER, GOOD START, PROTECT PLUS, ready-to-feed	30.4	1 fl oz	20	2.18
Infant formula, MEAD JOHNSON, Enfamil 24, ready to feed, with ARA and DHA	30.5	1 fl oz	22	2.11
Infant formula, MEAD JOHNSON, Enfamil Enspire Powder, with ARA and DHA, not reconstituted	8.8	1 scoop	45	5.03
Infant formula, MEAD JOHNSON, Enfamil for Supplementing, powder, with ARA and DHA, not reconstituted	8.7	1 serv	45	4.85
Infant formula, MEAD JOHNSON, Enfamil for Supplementing, ready to feed, with ARA and DHA	103	100.0 ml	70	7.83
Infant Formula, MEAD JOHNSON, ENFAMIL GENTLEASE, with iron, prepared from powder	30.5	1 fl oz	21	2.32
Infant formula, MEAD JOHNSON, ENFAMIL LIPIL, with iron, ready-to-feed, with ARA and DHA	106	100 ml	68	7.53
Infant formula, MEAD JOHNSON, Enfamil Premature 30 Calories, ready to feed, with ARA and DHA	30.5	1 fl oz	31	3.39

Food Name ---> per serving	Weight (g)	Measure	Calories	Net Carb (g)
Infant formula, MEAD JOHNSON, Enfamil Premature High Protein 24 Calories, ready to feed, with ARA and DHA	30.4	1 fl oz	25	2.63
Infant formula, MEAD JOHNSON, Enfamil Reguline Powder, with ARA and DHA, not reconstituted	8.7	1 scoop	45	4.86
Infant formula, MEAD JOHNSON, Enfamil Reguline, ready to feed, with ARA and DHA	30.5	1 fl oz	21	2.32
Infant formula, MEAD JOHNSON, ENFAMIL, AR, powder, with ARA and DHA	9	1 scoop	45	5.17
Infant formula, MEAD JOHNSON, ENFAMIL, AR, ready-to-feed, with ARA and DHA	106	100 ml	75	8.85
Infant Formula, MEAD JOHNSON, ENFAMIL, ENFACARE, ready-to-feed, with ARA and DHA	30.8	1 fl oz	22	2.38
Infant formula, MEAD JOHNSON, ENFAMIL, ENFACARE, with iron, powder, with ARA and DHA	9.9	1 scoop	50	5.33
Infant formula, MEAD JOHNSON, ENFAMIL, ENFAGROW, GENTLEASE, Toddler transitions, with ARA and DHA, powder	9	1 scoop	45	4.82
Infant formula, MEAD JOHNSON, ENFAMIL, Enfagrow, Soy, Toddler ready-to-feed	30.4	1 fl oz	20	2.32
Infant formula, MEAD JOHNSON, ENFAMIL, ENFAGROW, Soy, Toddler transitions, with ARA and DHA, powder	9.4	1 scoop	45	5.26
Infant Formula, MEAD JOHNSON, ENFAMIL, GENTLEASE, with ARA and DHA powder not reconstituted	8.7	1 scoop	45	4.92
Infant formula, MEAD JOHNSON, ENFAMIL, Infant, ready-to-feed, with ARA and DHA	106	100 ml	72	8.33
Infant formula, MEAD JOHNSON, ENFAMIL, Infant, with iron, liquid concentrate, with ARA and DHA, reconstituted	31.3	1 fl oz	21	2.46
Infant formula, MEAD JOHNSON, ENFAMIL, Infant, with iron, powder, with ARA and DHA	8.8	1 scope	45	4.95
Infant formula, MEAD JOHNSON, ENFAMIL, LIPIL, low iron, liquid concentrate, with ARA and DHA	31.3	1 fl oz	41	4.46

Food Name ---> per serving	Weight (g)	Measure	Calories	Net Carb (g)
Infant formula, MEAD JOHNSON, ENFAMIL, LIPIL, low iron, ready to feed, with ARA and DHA	106	100 ml	68	7.61
Infant Formula, MEAD JOHNSON, ENFAMIL, Newborn, with ARA and DHA, powder	8.7	1 scoop	45	5.01
Infant Formula, MEAD JOHNSON, ENFAMIL, Newborn, with DHA and ARA, ready-to-feed	30.5	1 fl oz	21	2.38
Infant formula, MEAD JOHNSON, ENFAMIL, NUTRAMIGEN AA, ready-to-feed	30.4	1 fl oz	20	2.06
Infant formula, MEAD JOHNSON, ENFAMIL, NUTRAMIGEN WITH LGG, with iron, powder, not reconstituted, with ARA and DHA	9	1 scoop	46	4.82
Infant formula, MEAD JOHNSON, ENFAMIL, NUTRAMIGEN, PurAmino, powder, not reconstituted	9.4	1 scoop	48	5.23
Infant formula, MEAD JOHNSON, ENFAMIL, NUTRAMIGEN, with iron, liquid concentrate not reconstituted, with ARA and DHA	31.6	1 fl oz	21	2.28
Infant formula, MEAD JOHNSON, ENFAMIL, NUTRAMIGEN, with iron, ready-to-feed, with ARA and DHA	107	100 ml	73	7.71
Infant formula, MEAD JOHNSON, ENFAMIL, Premature, 20 calories ready-to-feed Low iron	30.4	1 fl oz	20	2.19
Infant formula, MEAD JOHNSON, ENFAMIL, Premature, 24 calories ready-to-feed Low iron	30	5.0 fl oz	20	2.16
Infant formula, MEAD JOHNSON, ENFAMIL, Premature, with iron, 20 calories, ready-to-feed	30.4	1 fl oz	19	1.88
Infant formula, MEAD JOHNSON, ENFAMIL, Premature, with iron, 24 calories, ready-to-feed	30.4	1 fl oz	25	2.7
Infant Formula, MEAD JOHNSON, ENFAMIL, Premium LIPIL, Infant, Liquid concentrate, not reconstituted	31.4	1 fl oz	41	4.53
Infant Formula, MEAD JOHNSON, ENFAMIL, Premium LIPIL, Infant, powder	8.7	1 scoop	44	4.96
Infant Formula, MEAD JOHNSON, ENFAMIL, Premium, Infant, Liquid concentrate, not reconstituted	31.4	1 fl oz	41	4.5
Infant Formula, MEAD JOHNSON, ENFAMIL, Premium, Infant, powder	8.7	1 scoop	44	4.96

Food Name ---> per serving	Weight (g)	Measure	Calories	Net Carb (g)
Infant Formula, MEAD JOHNSON, ENFAMIL, Premium, Infant, ready-to-feed	30.5	1 fl oz	20	2.25
Infant formula, MEAD JOHNSON, ENFAMIL, PROSOBEE, liquid concentrate, reconstituted, with ARA and DHA	31.3	1 fl oz	21	2.37
Infant formula, MEAD JOHNSON, ENFAMIL, PROSOBEE, with iron, powder, not reconstituted, with ARA and DHA	8.8	1 scoop	45	4.8
Infant formula, MEAD JOHNSON, ENFAMIL, with iron, powder	8.3	1 scoop	43	4.66
Infant formula, MEAD JOHNSON, Gentlease, ready to feed, with ARA and DHA	30	1 fl oz	20	2.28
Infant formula, MEAD JOHNSON, NEXT STEP PROSOBEE, powder, not reconstituted	9.3	1 scoop	45	5.31
Infant formula, MEAD JOHNSON, NEXT STEP, PROSOBEE LIPIL, powder, with ARA and DHA	28	3 scoop	134	15.99
Infant formula, MEAD JOHNSON, NEXT STEP, PROSOBEE, LIPIL, ready to feed, with ARA and DHA	103	100 ml	69	8.33
Infant formula, MEAD JOHNSON, Pregestimil 20 Calories, ready to feed, with ARA and DHA	1	100.0 ml	1	0.07
Infant formula, MEAD JOHNSON, Pregestimil 24 Calories, ready to feed, with ARA and DHA	104	100.0 ml	75	6.19
Infant formula, MEAD JOHNSON, PREGESTIMIL, with iron, powder, with ARA and DHA, not reconstituted	8.8	1 scoop	45	4.59
Infant formula, MEAD JOHNSON, PREGESTIMIL, with iron, with ARA and DHA, prepared from powder	104	1 serv 100 ml	70	6.8
Infant formula, MEAD JOHNSON, PROSOBEE, with iron, ready to feed, with ARA and DHA	106	1 serv 100 ml	68	6.86
Infant formula, MEAD JOHNSON, PROSOBEE, with iron, ready-to-feed	106	1 Serv 100 ml	67	6.48
Infant formula, MEAD JOHNSON,NEXT STEP PROSOBEE, prepared from powder	30.5	1 fl oz	20	2.46
Infant formula, NESTLE, GOOD START ESSENTIALS SOY, with iron, powder	8.5	1 scoop	43	4.73
Infant formula, NESTLE, GOOD START SOY, with ARA and DHA, powder	9.4	1 scoop	47	5.23

Food Name ---> per serving	Weight (g)	Measure	Calories	Net Carb (g)
Infant formula, NESTLE, GOOD START SOY, with DHA and ARA, liquid concentrate	29.2	1 fl oz	39	4.3
Infant formula, NESTLE, GOOD START SOY, with DHA and ARA, ready-to-feed	29	1 oz	19	2.07
Infant formula, NESTLE, GOOD START SUPREME, with iron, DHA and ARA, prepared from liquid concentrate	31.4	1 fl oz	21	2.32
Infant formula, NESTLE, GOOD START SUPREME, with iron, DHA and ARA, ready-to-feed	30.5	1 fl oz	20	2.25
Infant formula, NESTLE, GOOD START SUPREME, with iron, liquid concentrate, not reconstituted	31.4	1 fl oz	40	4.46
Infant formula, NESTLE, GOOD START SUPREME, with iron, powder	8.7	1 scoop	44	4.99
Infant formula, PBM PRODUCTS, store brand, liquid concentrate, not reconstituted	31.4	1 fl oz	41	4.36
Infant formula, PBM PRODUCTS, store brand, powder	8.4	1 scoop	44	4.7
Infant formula, PBM PRODUCTS, store brand, ready-to-feed	30.4	1 fl oz	19	1.94
Infant formula, PBM PRODUCTS, store brand, soy, liquid concentrate, not reconstituted	31.4	1 fl oz	40	3.82
Infant formula, PBM PRODUCTS, store brand, soy, powder	8.7	1 scoop	44	4.54
Infant formula, PBM PRODUCTS, store brand, soy, ready-to-feed	30.4	1 fl oz	19	1.85
Toddler drink, MEAD JOHNSON, PurAmino Toddler Powder, with ARA and DHA, not reconstituted	7.2	1 scoop	37	4.01
Toddler formula, MEAD JOHNSON, ENFAGROW PREMIUM (formerly ENFAMIL, LIPIL, NEXT STEP), ready-to-feed	29.2	1 fl oz	19	2.1
Toddler formula, MEAD JOHNSON, ENFAGROW, Toddler Transitions, with ARA and DHA, powder	9	1 scoop	45	4.75
Toddler formula, MEAD JOHNSON, Nutramigen Toddler with LGG Powder, with ARA and DHA, not reconstituted	9.3	1 scoop	45	5.76
Zwieback	28.35	1 oz	121	20.34

Beef and Beef Products

Food Name ---> per 100 g	Protein (g)	Fat (g)	Calories	Net Carb (g)
Beef, grass-fed, strip steaks, lean only, raw	23.07	2.69	117	0
Beef, carcass, separable lean and fat, choice, raw	17.32	24.05	291	0
Beef, carcass, separable lean and fat, select, raw	17.48	22.55	278	0
Beef, retail cuts, separable fat, raw	8.21	70.89	674	0
Beef, retail cuts, separable fat, cooked	10.65	70.33	680	0
Beef, brisket, whole, separable lean only, all grades, raw	20.72	7.37	155	0
Beef, grass-fed, ground, raw	19.42	12.73	198	0
Beef, brisket, flat half, separable lean and fat, trimmed to 1/8" fat, select, cooked, braised	28.97	17.37	280	0
Beef, flank, steak, separable lean and fat, trimmed to 0" fat, choice, raw	21.22	8.29	165	0
Beef, flank, steak, separable lean and fat, trimmed to 0" fat, choice, cooked, braised	26.98	16.44	263	0
Beef, flank, steak, separable lean and fat, trimmed to 0" fat, choice, cooked, broiled	27.55	9.31	202	0
Beef, flank, steak, separable lean only, trimmed to 0" fat, choice, raw	21.72	6.29	149	0
Beef, flank, steak, separable lean only, trimmed to 0" fat, choice, cooked, braised	28.02	13	237	0
Beef, flank, steak, separable lean only, trimmed to 0" fat, choice, cooked, broiled	27.82	8.32	194	0
Beef, rib, eye, small end (ribs 10-12), separable lean and fat, trimmed to 0" fat, choice, raw	17.51	22.07	274	0
Beef, rib, eye, small end (ribs 10-12), separable lean and fat, trimmed to 0" fat, choice, cooked, broiled	26.58	16.76	265	0
Beef, rib, eye, small end (ribs 10-12), separable lean only, trimmed to 0" fat, choice, raw	20.13	8.3	161	0
Beef, rib, eye, small end (ribs 10-12), separable lean only, trimmed to 0" fat, choice, cooked, broiled	28.88	9.01	205	0
Beef, rib, shortribs, separable lean and fat, choice, raw	14.4	36.23	388	0
Beef, rib, shortribs, separable lean and fat, choice, cooked, braised	21.57	41.98	471	0

Food Name ---> per 100 g	Protein (g)	Fat (g)	Calories	Net Carb (g)
Beef, rib, shortribs, separable lean only, choice, raw	19.05	10.19	173	0
Beef, rib, shortribs, separable lean only, choice, cooked, braised	30.76	18.13	295	0
Beef, round, full cut, separable lean only, trimmed to 1/4" fat, choice, cooked, broiled	29.21	7.31	191	0
Beef, round, full cut, separable lean only, trimmed to 1/4" fat, select, cooked, broiled	29.25	5.22	172	0
Beef, brisket, flat half, separable lean and fat, trimmed to 0" fat, choice, cooked, braised	32.21	9.24	221	0
USDA Commodity, beef, canned	20.52	17.57	246	0
Beef, shank crosscuts, separable lean only, trimmed to 1/4" fat, choice, raw	21.75	3.85	128	0
Beef, shank crosscuts, separable lean only, trimmed to 1/4" fat, choice, cooked, simmered	33.68	6.36	201	0
Beef, short loin, porterhouse steak, separable lean only, trimmed to 1/8" fat, choice, raw	22.13	7.39	161	0
Beef, short loin, porterhouse steak, separable lean only, trimmed to 1/8" fat, choice, cooked, grilled	27.65	11.36	221	0
Beef, short loin, t-bone steak, bone-in, separable lean only, trimmed to 1/8" fat, choice, raw	22.1	7.27	160	0
Beef, short loin, t-bone steak, bone-in, separable lean only, trimmed to 1/8" fat, choice, cooked, grilled	27.48	11.05	217	0
Beef, rib eye, small end (ribs 10-12), separable lean only, trimmed to 0" fat, select, raw	21.17	6.57	149	0
Beef, chuck, under blade pot roast, boneless, separable lean only, trimmed to 0" fat, all grades, cooked, braised	30.54	10.46	216	0
Beef, chuck, under blade pot roast or steak, boneless, separable lean only, trimmed to 0" fat, all grades, raw	21.13	6.07	140	0.31
Beef, chuck, under blade pot roast or steak, boneless, separable lean only, trimmed to 0" fat, choice, raw	21.19	6.51	145	0.39
Beef, ground, patties, frozen, cooked, broiled	23.05	21.83	295	0
Beef, variety meats and by-products, brain, raw	10.86	10.3	143	1.05
Beef, variety meats and by-products, brain, cooked, pan-fried	12.57	15.83	196	0
Beef, variety meats and by-products, brain, cooked, simmered	11.67	10.53	151	1.48
Beef, variety meats and by-products, heart, raw	17.72	3.94	112	0.14
Beef, variety meats and by-products, heart, cooked, simmered	28.48	4.73	165	0.15
Beef, variety meats and by-products, kidneys, raw	17.4	3.09	99	0.29

Food Name ---> per 100 g	Protein (g)	Fat (g)	Calories	Net Carb (g)
Beef, variety meats and by-products, kidneys, cooked, simmered	27.27	4.65	158	0
Beef, variety meats and by-products, liver, raw	20.36	3.63	135	3.89
Beef, variety meats and by-products, liver, cooked, braised	29.08	5.26	191	5.13
Beef, variety meats and by-products, liver, cooked, pan-fried	26.52	4.68	175	5.16
Beef, variety meats and by-products, lungs, raw	16.2	2.5	92	0
Beef, variety meats and by-products, lungs, cooked, braised	20.4	3.7	120	0
Beef, variety meats and by-products, mechanically separated beef, raw	14.97	23.52	276	0
Beef, variety meats and by-products, pancreas, raw	15.7	18.6	235	0
Beef, variety meats and by-products, pancreas, cooked, braised	27.1	17.2	271	0
Beef, variety meats and by-products, spleen, raw	18.3	3	105	0
Beef, variety meats and by-products, spleen, cooked, braised	25.1	4.2	145	0
Beef, variety meats and by-products, suet, raw	1.5	94	854	0
Beef, variety meats and by-products, thymus, raw	12.18	20.35	236	0
Beef, variety meats and by-products, thymus, cooked, braised	21.85	24.98	319	0
Beef, variety meats and by-products, tongue, raw	14.9	16.09	224	3.68
Beef, variety meats and by-products, tongue, cooked, simmered	19.29	22.3	284	0
Beef, variety meats and by-products, tripe, raw	12.07	3.69	85	0
Beef, sandwich steaks, flaked, chopped, formed and thinly sliced, raw	16.5	27	309	0
Beef, brisket, flat half, separable lean only, trimmed to 0" fat, choice, cooked, braised	32.62	8.07	212	0
Beef, cured, breakfast strips, raw or unheated	12.5	38.8	406	0.7
Beef, cured, breakfast strips, cooked	31.3	34.4	449	1.4
Beef, cured, corned beef, brisket, raw	14.68	14.9	198	0.14
Beef, cured, corned beef, brisket, cooked	18.17	18.98	251	0.47
Beef, chuck, under blade pot roast or steak, boneless, separable lean only, trimmed to 0" fat, select, raw	21.03	5.41	134	0.19
Beef, chuck, under blade center steak, boneless, Denver Cut, separable lean only, trimmed to 0" fat, all grades, cooked, grilled	26.5	12.64	220	0.14
Beef, chuck, under blade center steak, boneless, Denver Cut, separable lean only, trimmed to 0" fat, choice, cooked, grilled	26.49	13.42	228	0.28
Beef, chuck, under blade center steak, boneless, Denver Cut, separable lean only, trimmed to 0" fat, select, cooked, grilled	26.53	11.46	209	0

Food Name ---> per 100 g	Protein (g)	Fat (g)	Calories	Net Carb (g)
Beef, chuck, under blade center steak, boneless, Denver Cut, separable lean only, trimmed to 0" fat, all grades, raw	19.42	9.99	170	0.49
Beef, chuck, under blade center steak, boneless, Denver Cut, separable lean only, trimmed to 0" fat, choice, raw	19.23	10.96	178	0.67
Beef, composite of trimmed retail cuts, separable lean and fat, trimmed to 0" fat, all grades, cooked	28.4	12.42	230	0
Beef, composite of trimmed retail cuts, separable lean and fat, trimmed to 0" fat, choice, cooked	28.17	12.53	233	0
Beef, composite of trimmed retail cuts, separable lean and fat, trimmed to 0" fat, select, cooked	28.61	9.18	203	0
Beef, composite of trimmed retail cuts, separable lean only, trimmed to 0" fat, all grades, cooked	29.9	8.37	203	0
Beef, composite of trimmed retail cuts, separable lean only, trimmed to 0" fat, choice, cooked	29.51	8.87	206	0
Beef, composite of trimmed retail cuts, separable lean only, trimmed to 0" fat, select, cooked	29.88	7.12	188	0
Beef, brisket, whole, separable lean and fat, trimmed to 0" fat, all grades, cooked, braised	26.79	19.52	291	0
Beef, brisket, whole, separable lean only, trimmed to 0" fat, all grades, cooked, braised	29.75	10.08	218	0
Beef, brisket, flat half, separable lean and fat, trimmed to 0" fat, all grades, cooked, braised	32.9	8.01	213	0
Beef, brisket, flat half, separable lean only, trimmed to 0" fat, all grades, cooked, braised	33.26	6.99	205	0
Beef, brisket, point half, separable lean and fat, trimmed to 0" fat, all grades, cooked, braised	23.53	28.5	358	0
Beef, brisket, point half, separable lean only, trimmed to 0" fat, all grades, cooked, braised	28.05	13.8	244	0
Beef, chuck, arm pot roast, separable lean and fat, trimmed to 0" fat, all grades, cooked, braised	28.94	19.17	297	0
Beef, chuck, arm pot roast, separable lean and fat, trimmed to 0" fat, select, cooked, braised	29.23	17.56	283	0
Beef, chuck, arm pot roast, separable lean only, trimmed to 0" fat, choice, cooked, braised	33.36	7.67	212	0
Beef, chuck, arm pot roast, separable lean only, trimmed to 0" fat, select, cooked, braised	33.37	5.8	195	0
Beef, chuck, blade roast, separable lean and fat, trimmed to 0" fat, all grades, cooked, braised	27.18	24.14	334	0

Food Name ---> per 100 g	Protein (g)	Fat (g)	Calories	Net Carb (g)
Beef, chuck, under blade pot roast, boneless, separable lean and fat, trimmed to 0" fat, choice, cooked, braised	26.39	21.48	306	0
Beef, chuck, under blade pot roast, boneless, separable lean and fat, trimmed to 0" fat, select, cooked, braised	27.17	19.02	288	0
Beef, chuck, blade roast, separable lean only, trimmed to 0" fat, all grades, cooked, braised	31.06	13.3	253	0
Beef, chuck, under blade pot roast, boneless, separable lean only, trimmed to 0" fat, choice, cooked, braised	30.45	11.14	231	0
Beef, chuck, under blade pot roast, boneless, separable lean only, trimmed to 0" fat, select, cooked, braised	30.68	9.44	216	0
Beef, rib, large end (ribs 6-9), separable lean and fat, trimmed to 0" fat, choice, cooked, roasted	22.8	30.49	372	0
Beef, rib, large end (ribs 6-9), separable lean and fat, trimmed to 0" fat, select, cooked, roasted	23.48	25.54	331	0
Beef, rib, large end (ribs 6-9), separable lean only, trimmed to 0" fat, all grades, cooked, roasted	27.53	13.4	238	0
Beef, rib, large end (ribs 6-9), separable lean only, trimmed to 0" fat, choice, cooked, roasted	27.53	15	253	0
Beef, rib, large end (ribs 6-9), separable lean only, trimmed to 0" fat, select, cooked, roasted	27.53	11.4	220	0
Beef, rib, small end (ribs 10-12), separable lean and fat, trimmed to 0" fat, all grades, cooked, broiled	27.27	14.74	249	0
Beef, rib, small end (ribs 10-12), separable lean and fat, trimmed to 0" fat, choice, cooked, broiled	24.73	22.84	312	0
Beef, rib, small end (ribs 10-12), separable lean and fat, trimmed to 0" fat, select, cooked, broiled	24.91	19.79	285	0
Beef, rib, small end (ribs 10-12), separable lean only, trimmed to 0" fat, all grades, cooked, broiled	29.41	7.53	193	0
Beef, rib, small end (ribs 10-12), separable lean only, trimmed to 0" fat, choice, cooked, broiled	28.04	11.7	225	0
Beef, rib, small end (ribs 10-12), separable lean only, trimmed to 0" fat, select, cooked, broiled	28.04	8.7	198	0
Beef, round, bottom round, steak, separable lean and fat, trimmed to 0" fat, all grades, cooked, braised	33.56	8.86	223	0
Beef, round, bottom round, roast, separable lean and fat, trimmed to 0" fat, all grades, cooked, roasted	27.42	7.72	187	0
Beef, round, bottom round, steak, separable lean and fat, trimmed to 0" fat, choice, cooked, braised	32.73	10	230	0

Food Name ---> per 100 g	Protein (g)	Fat (g)	Calories	Net Carb (g)
Beef, round, bottom round, roast, separable lean and fat, trimmed to 0" fat, choice, cooked, roasted	26.76	9.37	199	0
Beef, round, bottom round, steak, separable lean and fat, trimmed to 0" fat, select, cooked, braised	34.39	7.72	217	0
Beef, round, bottom round, roast, separable lean and fat, trimmed to 0" fat, select, cooked, roasted	28.08	6.06	175	0
Beef, round, bottom round, steak, separable lean only, trimmed to 0" fat, all grades, cooked, braised	34	7.67	214	0
Beef, round, bottom round, roast, separable lean only, trimmed to 0" fat, all grades, cooked, roasted	27.76	6.48	177	0
Beef, round, bottom round, steak, separable lean only, trimmed to 0" fat, choice, cooked, braised	33.08	9.03	223	0
Beef, round, bottom round, roast, separable lean only, trimmed to 0" fat, choice, cooked, roasted	27.23	7.63	185	0
Beef, round, bottom round, steak, separable lean only, trimmed to 0" fat, select, cooked, braised	34.93	6.3	206	0
Beef, round, bottom round roast, separable lean only, trimmed to 0" fat, select, cooked, roasted	28.29	5.33	169	0
Beef, round, eye of round roast, boneless, separable lean and fat, trimmed to 0" fat, all grades, cooked, roasted	29.66	4.46	167	0
Beef, round, eye of round roast, boneless, separable lean and fat, trimmed to 0" fat, choice, cooked, roasted	29.79	4.83	171	0
Beef, round, eye of round roast, boneless, separable lean and fat, trimmed to 0" fat, select, cooked, roasted	29.45	3.97	162	0
Beef, round, eye of round roast, boneless, separable lean only, trimmed to 0" fat, all grades, cooked, roasted	29.85	3.9	163	0
Beef, round, eye of round roast, boneless, separable lean only, trimmed to 0" fat, choice, cooked, roasted	29.94	4.26	166	0
Beef, round, eye of round roast, boneless, separable lean only, trimmed to 0" fat, select, cooked, roasted	29.52	3.43	157	0
Beef, round, tip round, roast, separable lean and fat, trimmed to 0" fat, all grades, cooked, roasted	26.79	8.21	188	0
Beef, round, tip round, roast, separable lean and fat, trimmed to 0" fat, choice, cooked, roasted	27.01	8.9	196	0
Beef, round, tip round, roast, separable lean and fat, trimmed to 0" fat, select, cooked, roasted	26.57	7.53	181	0
Beef, round, tip round, roast, separable lean only, trimmed to 0" fat, all grades, cooked, roasted	27.53	6.2	174	0

Food Name ---> per 100 g	Protein (g)	Fat (g)	Calories	Net Carb (g)
Beef, round, tip round, roast, separable lean only, trimmed to 0" fat, choice, cooked, roasted	27.68	6.42	176	0
Beef, round, tip round, roast, separable lean only, trimmed to 0" fat, select, cooked, roasted	27.37	4.38	149	0
Beef, round, top round, separable lean and fat, trimmed to 0" fat, all grades, cooked, braised	35.62	6.31	209	0
Beef, round, top round, separable lean and fat, trimmed to 0" fat, choice, cooked, braised	35.62	7.09	216	0
Beef, round, top round, separable lean and fat, trimmed to 0" fat, select, cooked, braised	35.62	5.33	200	0
Beef, round, top round, separable lean only, trimmed to 0" fat, choice, cooked, braised	36.12	5.8	207	0
Beef, round, top round, separable lean only, trimmed to 0" fat, select, cooked, braised	36.12	4	190	0
Beef, loin, tenderloin steak, boneless, separable lean and fat, trimmed to 0" fat, all grades, cooked, grilled	30.5	8.91	211	0
Beef, loin, tenderloin steak, boneless, separable lean and fat, trimmed to 0" fat, choice, cooked, grilled	30.21	9.71	217	0
Beef, loin, tenderloin steak, boneless, separable lean and fat, trimmed to 0" fat, select, cooked, grilled	30.93	7.7	202	0
Beef, loin, tenderloin steak, boneless, separable lean only, trimmed to 0" fat, all grades, cooked, grilled	30.7	8.32	198	0
Beef, loin, tenderloin steak, boneless, separable lean only, trimmed to 0" fat, choice, cooked, grilled	30.45	9.03	211	0
Beef, loin, tenderloin steak, boneless, separable lean only, trimmed to 0" fat, select, cooked, grilled	31.09	7.25	198	0
Beef, loin, top loin steak, boneless, lip off, separable lean and fat, trimmed to 0" fat, all grades, cooked, grilled	28.57	11.15	223	0
Beef, loin, top loin steak, boneless, lip off, separable lean and fat, trimmed to 0" fat, choice, cooked, grilled	28.19	12.51	233	0
Beef, loin, top loin steak, boneless, lip off, separable lean and fat, trimmed to 0" fat, select, cooked, grilled	29.16	9.12	207	0
Beef, loin, top loin steak, boneless, lip off, separable lean only, trimmed to 0" fat, all grades, cooked, grilled	29.53	8.41	202	0
Beef, loin, top loin steak, boneless, lip off, separable lean only, trimmed to 0" fat, choice, cooked, grilled	29.22	9.52	211	0
Beef, loin, top loin steak, boneless, lip off, separable lean only, trimmed to 0" fat, select, cooked, grilled	29.99	6.74	189	0

Food Name ---> per 100 g	Protein (g)	Fat (g)	Calories	Net Carb (g)
Beef, top sirloin, steak, separable lean and fat, trimmed to 0" fat, all grades, cooked, broiled	29.33	9.67	212	0
Beef, top sirloin, steak, separable lean and fat, trimmed to 0" fat, choice, cooked, broiled	29.02	10.54	219	0
Beef, top sirloin, steak, separable lean and fat, trimmed to 0" fat, select, cooked, broiled	29.65	8.8	206	0
Beef, top sirloin, steak, separable lean only, trimmed to 0" fat, all grades, cooked, broiled	30.55	5.79	183	0
Beef, top sirloin, steak, separable lean only, trimmed to 0" fat, choice, cooked, broiled	30.29	6.55	188	0
Beef, top sirloin, steak, separable lean only, trimmed to 0" fat, select, cooked, broiled	30.8	5.03	177	0
Beef, short loin, porterhouse steak, separable lean and fat, trimmed to 0" fat, all grades, cooked, broiled	23.96	19.27	276	0
Beef, short loin, porterhouse steak, separable lean and fat, trimmed to 0" fat, USDA choice, cooked, broiled	23.61	20.15	283	0
Beef, short loin, porterhouse steak, separable lean and fat, trimmed to 0" fat, USDA select, cooked, broiled	24.47	17.98	267	0
Beef, short loin, porterhouse steak, separable lean only, trimmed to 1/8" fat, all grades, raw	22.32	6.6	155	0
Beef, short loin, porterhouse steak, separable lean only, trimmed to 1/8" fat, all grades, cooked, grilled	28.16	10.32	213	0
Beef, short loin, porterhouse steak, separable lean only, trimmed to 0" fat, all grades, cooked, broiled	26.07	11.18	212	0
Beef, short loin, porterhouse steak, separable lean only, trimmed to 0" fat, choice, cooked, broiled	25.51	12.8	224	0
Beef, short loin, porterhouse steak, separable lean only, trimmed to 1/8" fat, select, raw	22.61	5.41	145	0
Beef, short loin, porterhouse steak, separable lean only, trimmed to 1/8" fat, select, cooked, grilled	28.92	8.76	203	0
Beef, short loin, porterhouse steak, separable lean only, trimmed to 0" fat, select, cooked, broiled	26.89	8.81	194	0
Beef, short loin, t-bone steak, separable lean and fat, trimmed to 0" fat, all grades, cooked, broiled	24.18	15.93	247	0
Beef, short loin, t-bone steak, separable lean and fat, trimmed to 0" fat, USDA choice, cooked, broiled	24.05	17.26	258	0
Beef, short loin, t-bone steak, separable lean and fat, trimmed to 0" fat, USDA select, cooked, broiled	24.38	14	230	0

Food Name ---> per 100 g	Protein (g)	Fat (g)	Calories	Net Carb (g)
Beef, short loin, t-bone steak, bone-in, separable lean only, trimmed to 1/8" fat, all grades, raw	22.22	6.5	153	0
Beef, short loin, t-bone steak, bone-in, separable lean only, trimmed to 1/8" fat, all grades, cooked, grilled	27.86	10.37	212	0
Beef, short loin, t-bone steak, separable lean only, trimmed to 0" fat, choice, cooked, broiled	25.98	9.61	198	0
Beef, short loin, t-bone steak, bone-in, separable lean only, trimmed to 1/8" fat, select, raw	22.41	5.34	144	0
Beef, short loin, t-bone steak, bone-in, separable lean only, trimmed to 1/8" fat, select, cooked, grilled	28.45	9.35	206	0
Beef, short loin, t-bone steak, separable lean only, trimmed to 0" fat, select, cooked, broiled	26	7.36	177	0
Beef, brisket, flat half, separable lean only, trimmed to 0" fat, select, cooked, braised	33.9	5.92	198	0
Beef, round, tip round, roast, separable lean and fat, trimmed to 0" fat, all grades, raw	20.48	7.01	151	0
Beef, round, tip round, roast, separable lean and fat, trimmed to 0" fat, choice, raw	20.16	7.73	156	0
Beef, round, tip round, roast, separable lean and fat, trimmed to 0" fat, select, raw	20.8	6.28	145	0
Beef, rib, eye, small end (ribs 10- 12) separable lean only, trimmed to 0" fat, select, cooked, broiled	29.93	6.05	182	0
Beef, round, top round steak, boneless, separable lean only, trimmed to 0" fat, all grades, cooked, grilled	30.09	3.77	162	0
Beef, round, top round steak, boneless, separable lean only, trimmed to 0" fat, choice, cooked, grilled	30.24	4.11	166	0
Beef, round, top round steak, boneless, separable lean only, trimmed to 0" fat, select, cooked, grilled	29.81	3.37	158	0
Beef, ground, 70% lean meat / 30% fat, crumbles, cooked, pan-browned	25.56	17.86	270	0
Beef, ground, 70% lean meat / 30% fat, loaf, cooked, baked	23.87	15.37	241	0
Beef, ground, 70% lean meat / 30% fat, patty cooked, pan-broiled	22.86	15.54	238	0
Beef, ground, 70% lean meat / 30% fat, patty, cooked, broiled	25.38	18.66	277	0
Beef, ground, 70% lean meat / 30% fat, raw	14.35	30	332	0
Beef, chuck, under blade center steak, boneless, Denver Cut, separable lean only, trimmed to 0" fat, select, raw	19.71	8.54	157	0.21
Beef, shoulder top blade steak, boneless, separable lean only, trimmed to 0" fat, all grades, cooked, grilled	28.15	9.23	196	0

Food Name ---> per 100 g	Protein (g)	Fat (g)	Calories	Net Carb (g)
Beef, shoulder top blade steak, boneless, separable lean only, trimmed to 0" fat, choice, cooked, grilled	28.28	9.83	202	0
Beef, shoulder top blade steak, boneless, separable lean only, trimmed to 0" fat, select, cooked, grilled	27.96	8.34	187	0
Beef, shoulder top blade steak, boneless, separable lean only, trimmed to 0" fat, all grades, raw	20.36	6.42	139	0
Beef, shoulder top blade steak, boneless, separable lean only, trimmed to 0" fat, choice, raw	20.35	6.88	143	0
Beef, shoulder top blade steak, boneless, separable lean only, trimmed to 0" fat, select, raw	20.39	5.73	133	0
Beef, brisket, flat half, boneless separable lean only, trimmed to 0" fat, all grades, raw	21.47	5.11	132	0
Beef, brisket, flat half, boneless, separable lean only, trimmed to 0" fat, choice, raw	21.28	5.75	137	0
Beef, brisket, flat half, boneless, separable lean only, trimmed to 0" fat, select, raw	21.74	4.14	124	0
Beef, shoulder top blade steak, boneless, separable lean and fat, trimmed to 0" fat, all grades, cooked, grilled	27.59	11.07	210	0
Beef, shoulder pot roast or steak, boneless, separable lean only, trimmed to 0" fat, all grades, raw	21.64	4.09	123	0
Beef, shoulder pot roast or steak, boneless, separable lean only, trimmed to 0" fat, choice, raw	21.45	4.35	125	0.11
Beef, shoulder pot roast or steak, boneless, separable lean only, trimmed to 0" fat, select, raw	21.93	3.7	121	0
Beef, shoulder top blade steak, boneless, separable lean and fat, trimmed to 0" fat, choice, cooked, grilled	27.51	12.26	220	0
Beef, chuck eye roast, boneless, America's Beef Roast, separable lean and fat, trimmed to 0" fat, all grades, raw	19.18	11.48	180	0
Beef, chuck eye roast, boneless, America's Beef Roast, separable lean and fat, trimmed to 0" fat, choice, raw	19.14	12.02	185	0
Beef, chuck eye roast, boneless, America's Beef Roast, separable lean and fat, trimmed to 0" fat, select, raw	19.25	10.67	173	0
Beef, composite of trimmed retail cuts, separable lean and fat, trimmed to 1/8" fat, all grades, raw	20.01	14.42	214	0
Beef, composite of trimmed retail cuts, separable lean and fat, trimmed to 1/8" fat, all grades, cooked	26.11	16.59	259	0
Beef, composite of trimmed retail cuts, separable lean and fat, trimmed to 1/8" fat, choice, raw	19.79	15.42	222	0

Food Name ---> per 100 g	Protein (g)	Fat (g)	Calories	Net Carb (g)
Beef, composite of trimmed retail cuts, separable lean and fat, trimmed to 1/8" fat, choice, cooked	25.85	17.68	268	0
Beef, composite of trimmed retail cuts, separable lean and fat, trimmed to 1/8" fat, select, raw	19.06	12.4	192	0
Beef, composite of trimmed retail cuts, separable lean and fat, trimmed to 1/8" fat, select, cooked	26.06	15.09	245	0
Beef, brisket, whole, separable lean and fat, trimmed to 1/8" fat, all grades, raw	18.42	19.06	251	0
Beef, brisket, whole, separable lean and fat, trimmed to 1/8" fat, all grades, cooked, braised	25.85	24.5	331	0
Beef, brisket, flat half, separable lean and fat, trimmed to 1/8" fat, all grades, raw	17.94	22.18	277	0
Beef, brisket, flat half, separable lean and fat, trimmed to 1/8" fat, all grades, cooked, braised	28.82	18.42	289	0
Beef, brisket, point half, separable lean and fat, trimmed to 1/8" fat, all grades, raw	17.65	20.98	265	0
Beef, brisket, point half, separable lean and fat, trimmed to 1/8" fat, all grades, cooked, braised	24.4	27.17	349	0
Beef, chuck, arm pot roast, separable lean and fat, trimmed to 1/8" fat, all grades, raw	19.23	17.98	244	0
Beef, chuck, arm pot roast, separable lean and fat, trimmed to 1/8" fat, all grades, cooked, braised	30.12	19.22	302	0
Beef, chuck, arm pot roast, separable lean and fat, trimmed to 1/8" fat, choice, raw	19.14	18.57	249	0
Beef, chuck, arm pot roast, separable lean and fat, trimmed to 1/8" fat, choice, cooked, braised	30.2	19.93	309	0
Beef, chuck, arm pot roast, separable lean and fat, trimmed to 1/8" fat, select, raw	19.33	17.39	239	0
Beef, chuck, arm pot roast, separable lean and fat, trimmed to 1/8" fat, select, cooked, braised	30.05	18.5	295	0
Beef, chuck, blade roast, separable lean and fat, trimmed to 1/8" fat, all grades, raw	17.16	19.41	248	0
Beef, chuck, blade roast, separable lean and fat, trimmed to 1/8" fat, all grades, cooked, braised	26.78	25.12	341	0
Beef, chuck, blade roast, separable lean and fat, trimmed to 1/8" fat, choice, raw	16.98	21.31	265	0
Beef, chuck, blade roast, separable lean and fat, trimmed to 1/8" fat, choice, cooked, braised	26.37	27.26	359	0

Food Name ---> per 100 g	Protein (g)	Fat (g)	Calories	Net Carb (g)
Beef, chuck, blade roast, separable lean and fat, trimmed to 1/8" fat, select, raw	17.37	17.33	230	0
Beef, chuck, blade roast, separable lean and fat, trimmed to 1/8" fat, select, cooked, braised	27.33	22.35	318	0
Beef, chuck eye roast, boneless, America's Beef Roast, separable lean only, trimmed to 0" fat, all grades, cooked, roasted	26.65	8.46	183	0
Beef, chuck eye roast, boneless, America's Beef Roast, separable lean only, trimmed to 0" fat, choice, cooked, roasted	26.41	9.36	190	0
Beef, chuck eye roast, boneless, America's Beef Roast, separable lean only, trimmed to 0" fat, select, cooked, roasted	27.02	7.12	172	0
Beef, rib, whole (ribs 6-12), separable lean and fat, trimmed to 1/8" fat, all grades, raw	16.53	26.1	306	0
Beef, rib, whole (ribs 6-12), separable lean and fat, trimmed to 1/8" fat, all grades, cooked, broiled	22.42	26.75	337	0
Beef, rib, whole (ribs 6-12), separable lean and fat, trimmed to 1/8" fat, all grades, cooked, roasted	22.77	28.11	351	0
Beef, rib, whole (ribs 6-12), separable lean and fat, trimmed to 1/8" fat, choice, raw	16.34	27.93	322	0
Beef, rib, whole (ribs 6-12), separable lean and fat, trimmed to 1/8" fat, choice, cooked, broiled	22.26	28.5	352	0
Beef, rib, whole (ribs 6-12), separable lean and fat, trimmed to 1/8" fat, choice, cooked, roasted	22.6	29.79	365	0
Beef, rib, whole (ribs 6-12), separable lean and fat, trimmed to 1/8" fat, select, raw	16.75	23.95	288	0
Beef, rib, whole (ribs 6-12), separable lean and fat, trimmed to 1/8" fat, select, cooked, broiled	22.73	24.2	315	0
Beef, rib, whole (ribs 6-12), separable lean and fat, trimmed to 1/8" fat, select, cooked, roasted	23.1	25.63	330	0
Beef, rib, whole (ribs 6-12), separable lean and fat, trimmed to 1/8" fat, prime, raw	16.15	31.66	355	0
Beef, rib, whole (ribs 6-12), separable lean and fat, trimmed to 1/8" fat, prime, cooked, broiled	21.95	32.38	386	0
Beef, rib, whole (ribs 6-12), separable lean and fat, trimmed to 1/8" fat, prime, cooked, roasted	22.57	33.7	400	0
Beef, rib, large end (ribs 6-9), separable lean and fat, trimmed to 1/8" fat, all grades, raw	16.26	27.29	316	0
Beef, rib, large end (ribs 6-9), separable lean and fat, trimmed to 1/8" fat, all grades, cooked, broiled	21.55	27.22	338	0

Food Name ---> per 100 g	Protein (g)	Fat (g)	Calories	Net Carb (g)
Beef, rib, large end (ribs 6-9), separable lean and fat, trimmed to 1/8" fat, all grades, cooked, roasted	23.01	28.51	355	0
Beef, rib, large end (ribs 6-9), separable lean and fat, trimmed to 1/8" fat, choice, raw	16.03	29.34	333	0
Beef, rib, large end (ribs 6-9), separable lean and fat, trimmed to 1/8" fat, choice, cooked, broiled	20.86	31.18	370	0
Beef, rib, large end (ribs 6-9), separable lean and fat, trimmed to 1/8" fat, choice, cooked, roasted	22.5	31.28	378	0
Beef, rib, large end (ribs 6-9), separable lean and fat, trimmed to 1/8" fat, select, raw	16.52	24.85	295	0
Beef, rib, large end (ribs 6-9), separable lean and fat, trimmed to 1/8" fat, select, cooked, broiled	21.55	25.71	324	0
Beef, rib, large end (ribs 6-9), separable lean and fat, trimmed to 1/8" fat, select, cooked, roasted	23.4	25.84	333	0
Beef, rib, large end (ribs 6-9), separable lean and fat, trimmed to 1/8" fat, prime, raw	15.77	33.26	367	0
Beef, rib, large end (ribs 6-9), separable lean and fat, trimmed to 1/8" fat, prime, cooked, broiled	20.65	34.97	404	0
Beef, rib, large end (ribs 6-9), separable lean and fat, trimmed to 1/8" fat, prime, cooked, roasted	22.86	32.74	393	0
Beef, rib, small end (ribs 10-12), separable lean and fat, trimmed to 1/8" fat, all grades, raw	19.33	19.06	254	0
Beef, rib, small end (ribs 10-12), separable lean and fat, trimmed to 1/8" fat, all grades, cooked, broiled	25.85	20.04	291	0
Beef, rib, small end (ribs 10-12), separable lean and fat, trimmed to 1/8" fat, all grades, cooked, roasted	22.54	27.14	341	0
Beef, rib, small end (ribs 10-12), separable lean and fat, trimmed to 1/8" fat, choice, raw	19.09	20.13	263	0
Beef, rib, small end (ribs 10-12), separable lean and fat, trimmed to 1/8" fat, choice, cooked, broiled	24.53	22.09	304	0
Beef, rib, small end (ribs 10-12), separable lean and fat, trimmed to 1/8" fat, choice, cooked, roasted	22.28	29.21	359	0
Beef, rib, small end (ribs 10-12), separable lean and fat, trimmed to 1/8" fat, select, raw	19.56	18	246	0
Beef, rib, small end (ribs 10-12), separable lean and fat, trimmed to 1/8" fat, select, cooked, broiled	27.17	18	278	0
Beef, rib, small end (ribs 10-12), separable lean and fat, trimmed to 1/8" fat, select, cooked, roasted	22.76	25.02	323	0

Food Name ---> per 100 g	Protein (g)	Fat (g)	Calories	Net Carb (g)
Beef, rib, small end (ribs 10-12), separable lean and fat, trimmed to 1/8" fat, prime, raw	16.74	29.18	335	0
Beef, rib, small end (ribs 10-12), separable lean and fat, trimmed to 1/8" fat, prime, cooked, broiled	24.13	27.86	354	0
Beef, rib, small end (ribs 10-12), separable lean and fat, trimmed to 1/8" fat, prime, cooked, roasted	22.15	35.12	411	0
Beef, shoulder top blade steak, boneless, separable lean and fat, trimmed to 0" fat, select, cooked, grilled	27.7	9.29	194	0
Beef, shoulder top blade steak, boneless, separable lean and fat, trimmed to 0" fat, all grades, raw	20.16	7.25	146	0
Beef, round, full cut, separable lean and fat, trimmed to 1/8" fat, choice, raw	20.56	11.92	195	0
Beef, round, full cut, separable lean and fat, trimmed to 1/8" fat, choice, cooked, broiled	27.54	12.98	235	0
Beef, round, full cut, separable lean and fat, trimmed to 1/8" fat, select, raw	20.56	10.68	184	0
Beef, round, full cut, separable lean and fat, trimmed to 1/8" fat, select, cooked, broiled	27.58	11.08	218	0
Beef, round, bottom round, steak, separable lean and fat, trimmed to 1/8" fat, all grades, raw	20.7	11.54	192	0
Beef, round, bottom round, steak, separable lean and fat, trimmed to 1/8" fat, all grades, cooked, braised	32.76	11.87	247	0
Beef, round, bottom round, roast, separable lean and fat, trimmed to 1/8" fat, all grades, cooked, roasted	26.41	11.64	218	0
Beef, round, bottom round, steak, separable lean and fat, trimmed to 1/8" fat, choice, raw	20.71	12.15	198	0
Beef, round, bottom round, steak, separable lean and fat, trimmed to 1/8" fat, choice, cooked, braised	32.85	12.56	254	0
Beef, round, bottom round, roast, separable lean and fat, trimmed to 1/8" fat, choice, cooked, roasted	26.05	12.44	223	0
Beef, round, bottom round, steak, separable lean and fat, trimmed to 1/8" fat, select, raw	20.68	10.93	187	0
Beef, round, bottom round, steak, separable lean and fat, trimmed to 1/8" fat, select, cooked, braised	32.67	11.19	240	0
Beef, round, bottom round, roast, separable lean and fat, trimmed to 1/8" fat, select, cooked, roasted	26.77	10.85	212	0
Beef, round, eye of round, roast, separable lean and fat, trimmed to 1/8" fat, all grades, raw	21.49	8.24	166	0

Food Name ---> per 100 g	Protein (g)	Fat (g)	Calories	Net Carb (g)
Beef, round, eye of round, roast, separable lean and fat, trimmed to 1/8" fat, all grades, cooked, roasted	28.31	9.65	208	0
Beef, round, eye of round, roast, separable lean and fat, trimmed to 1/8" fat, choice, raw	21.68	8.91	173	0
Beef, round, eye of round, roast, separable lean and fat, trimmed to 1/8" fat, choice, cooked, roasted	28.48	10.05	212	0
Beef, round, eye of round, roast, separable lean and fat, trimmed to 1/8" fat, select, raw	21.3	7.57	159	0
Beef, round, eye of round, roast, separable lean and fat, trimmed to 1/8" fat, select, cooked, roasted	28.13	9.26	204	0
Beef, round, tip round, separable lean and fat, trimmed to 1/8" fat, all grades, raw	19.6	11.67	189	0
Beef, round, tip round, roast, separable lean and fat, trimmed to 1/8" fat, all grades, cooked, roasted	27.45	11.34	219	0
Beef, round, tip round, separable lean and fat, trimmed to 1/8" fat, choice, raw	19.48	12.83	199	0
Beef, round, tip round, roast, separable lean and fat, trimmed to 1/8" fat, choice, cooked, roasted	27.27	12.34	228	0
Beef, round, tip round, separable lean and fat, trimmed to 1/8" fat, select, raw	19.74	10.39	178	0
Beef, round, tip round, roast, separable lean and fat, trimmed to 1/8" fat, select, cooked, roasted	27.63	10.24	210	0
Beef, shoulder top blade steak, boneless, separable lean and fat, trimmed to 0" fat, choice, raw	20.07	7.94	152	0
Beef, round, top round, separable lean only, trimmed to 1/8" fat, choice, cooked, pan-fried	33.93	8.33	228	2.03
Beef, round, top round, steak, separable lean and fat, trimmed to 1/8" fat, all grades, raw	22.06	7.93	166	0
Beef, round, top round, separable lean and fat, trimmed to 1/8" fat, all grades, cooked, braised	34.34	10.13	238	0
Beef, round, top round steak, separable lean and fat, trimmed to 1/8" fat, all grades, cooked, broiled	30.67	9	204	0
Beef, round, top round, steak, separable lean and fat, trimmed to 1/8" fat, choice, raw	21.94	8.19	168	0
Beef, round, top round, separable lean and fat, trimmed to 1/8" fat, choice, cooked, braised	34.09	11.61	250	0
Beef, round, top round, steak, separable lean and fat, trimmed to 1/8" fat, choice, cooked, broiled	30.7	10.27	224	0

Food Name ---> per 100 g	Protein (g)	Fat (g)	Calories	Net Carb (g)
Beef, round, top round, separable lean and fat, trimmed to 1/8" fat, choice, cooked, pan-fried	32.99	13.83	266	0
Beef, round, top round, steak, separable lean and fat, trimmed to 1/8" fat, select, raw	22.18	7.68	164	0
Beef, round, top round, separable lean and fat, trimmed to 1/8" fat, select, cooked, braised	34.6	8.54	225	0
Beef, round, top round, steak, separable lean and fat, trimmed to 1/8" fat, select, cooked, broiled	30.63	7.73	201	0
Beef, round, top round, separable lean and fat, trimmed to 1/8" fat, prime, raw	22.24	8.67	173	0
Beef, round, top round, steak, separable lean and fat, trimmed to 1/8" fat, prime, cooked, broiled	31.27	10.1	225	0
Beef, shoulder top blade steak, boneless, separable lean and fat, trimmed to 0" fat, select, raw	20.28	6.21	137	0
Beef, brisket, flat half, boneless, separable lean and fat, trimmed to 0" fat, all grades, raw	20.32	9.29	165	0
Beef, short loin, porterhouse steak, separable lean and fat, trimmed to 1/8" fat, choice, raw	20.36	14.58	218	0
Beef, short loin, porterhouse steak, separable lean and fat, trimmed to 1/8" fat, choice, cooked, grilled	24.85	19.78	284	0
Beef, short loin, t-bone steak, separable lean and fat, trimmed to 1/8" fat, choice, raw	20	15.83	228	0
Beef, short loin, t-bone steak, separable lean and fat, trimmed to 1/8" fat, choice, cooked, grilled	24.21	21.13	294	0
Beef, short loin, top loin, steak, separable lean and fat, trimmed to 1/8" fat, all grades, raw	20.61	15.49	228	0
Beef, loin, top loin, separable lean and fat, trimmed to 1/8" fat, all grades, cooked, grilled	26.44	16.78	264	0
Beef, loin, top loin, separable lean and fat, trimmed to 1/8" fat, choice, raw	19.32	17.1	237	0
Beef, short loin, top loin, steak, separable lean and fat, trimmed to 1/8" fat, choice, cooked, grilled	26.16	18.45	278	0
Beef, loin, top loin, separable lean and fat, trimmed to 1/8" fat, select, raw	20.59	15.04	224	0
Beef, loin, top loin, separable lean and fat, trimmed to 1/8" fat, select, cooked, grilled	26.72	15.11	250	0
Beef, short loin, top loin, steak, separable lean and fat, trimmed to 1/8" fat, prime, raw	19	22.17	281	0

Food Name ---> per 100 g	Protein (g)	Fat (g)	Calories	Net Carb (g)
Beef, short loin, top loin, separable lean and fat, trimmed to 1/8" fat, prime, cooked, broiled	25.92	22.12	310	0
Beef, tenderloin, steak, separable lean and fat, trimmed to 1/8" fat, all grades, raw	19.61	18.16	247	0
Beef, tenderloin, steak, separable lean and fat, trimmed to 1/8" fat, all grades, cooked, broiled	26.46	17.12	267	0
Beef, tenderloin, roast, separable lean and fat, trimmed to 1/8" fat, all grades, cooked, roasted	23.9	24.6	324	0
Beef, tenderloin, steak, separable lean and fat, trimmed to 1/8" fat, choice, raw	19.82	17.88	246	0
Beef, tenderloin, steak, separable lean and fat, trimmed to 1/8" fat, choice, cooked, broiled	26.43	17.78	273	0
Beef, tenderloin, roast, separable lean and fat, trimmed to 1/8" fat, choice, cooked, roasted	23.9	25.39	331	0
Beef, tenderloin, steak, separable lean and fat, trimmed to 1/8" fat, select, raw	19.37	18.46	249	0
Beef, tenderloin, steak, separable lean and fat, trimmed to 1/8" fat, select, cooked, broiled	26.48	16.53	262	0
Beef, tenderloin, roast, separable lean and fat, trimmed to 1/8" fat, select, cooked, roasted	23.9	23.7	316	0
Beef, tenderloin, separable lean and fat, trimmed to 1/8" fat, prime, raw	18.15	21.83	274	0
Beef, tenderloin, steak, separable lean and fat, trimmed to 1/8" fat, prime, cooked, broiled	25.26	22.21	308	0
Beef, tenderloin, roast, separable lean and fat, trimmed to 1/8" fat, prime, cooked, roasted	24.04	26.67	343	0
Beef, top sirloin, steak, separable lean and fat, trimmed to 1/8" fat, all grades, raw	20.3	12.71	201	0
Beef, top sirloin, steak, separable lean and fat, trimmed to 1/8" fat, all grades, cooked, broiled	26.96	14.23	243	0
Beef, top sirloin, steak, separable lean and fat, trimmed to 1/8" fat, choice, raw	19.92	14.28	214	0
Beef, top sirloin, steak, separable lean and fat, trimmed to 1/8" fat, choice, cooked, broiled	26.8	15.75	257	0
Beef, top sirloin, steak, separable lean and fat, trimmed to 1/8" fat, choice, cooked, pan-fried	28.77	21.06	313	0
Beef, top sirloin, steak, separable lean and fat, trimmed to 1/8" fat, select, raw	20.68	11.13	189	0

Food Name ---> per 100 g	Protein (g)	Fat (g)	Calories	Net Carb (g)
Beef, top sirloin, steak, separable lean and fat, trimmed to 1/8" fat, select, cooked, broiled	27.12	12.71	230	0
Beef, chuck, clod roast, separable lean only, trimmed to 0" fat, choice, cooked, roasted	25.95	6.69	171	0
Beef, chuck, clod roast, separable lean only, trimmed to 0" fat, select, cooked, roasted	28.09	5.82	172	0
Beef, shoulder steak, boneless, separable lean only, trimmed to 0" fat, choice, cooked, grilled	28.54	6.25	178	0
Beef, shoulder steak, boneless, separable lean only, trimmed to 0" fat, select, cooked, grilled	28.71	5.17	169	0
Beef, flank, steak, separable lean and fat, trimmed to 0" fat, all grades, cooked, broiled	27.66	8.23	192	0
Beef, flank, steak, separable lean and fat, trimmed to 0" fat, select, cooked, broiled	27.78	7.15	183	0
Beef, brisket, flat half, separable lean and fat, trimmed to 0" fat, select, cooked, braised	33.59	6.77	205	0
Beef, rib eye, small end (ribs 10-12), separable lean and fat, trimmed to 0" fat, select, cooked, broiled	27.95	12.71	234	0
Beef, rib eye, small end (ribs 10-12), separable lean and fat, trimmed to 0" fat, all grades, cooked, broiled	27.27	14.74	249	0
Beef, bottom sirloin, tri-tip roast, separable lean and fat, trimmed to 0" fat, all grades, cooked, roasted	26.05	11.07	211	0
Beef, bottom sirloin, tri-tip roast, separable lean and fat, trimmed to 0" fat, all grades, raw	20.64	8.55	165	0
Beef, bottom sirloin, tri-tip roast, separable lean and fat, trimmed to 0" fat, choice, cooked, roasted	25.66	12.36	221	0
Beef, bottom sirloin, tri-tip roast, separable lean and fat, trimmed to 0" fat, choice, raw	20.64	9.51	174	0
Beef, bottom sirloin, tri-tip roast, separable lean and fat, trimmed to 0" fat, select, cooked, roasted	26.44	9.78	201	0
Beef, bottom sirloin, tri-tip roast, separable lean and fat, trimmed to 0" fat, select, raw	20.64	7.68	157	0
Beef, round, top round steak, boneless, separable lean and fat, trimmed to 0" fat, all grades, cooked, grilled	29.96	4.28	167	0
Beef, chuck, mock tender steak, separable lean only, trimmed to 0" fat, choice, cooked, broiled	25.74	5.69	161	0
Beef, chuck, mock tender steak, separable lean only, trimmed to 0" fat, select, cooked, broiled	26.13	5.02	157	0

Food Name ---> per 100 g	Protein (g)	Fat (g)	Calories	Net Carb (g)
Beef, chuck, top blade, separable lean only, trimmed to 0" fat, choice, cooked, broiled	26.11	11.65	217	0
Beef, chuck, top blade, separable lean only, trimmed to 0" fat, select, cooked, broiled	26.16	8	184	0
Beef, round, top round steak, boneless, separable lean and fat, trimmed to 0" fat, choice, cooked, grilled	30.12	4.62	170	0
Beef, round, top round steak, boneless, separable lean and fat, trimmed to 0" fat, select, cooked, grilled	29.7	3.85	162	0
Beef, flank, steak, separable lean and fat, trimmed to 0" fat, all grades, raw	21.22	7.17	155	0
Beef, flank, steak, separable lean and fat, trimmed to 0" fat, select, raw	21.22	6.06	145	0
Beef, chuck eye roast, boneless, America's Beef Roast, separable lean only, trimmed to 0" fat, all grades, raw	20.61	6.01	137	0
Beef, chuck eye roast, boneless, America's Beef Roast, separable lean only, trimmed to 0" fat, choice, raw	20.67	6.21	139	0
Beef, chuck eye roast, boneless, America's Beef Roast, separable lean only, trimmed to 0" fat, select, raw	20.52	5.71	133	0
Beef, brisket, flat half, boneless, separable lean and fat, trimmed to 0" fat, choice, raw	20.15	9.86	169	0
Beef, plate, inside skirt steak, separable lean only, trimmed to 0" fat, all grades, cooked, broiled	26.66	10.06	205	0
Beef, plate, outside skirt steak, separable lean only, trimmed to 0" fat, all grades, cooked, broiled	24.18	14.37	233	0
Beef, chuck, short ribs, boneless, separable lean only, trimmed to 0" fat, choice, cooked, braised	28.84	14.95	250	0
Beef, chuck, short ribs, boneless, separable lean only, trimmed to 0" fat, select, cooked, braised	28.79	12.08	224	0
Beef, chuck, short ribs, boneless, separable lean only, trimmed to 0" fat, all grades, cooked, braised	28.82	13.8	240	0
Beef, brisket, flat half, boneless, separable lean and fat, trimmed to 0" fat, select, raw	20.57	8.45	158	0
Beef, loin, bottom sirloin butt, tri-tip roast, separable lean only, trimmed to 0" fat, all grades, cooked, roasted	26.75	8.34	182	0
Beef, shoulder pot roast or steak, boneless, separable lean and fat, trimmed to 0" fat, all grades, raw	21.39	4.97	130	0
Beef, short loin, porterhouse steak, separable lean and fat, trimmed to 1/8" fat, all grades, raw	20.49	14.06	214	0

Food Name ---> per 100 g	Protein (g)	Fat (g)	Calories	Net Carb (g)
Beef, short loin, porterhouse steak, separable lean and fat, trimmed to 1/8" fat, all grades, cooked, grilled	25.4	18.57	276	0
Beef, short loin, porterhouse steak, separable lean and fat, trimmed to 1/8" fat, select, raw	20.69	13.27	208	0
Beef, short loin, porterhouse steak, separable lean and fat, trimmed to 1/8" fat, select, cooked, grilled	26.21	16.75	263	0
Beef, short loin, t-bone steak, separable lean and fat, trimmed to 1/8" fat, all grades, raw	20.11	15.18	223	0
Beef, short loin, t-bone steak, separable lean and fat, trimmed to 1/8" fat, all grades, cooked, grilled	24.6	20.36	289	0
Beef, short loin, t-bone steak, separable lean and fat, trimmed to 1/8" fat, select, raw	20.28	14.19	215	0
Beef, short loin, t-bone steak, separable lean and fat, trimmed to 1/8" fat, select, cooked, grilled	25.18	19.22	281	0
Beef, round, knuckle, tip side, steak, separable lean and fat, trimmed to 0" fat, choice, raw	21.41	4.66	133	0
Beef, round, knuckle, tip side, steak, separable lean and fat, trimmed to 0" fat, choice, cooked, grilled	28.79	5.71	174	0
Beef, round, knuckle, tip side, steak, separable lean and fat, trimmed to 0" fat, select, raw	21.96	3.24	124	0
Beef, round, knuckle, tip side, steak, separable lean and fat, trimmed to 0" fat, select, cooked, grilled	29.24	3.91	160	0
Beef, chuck, shoulder clod, shoulder tender, medallion, separable lean and fat, trimmed to 0" fat, choice, raw	20.51	6.36	145	0
Beef, chuck, shoulder clod, shoulder tender, medallion, separable lean and fat, trimmed to 0" fat, choice, cooked, grilled	26.07	7.68	181	0
Beef, chuck, shoulder clod, shoulder tender, medallion, separable lean and fat, trimmed to 0" fat, select, raw	20.93	5.79	142	0
Beef, chuck, shoulder clod, shoulder top and center steaks, separable lean and fat, trimmed to 0" fat, choice, raw	20.39	6.12	143	0
Beef, chuck, shoulder clod, shoulder top and center steaks, separable lean and fat, trimmed to 0" fat, choice, cooked, grilled	26.07	8.11	184	0
Beef, chuck, shoulder clod, shoulder top and center steaks, separable lean and fat, trimmed to 0" fat, select, raw	21.13	5.51	140	0
Beef, chuck, shoulder clod, shoulder top and center steaks, separable lean and fat, trimmed to 0" fat, select, cooked, grilled	26.66	6.94	176	0
Beef, chuck, shoulder clod, top blade, steak, separable lean and fat, trimmed to 0" fat, choice, raw	18.75	11.33	182	0

Food Name ---> per 100 g	Protein (g)	Fat (g)	Calories	Net Carb (g)
Beef, chuck, shoulder clod, top blade, steak, separable lean and fat, trimmed to 0" fat, choice, cooked, grilled	24.7	13.59	228	0
Beef, chuck, shoulder clod, top blade, steak, separable lean and fat, trimmed to 0" fat, select, raw	19.38	9.22	166	0
Beef, chuck, shoulder clod, top blade, steak, separable lean and fat, trimmed to 0" fat, select, cooked, grilled	25.29	11.52	212	0
Beef, round, knuckle, tip center, steak, separable lean and fat, trimmed to 0" fat, choice, raw	20.74	6.85	150	0
Beef, round, knuckle, tip center, steak, separable lean and fat, trimmed to 0" fat, choice, cooked, grilled	26.88	8.13	188	0
Beef, round, knuckle, tip center, steak, separable lean and fat, trimmed to 0" fat, select, raw	20.98	5.21	137	0
Beef, round, knuckle, tip center, steak, separable lean and fat, trimmed to 0" fat, select, cooked, grilled	26.61	5.32	162	0
Beef, round, outside round, bottom round, steak, separable lean and fat, trimmed to 0" fat, choice, raw	21.24	6.59	150	0
Beef, round, outside round, bottom round, steak, separable lean and fat, trimmed to 0" fat, choice, cooked, grilled	27.22	8.3	191	0
Beef, round, outside round, bottom round, steak, separable lean and fat, trimmed to 0" fat, select, raw	22.15	3.83	129	0
Beef, round, outside round, bottom round, steak, separable lean and fat, trimmed to 0" fat, select, cooked, grilled	28.01	5.17	166	0
Beef, chuck, shoulder clod, shoulder tender, medallion, separable lean and fat, trimmed to 0" fat, all grades, raw	20.54	6.22	144	0
Beef, chuck, shoulder clod, shoulder tender, medallion, separable lean and fat, trimmed to 0" fat, all grades, cooked, grilled	26.22	7.2	177	0
Beef, round, knuckle, tip side, steak, separable lean and fat, trimmed to 0" fat, all grades, raw	21.69	4	129	0
Beef, round, knuckle, tip side, steak, separable lean and fat, trimmed to 0" fat, all grades, cooked, grilled	29.08	4.84	168	0
Beef, chuck, shoulder clod, shoulder top and center steaks, separable lean and fat, trimmed to 0" fat, all grades, raw	20.67	5.88	141	0
Beef, chuck, shoulder clod, shoulder top and center steaks, separable lean and fat, trimmed to 0" fat, all grades, cooked, grilled	26.3	7.66	182	0
Beef, chuck, shoulder clod, top blade, steak, separable lean and fat, trimmed to 0" fat, all grades, raw	18.99	10.52	176	0
Beef, chuck, shoulder clod, top blade, steak, separable lean and fat, trimmed to 0" fat, all grades, cooked, grilled	24.93	12.79	222	0

Food Name ---> per 100 g	Protein (g)	Fat (g)	Calories	Net Carb (g)
Beef, round, knuckle, tip center, steak, separable lean and fat, trimmed to 0" fat, all grades, raw	20.93	5.89	143	0
Beef, round, knuckle, tip center, steak, separable lean and fat, trimmed to 0" fat, all grades, cooked, grilled	27.12	6.78	177	0
Beef, round, outside round, bottom round, steak, separable lean and fat, trimmed to 0" fat, all grades, raw	21.59	5.53	142	0
Beef, round, outside round, bottom round, steak, separable lean and fat, trimmed to 0" fat, all grades, cooked, grilled	27.52	7.1	182	0
Beef, chuck, shoulder clod, shoulder tender, medallion, separable lean and fat, trimmed to 0" fat, select, cooked, grilled	26.45	6.43	172	0
Beef, chuck, short ribs, boneless, separable lean only, trimmed to 0" fat, choice, raw	19.38	10.7	175	0.29
Beef, chuck, short ribs, boneless, separable lean only, trimmed to 0" fat, select, raw	20.14	8.99	161	0
Beef, chuck, short ribs, boneless, separable lean only, trimmed to 0" fat, all grades, raw	19.68	10.02	169	0.05
Beef, chuck eye Country-Style ribs, boneless, separable lean only, trimmed to 0" fat, choice, cooked, braised	30.95	12.22	234	0
Beef, chuck eye Country-Style ribs, boneless, separable lean only, trimmed to 0" fat, select, cooked, braised	32.1	10.24	221	0
Beef, chuck eye Country-Style ribs, boneless, separable lean only, trimmed to 0" fat, all grades, cooked, braised	31.41	11.43	228	0
Beef, chuck eye Country-Style ribs, boneless, separable lean only, trimmed to 0" fat, choice, raw	20.87	7.67	152	0
Beef, chuck eye Country-Style ribs, boneless, separable lean only, trimmed to 0" fat, select, raw	21.1	5.89	137	0
Beef, chuck eye Country-Style ribs, boneless, separable lean only, trimmed to 0" fat, all grades, raw	20.96	6.95	146	0
Beef, chuck eye steak, boneless, separable lean only, trimmed to 0" fat, choice, cooked, grilled	27.97	11.47	215	0
Beef, chuck eye steak, boneless, separable lean only, trimmed to 0" fat, select, cooked, grilled	27.88	9.77	199	0
Beef, chuck eye steak, boneless, separable lean only, trimmed to 0" fat, all grades, cooked, grilled	27.94	10.79	209	0
Beef, chuck eye steak, boneless, separable lean only, trimmed to 0" fat, choice, raw	21.31	8.29	160	0
Beef, chuck eye steak, boneless, separable lean only, trimmed to 0" fat, select, raw	21.28	6.47	143	0

Food Name ---> per 100 g	Protein (g)	Fat (g)	Calories	Net Carb (g)
Beef, chuck eye steak, boneless, separable lean only, trimmed to 0" fat, all grades, raw	21.29	7.56	153	0
Beef, shoulder pot roast, boneless, separable lean only, trimmed to 0" fat, choice, cooked, braised	31.32	8.3	200	0
Beef, shoulder pot roast, boneless, separable lean only, trimmed to 0" fat, select, cooked, braised	31.71	7.02	190	0
Beef, shoulder pot roast, boneless, separable lean only, trimmed to 0" fat, all grades, cooked, braised	31.48	7.78	196	0
Beef, chuck, mock tender steak, boneless, separable lean only, trimmed to 0" fat, choice, cooked, braised	33.55	6.94	197	0
Beef, chuck, mock tender steak, boneless, separable lean only, trimmed to 0" fat, select, cooked, braised	32.96	5.44	181	0
Beef, chuck, mock tender steak, boneless, separable lean only, trimmed to 0" fat, all grades, cooked, braised	33.31	6.34	190	0
Beef, chuck, mock tender steak, boneless, separable lean only, trimmed to 0" fat, choice, raw	21.36	4.6	127	0
Beef, chuck, mock tender steak, boneless, separable lean only, trimmed to 0" fat, select, raw	21.22	3.53	117	0
Beef, chuck, mock tender steak, boneless, separable lean only, trimmed to 0" fat, all grades, raw	21.3	4.17	123	0
Beef, chuck for stew, separable lean and fat, all grades, cooked, braised	32.41	6.82	191	0
Beef, chuck for stew, separable lean and fat, select, cooked, braised	32.29	6.34	186	0
Beef, chuck for stew, separable lean and fat, choice, cooked, braised	32.49	7.14	194	0
Beef, chuck for stew, separable lean and fat, all grades, raw	21.75	4.48	128	0.16
Beef, chuck for stew, separable lean and fat, select, raw	21.9	3.99	124	0.21
Beef, chuck for stew, separable lean and fat, choice, raw	21.64	4.81	130	0.12
Beef, chuck, under blade steak, boneless, separable lean only, trimmed to 0" fat, choice, cooked, braised	30.91	10.91	222	0
Beef, chuck, under blade steak, boneless, separable lean only, trimmed to 0" fat, select, cooked, braised	32.01	9.66	215	0
Beef, chuck, under blade steak, boneless, separable lean only, trimmed to 0" fat, all grades, cooked, braised	31.35	10.41	219	0
Beef, chuck, under blade pot roast, boneless, separable lean and fat, trimmed to 0" fat, all grades, cooked, braised	26.7	20.49	291	0

Food Name ---> per 100 g	Protein (g)	Fat (g)	Calories	Net Carb (g)
Beef, rib eye steak, boneless, lip-on, separable lean only, trimmed to 1/8" fat, all grades, cooked, grilled	27.97	10.57	207	0
Beef, rib eye roast, bone-in, lip-on, separable lean only, trimmed to 1/8" fat, choice, cooked, roasted	27.18	14.55	240	0
Beef, chuck, under blade pot roast or steak, boneless, separable lean and fat, trimmed to 0" fat, all grades, raw	19.17	13.26	196	0
Beef, chuck, under blade pot roast or steak, boneless, separable lean and fat, trimmed to 0" fat, choice, raw	19.15	13.93	202	0
Beef, chuck, under blade pot roast or steak, boneless, separable lean and fat, trimmed to 0" fat, select, raw	19.2	12.27	187	0
Beef, chuck, under blade center steak, boneless, Denver Cut, separable lean and fat, trimmed to 0" fat, all grades, cooked, grilled	26.18	13.54	227	0.21
Beef, chuck, under blade center steak, boneless, Denver Cut, separable lean and fat, trimmed to 0" fat, choice, cooked, grilled	26.1	14.41	236	0.4
Beef, chuck, under blade center steak, boneless, Denver Cut, separable lean and fat, trimmed to 0" fat, select, cooked, grilled	26.3	12.25	215	0
Beef, chuck, under blade center steak, boneless, Denver Cut, separable lean and fat, trimmed to 0" fat, all grades, raw	18.99	11.64	182	0.36
Beef, chuck, under blade center steak, boneless, Denver Cut, separable lean and fat, trimmed to 0" fat, choice, raw	18.85	12.4	189	0.53
Beef, chuck, under blade center steak, boneless, Denver Cut, separable lean and fat, trimmed to 0" fat, select, raw	19.2	10.5	172	0.09
Beef, shoulder pot roast or steak, boneless, separable lean and fat, trimmed to 0" fat, choice, raw	21.17	5.33	133	0.07
Beef, shoulder pot roast or steak, boneless, separable lean and fat, trimmed to 0" fat, select, raw	21.72	4.44	127	0
Beef, chuck eye roast, boneless, America's Beef Roast, separable lean and fat, trimmed to 0" fat, all grades, cooked, roasted	24.63	15.29	236	0
Beef, chuck eye roast, boneless, America's Beef Roast, separable lean and fat, trimmed to 0" fat, choice, cooked, roasted	24.47	15.87	241	0
Beef, chuck eye roast, boneless, America's Beef Roast, separable lean and fat, trimmed to 0" fat, select, cooked, roasted	24.86	14.41	229	0
Beef, chuck, under blade steak, boneless, separable lean and fat, trimmed to 0" fat, all grades, cooked, braised	28.23	18	275	0
Beef, chuck, under blade steak, boneless, separable lean and fat, trimmed to 0" fat, choice, cooked, braised	27.6	19.3	284	0
Beef, chuck, under blade steak, boneless, separable lean and fat, trimmed to 0" fat, select, cooked, braised	29.18	16.05	261	0

Food Name ---> per 100 g	Protein (g)	Fat (g)	Calories	Net Carb (g)
Beef, chuck, mock tender steak, boneless, separable lean and fat, trimmed to 0" fat, all grades, cooked, braised	32.07	10.18	220	0
Beef, chuck, mock tender steak, boneless, separable lean and fat, trimmed to 0" fat, choice, cooked, braised	32.21	10.74	225	0
Beef, chuck, mock tender steak, boneless, separable lean and fat, trimmed to 0" fat, select, cooked, braised	31.86	9.34	211	0
Beef, chuck, mock tender steak, boneless, separable lean and fat, trimmed to 0" fat, all grades, raw	21.13	4.79	128	0
Beef, chuck, mock tender steak, boneless, separable lean and fat, trimmed to 0" fat, choice, raw	21.19	5.18	131	0
Beef, chuck, mock tender steak, boneless, separable lean and fat, trimmed to 0" fat, select, raw	21.05	4.2	122	0
Beef, chuck, short ribs, boneless, separable lean and fat, trimmed to 0" fat, all grades, cooked, braised	25.48	22.58	305	0
Beef, chuck, short ribs, boneless, separable lean and fat, trimmed to 0" fat, choice, cooked, braised	25.26	24.05	317	0
Beef, chuck, short ribs, boneless, separable lean and fat, trimmed to 0" fat, select, cooked, braised	25.81	20.38	287	0
Beef, chuck, short ribs, boneless, separable lean and fat, trimmed to 0" fat, all grades, raw	17.48	18.33	235	0
Beef, chuck, short ribs, boneless, separable lean and fat, trimmed to 0" fat, choice, raw	17.22	19.03	240	0
Beef, chuck, short ribs, boneless, separable lean and fat, trimmed to 0" fat, select, raw	17.87	17.28	227	0
Beef, shoulder pot roast, boneless, separable lean and fat, trimmed to 0" fat, all grades, cooked, braised	31.03	8.92	204	0
Beef, shoulder pot roast, boneless, separable lean and fat, trimmed to 0" fat, choice, cooked, braised	30.93	9.25	207	0
Beef, shoulder pot roast, boneless, separable lean and fat, trimmed to 0" fat, select, cooked, braised	31.18	8.41	200	0
Beef, chuck eye Country-Style ribs, boneless, separable lean and fat, trimmed to 0" fat, all grades, cooked, braised	27.69	20.55	296	0
Beef, chuck eye Country-Style ribs, boneless, separable lean and fat, trimmed to 0" fat, choice, cooked, braised	27.16	21.56	303	0
Beef, chuck eye Country-Style ribs, boneless, separable lean and fat, trimmed to 0" fat, select, cooked, braised	28.47	19.03	285	0
Beef, chuck eye Country-Style ribs, boneless, separable lean and fat, trimmed to 0" fat, all grades, raw	18.97	14.32	205	0

Food Name ---> per 100 g	Protein (g)	Fat (g)	Calories	Net Carb (g)
Beef, chuck eye Country-Style ribs, boneless, separable lean and fat, trimmed to 0" fat, choice, raw	18.87	14.99	210	0
Beef, chuck eye Country-Style ribs, boneless, separable lean and fat, trimmed to 0" fat, select, raw	19.1	13.33	196	0
Beef, chuck eye steak, boneless, separable lean and fat, trimmed to 0" fat, all grades, cooked, grilled	24.98	19.64	277	0
Beef, chuck eye steak, boneless, separable lean and fat, trimmed to 0" fat, choice, cooked, grilled	24.95	20.35	283	0
Beef, chuck eye steak, boneless, separable lean and fat, trimmed to 0" fat, select, cooked, grilled	25.03	18.57	267	0
Beef, chuck eye steak, boneless, separable lean and fat, trimmed to 0" fat, all grades, raw	18.86	16.35	223	0
Beef, chuck eye steak, boneless, separable lean and fat, trimmed to 0" fat, choice, raw	18.86	16.85	227	0
Beef, chuck eye steak, boneless, separable lean and fat, trimmed to 0" fat, select, raw	18.86	15.6	216	0
Beef, rib eye roast, bone-in, lip-on, separable lean only, trimmed to 1/8" fat, all grades, cooked, roasted	27.12	13.64	231	0
Beef, rib eye roast, bone-in, lip-on, separable lean only, trimmed to 1/8" fat, select, cooked, roasted	27.03	12.29	219	0
Beef, rib eye steak, boneless, lip-on, separable lean only, trimmed to 1/8" fat, choice, cooked, grilled	27.3	11.97	217	0
Beef, rib eye steak, boneless, lip-on, separable lean only, trimmed to 1/8" fat, select, cooked, grilled	28.98	8.48	192	0
Beef, rib eye steak/roast, bone-in, lip-on, separable lean only, trimmed to 1/8" fat, all grades, raw	21.22	9.04	166	0
Beef, rib eye steak/roast, bone-in, lip-on, separable lean only, trimmed to 1/8" fat, choice, raw	20.93	9.97	173	0
Beef, rib eye steak/roast, bone-in, lip-on, separable lean only, trimmed to 1/8" fat, select, raw	21.65	7.64	155	0
Beef, rib eye steak/roast, boneless, lip-on, separable lean only, trimmed to 1/8" fat, all grades, raw	21.99	7.54	156	0
Beef, rib eye steak/roast, boneless, lip-on, separable lean only, trimmed to 1/8" fat, choice, raw	21.62	8.29	161	0
Beef, rib eye steak/roast, boneless, lip-on, separable lean only, trimmed to 1/8" fat, select, raw	22.55	6.41	148	0
Beef, rib eye steak, bone-in, lip-on, separable lean only, trimmed to 1/8" fat, all grades, cooked, grilled	27.4	12.43	221	0

Food Name ---> per 100 g	Protein (g)	Fat (g)	Calories	Net Carb (g)
Beef, rib eye steak, bone-in, lip-on, separable lean only, trimmed to 1/8" fat, choice, cooked, grilled	27.03	13.44	229	0
Beef, rib eye steak, bone-in, lip-on, separable lean only, trimmed to 1/8" fat, select, cooked, grilled	27.96	10.91	210	0
Beef, rib eye roast, boneless, lip-on, separable lean only, trimmed to 1/8" fat, all grades, cooked, roasted	28.21	11.68	218	0
Beef, rib eye roast, boneless, lip-on, separable lean only, trimmed to 1/8" fat, choice, cooked, roasted	27.87	13.01	229	0
Beef, rib eye roast, boneless, lip-on, separable lean only, trimmed to 1/8" fat, select, cooked, roasted	28.72	9.68	202	0
Beef, plate steak, boneless, inside skirt, separable lean only, trimmed to 0" fat, all grades, cooked, grilled	29.99	12.69	234	0
Beef, plate steak, boneless, inside skirt, separable lean only, trimmed to 0" fat, all grades, raw	21.17	8.82	164	0
Beef, plate steak, boneless, inside skirt, separable lean only, trimmed to 0" fat, choice, cooked, grilled	29.56	13.72	242	0
Beef, plate steak, boneless, inside skirt, separable lean only, trimmed to 0" fat, choice, raw	20.89	9.76	171	0
Beef, plate steak, boneless, inside skirt, separable lean only, trimmed to 0" fat, select, cooked, grilled	30.64	11.16	223	0
Beef, plate steak, boneless, inside skirt, separable lean only, trimmed to 0" fat, select, raw	21.61	7.41	153	0
Beef, plate steak, boneless, outside skirt, separable lean only, trimmed to 0" fat, all grades, cooked, grilled	27.68	19.01	282	0
Beef, plate steak, boneless, outside skirt, separable lean only, trimmed to 0" fat, all grades, raw	18.74	14.53	206	0.19
Beef, plate steak, boneless, outside skirt, separable lean only, trimmed to 0" fat, choice, cooked, grilled	27.03	20.28	291	0
Beef, plate steak, boneless, outside skirt, separable lean only, trimmed to 0" fat, choice, raw	18.47	15.26	212	0.17
Beef, plate steak, boneless, outside skirt, separable lean only, trimmed to 0" fat, select, cooked, grilled	28.65	17.1	268	0
Beef, plate steak, boneless, outside skirt, separable lean only, trimmed to 0" fat, select, raw	19.14	13.44	198	0.23
Beef, rib eye steak, boneless, lip off, separable lean only, trimmed to 0" fat, all grades, cooked, grilled	28.11	10.37	206	0
Beef, rib eye steak, boneless, lip off, separable lean only, trimmed to 0" fat, all grades, raw	21.85	7.41	154	0

Food Name ---> per 100 g	Protein (g)	Fat (g)	Calories	Net Carb (g)
Beef, rib eye steak, boneless, lip off, separable lean only, trimmed to 0" fat, choice, cooked, grilled	27.39	11.75	215	0
Beef, rib eye steak, boneless, lip off, separable lean only, trimmed to 0" fat, choice, raw	21.44	8.5	162	0
Beef, rib eye steak, boneless, lip off, separable lean only, trimmed to 0" fat, select, cooked, grilled	29.18	8.31	191	0
Beef, rib eye steak, boneless, lip off, separable lean only, trimmed to 0" fat, select, raw	22.46	5.78	142	0
Beef, rib, back ribs, bone-in, separable lean only, trimmed to 0" fat, all grades, cooked, braised	28.36	20.57	299	0
Beef, rib, back ribs, bone-in, separable lean only, trimmed to 0" fat, all grades, raw	19.11	17.91	239	0.46
Beef, rib, back ribs, bone-in, separable lean only, trimmed to 0" fat, choice, cooked, braised	27.75	21.72	306	0
Beef, rib, back ribs, bone-in, separable lean only, trimmed to 0" fat, choice, raw	18.72	19.36	252	0.64
Beef, rib, back ribs, bone-in, separable lean only, trimmed to 0" fat, select, cooked, braised	29.28	18.84	287	0
Beef, rib, back ribs, bone-in, separable lean only, trimmed to 0" fat, select, raw	19.71	15.73	221	0.2
Beef, rib eye steak, bone-in, lip-on, separable lean and fat, trimmed to 1/8" fat, choice, cooked, grilled	22.71	24.7	313	0
Beef, rib eye steak, bone-in, lip-on, separable lean and fat, trimmed to 1/8" fat, select, cooked, grilled	23.19	23.47	304	0
Beef, rib eye steak, bone-in, lip-on, separable lean and fat, trimmed to 1/8" fat, all grades, cooked, grilled	22.9	24.2	309	0
Beef, rib eye roast, bone-in, lip-on, separable lean and fat, trimmed to 1/8" fat, choice, cooked, roasted	23.53	23.61	307	0
Beef, rib eye roast, bone-in, lip-on, separable lean and fat, trimmed to 1/8" fat, select, cooked, roasted	23.36	21.85	290	0
Beef, rib eye roast, bone-in, lip-on, separable lean and fat, trimmed to 1/8" fat, all grades, cooked, roasted	23.47	22.91	300	0
Beef, rib eye steak/roast, bone-in, lip-on, separable lean and fat, trimmed to 1/8" fat, all grades, raw	18.13	20.31	255	0
Beef, rib eye steak/roast, bone-in, lip-on, separable lean and fat, trimmed to 1/8" fat, choice, raw	17.92	20.96	260	0
Beef, rib eye steak/roast, bone-in, lip-on, separable lean and fat, trimmed to 1/8" fat, select, raw	18.44	19.34	248	0

Food Name ---> per 100 g	Protein (g)	Fat (g)	Calories	Net Carb (g)
Beef, rib eye steak, boneless, lip-on, separable lean and fat, trimmed to 1/8" fat, choice, cooked, grilled	22.92	23.52	303	0
Beef, rib eye steak, boneless, lip-on, separable lean and fat, trimmed to 1/8" fat, select, cooked, grilled	24.83	19.25	273	0
Beef, rib eye steak, boneless, lip-on, separable lean and fat, trimmed to 1/8" fat, all grades, cooked, grilled	23.69	21.81	291	0
Beef, rib eye roast, boneless, lip-on, separable lean and fat, trimmed to 1/8" fat, all grades, cooked, roasted	24.3	21.66	292	0
Beef, rib eye roast, boneless, lip-on, separable lean and fat, trimmed to 1/8" fat, choice, cooked, roasted	23.92	22.98	303	0
Beef, rib eye roast, boneless, lip-on, separable lean and fat, trimmed to 1/8" fat, select, cooked, roasted	24.85	19.68	277	0
Beef, rib eye steak/roast, boneless, lip-on, separable lean and fat, trimmed to 1/8" fat, all grades, raw	18.85	18.73	244	0
Beef, rib eye steak/roast, boneless, lip-on, separable lean and fat, trimmed to 1/8" fat, choice, raw	18.39	19.95	253	0
Beef, rib eye steak/roast, boneless, lip-on, separable lean and fat, trimmed to 1/8" fat, select, raw	19.55	16.9	230	0
Beef, plate steak, boneless, inside skirt, separable lean and fat, trimmed to 0" fat, all grades, cooked, grilled	29.36	14.2	245	0
Beef, plate steak, boneless, inside skirt, separable lean and fat, trimmed to 0" fat, choice, cooked, grilled	28.9	15.3	253	0
Beef, plate steak, boneless, inside skirt, separable lean and fat, trimmed to 0" fat, select, cooked, grilled	30.06	12.54	233	0
Beef, plate steak, boneless, inside skirt, separable lean and fat, trimmed to 0" fat, all grades, raw	20.38	11.71	187	0
Beef, plate steak, boneless, inside skirt, separable lean and fat, trimmed to 0" fat, choice, raw	20.06	12.78	195	0
Beef, plate steak, boneless, inside skirt, separable lean and fat, trimmed to 0" fat, select, raw	20.87	10.11	174	0
Beef, ground, unspecified fat content, cooked	25.07	14.53	240	0.62
Beef, plate steak, boneless, outside skirt, separable lean and fat, trimmed to 0" fat, all grades, cooked, grilled	27.06	20.47	292	0
Beef, plate steak, boneless, outside skirt, separable lean and fat, trimmed to 0" fat, choice, cooked, grilled	26.46	21.62	300	0
Beef, plate steak, boneless, outside skirt, separable lean and fat, trimmed to 0" fat, select, cooked, grilled	27.95	18.75	281	0

Food Name ---> per 100 g	Protein (g)	Fat (g)	Calories	Net Carb (g)
Beef, plate steak, boneless, outside skirt, separable lean and fat, trimmed to 0" fat, all grades, raw	17.98	17.59	232	0.35
Beef, plate steak, boneless, outside skirt, separable lean and fat, trimmed to 0" fat, choice, raw	17.69	18.44	238	0.35
Beef, plate steak, boneless, outside skirt, separable lean and fat, trimmed to 0" fat, select, raw	18.43	16.31	222	0.36
Beef, rib eye steak, boneless, lip off, separable lean and fat, trimmed to 0" fat, all grades, cooked, grilled	24.85	19.02	271	0
Beef, rib eye steak, boneless, lip off, separable lean and fat, trimmed to 0" fat, choice, cooked, grilled	23.89	21.1	285	0
Beef, rib eye steak, boneless, lip off, separable lean and fat, trimmed to 0" fat, select, cooked, grilled	26.29	15.9	248	0
Beef, rib eye steak, boneless, lip off, separable lean and fat, trimmed to 0" fat, all grades, raw	19.26	16.71	228	0.12
Beef, rib eye steak, boneless, lip off, separable lean and fat, trimmed to 0" fat, choice, raw	18.69	18.43	241	0.2
Beef, rib eye steak, boneless, lip off, separable lean and fat, trimmed to 0" fat, select, raw	20.12	14.14	208	0
Beef, rib, back ribs, bone-in, separable lean and fat, trimmed to 0" fat, all grades, cooked, braised	24.23	29.21	360	0
Beef, rib, back ribs, bone-in, separable lean and fat, trimmed to 0" fat, choice, cooked, braised	23.34	30.95	372	0
Beef, rib, back ribs, bone-in, separable lean and fat, trimmed to 0" fat, select, cooked, braised	25.56	26.59	341	0
Beef, rib, back ribs, bone-in, separable lean and fat, trimmed to 0" fat, all grades, raw	16.15	28.42	324	0.78
Beef, rib, back ribs, bone-in, separable lean and fat, trimmed to 0" fat, choice, raw	15.75	29.89	336	0.9
Beef, rib, back ribs, bone-in, separable lean and fat, trimmed to 0" fat, select, raw	16.75	26.23	305	0.6
Beef, loin, top sirloin petite roast, boneless, separable lean only, trimmed to 0" fat, choice, cooked, roasted	28.97	6.37	173	0
Beef, loin, top sirloin petite roast/filet, boneless, separable lean only, trimmed to 0" fat, choice, raw	23.03	4.4	132	0
Beef, loin, top sirloin cap steak, boneless, separable lean only, trimmed to 1/8" fat, all grades, cooked, grilled	28.26	7.23	181	0.73
Beef, loin, top sirloin cap steak, boneless, separable lean only, trimmed to 1/8" fat, choice, cooked, grilled	28.19	7.96	189	1.07

Food Name ---> per 100 g	Protein (g)	Fat (g)	Calories	Net Carb (g)
Beef, loin, top sirloin cap steak, boneless, separable lean only, trimmed to 1/8" fat, select, cooked, grilled	28.36	6.14	170	0.22
Beef, loin, top sirloin cap steak, boneless, separable lean only, trimmed to 1/8" fat, all grades, raw	21.38	5.36	134	0
Beef, loin, top sirloin cap steak, boneless, separable lean only, trimmed to 1/8" fat, choice, raw	21.34	5.82	138	0
Beef, loin, top sirloin cap steak, boneless, separable lean only, trimmed to 1/8" fat, select, raw	21.44	4.68	128	0
Beef, top loin filet, boneless, separable lean only, trimmed to 1/8" fat, all grades, cooked, grilled	29.33	8.54	195	0.3
Beef, top loin filet, boneless, separable lean only, trimmed to 1/8" fat, choice, cooked, grilled	28.99	9.48	203	0.36
Beef, top loin filet, boneless, separable lean only, trimmed to 1/8" fat, select, cooked, grilled	29.85	7.12	184	0.2
Beef, top loin petite roast, boneless, separable lean only, trimmed to 1/8" fat, all grades, cooked, roasted	28.33	8.76	195	0.82
Beef, top loin petite roast, boneless, separable lean only, trimmed to 1/8" fat, choice, cooked, roasted	28.24	9.97	206	0.88
Beef, top loin petite roast, boneless, separable lean only, trimmed to 1/8" fat, select, cooked, roasted	28.48	6.95	179	0.74
Beef, top loin petite roast/filet, boneless, separable lean only, trimmed to 1/8" fat, all grades, raw	22.61	5.84	143	0
Beef, top loin petite roast/filet, boneless, separable lean only, trimmed to 1/8" fat, choice, raw	22.5	6.48	149	0.23
Beef, top loin petite roast/filet, boneless, separable lean only, trimmed to 1/8" fat, select, raw	22.77	4.88	135	0
Beef, loin, top sirloin filet, boneless, separable lean only, trimmed to 0" fat, all grades, cooked, grilled	30.58	5.37	171	0
Beef, loin, top sirloin filet, boneless, separable lean only, trimmed to 0" fat, choice, cooked, grilled	30.45	5.83	174	0
Beef, loin, top sirloin filet, boneless, separable lean only, trimmed to 0" fat, select, cooked, grilled	30.78	4.68	165	0
Beef, loin, top sirloin petite roast, boneless, separable lean only, trimmed to 0" fat, all grades, cooked, roasted	29.12	5.92	170	0
Beef, loin, top sirloin petite roast, boneless, separable lean only, trimmed to 0" fat, select, cooked, roasted	29.35	5.25	165	0
Beef, loin, top sirloin petite roast/filet, boneless, separable lean only, trimmed to 0" fat, all grades, raw	23.04	3.98	128	0

Food Name ---> per 100 g	Protein (g)	Fat (g)	Calories	Net Carb (g)
Beef, loin, top sirloin petite roast/filet, boneless, separable lean only, trimmed to 0" fat, select, raw	23.05	3.35	122	0
Beef, ribeye petite roast/filet, boneless, separable lean only, trimmed to 0" fat, all grades, raw	22.66	4.66	133	0.04
Beef, ribeye petite roast/filet, boneless, separable lean only, trimmed to 0" fat, choice, raw	22.52	5.29	138	0.18
Beef, ribeye petite roast/filet, boneless, separable lean only, trimmed to 0" fat, select, raw	22.89	3.72	125	0
Beef, ribeye cap steak, boneless, separable lean only, trimmed to 0" fat, all grades, cooked, grilled	24.66	15.7	246	1.53
Beef, ribeye cap steak, boneless, separable lean only, trimmed to 0" fat, choice, cooked, grilled	24.24	17.21	259	1.81
Beef, ribeye cap steak, boneless, separable lean only, trimmed to 0" fat, select, cooked, grilled	25.28	13.43	226	1.1
Beef, ribeye cap steak, boneless, separable lean only, trimmed to 0" fat, all grades, raw	19.7	10.6	180	1.51
Beef, ribeye cap steak, boneless, separable lean only, trimmed to 0" fat, choice, raw	19.46	11.4	187	1.75
Beef, ribeye cap steak, boneless, separable lean only, trimmed to 0" fat, select, raw	20.05	9.39	169	1.15
Beef, ribeye filet, boneless, separable lean only, trimmed to 0" fat, all grades, cooked, grilled	28.77	9.2	199	0.17
Beef, ribeye filet, boneless, separable lean only, trimmed to 0" fat, choice, cooked, grilled	28.35	10.26	208	0.51
Beef, ribeye filet, boneless, separable lean only, trimmed to 0" fat, select, cooked, grilled	29.39	7.61	186	0
Beef, ribeye petite roast, boneless, separable lean only, trimmed to 0" fat, all grades, cooked, roasted	28.15	7.31	178	0
Beef, ribeye petite roast, boneless, separable lean only, trimmed to 0" fat, choice, cooked, roasted	28	8.42	188	0
Beef, ribeye petite roast, boneless, separable lean only, trimmed to 0" fat, select, cooked, roasted	28.37	5.65	164	0
Beef, loin, top sirloin cap steak, boneless, separable lean and fat, trimmed to 1/8" fat, all grades, cooked, grilled	26	15	242	0.8
Beef, loin, top sirloin cap steak, boneless, separable lean and fat, trimmed to 1/8" fat, choice, cooked, grilled	26.3	14.3	238	1.1
Beef, loin, top sirloin cap steak, boneless, separable lean and fat, trimmed to 1/8" fat, select, cooked, grilled	25.5	16.1	249	0.4

Food Name ---> per 100 g	Protein (g)	Fat (g)	Calories	Net Carb (g)
Beef, loin, top sirloin cap steak, boneless, separable lean and fat, trimmed to 1/8" fat, all grades, raw	19.9	12.4	191	0
Beef, loin, top sirloin cap steak, boneless, separable lean and fat, trimmed to 1/8" fat, choice, raw	19.7	13.4	199	0
Beef, loin, top sirloin cap steak, boneless, separable lean and fat, trimmed to 1/8" fat, select, raw	20.1	10.9	179	0
Beef, top loin filet, boneless, separable lean and fat, trimmed to 1/8" fat, all grades, cooked, grilled	27.4	14.1	239	0.6
Beef, top loin filet, boneless, separable lean and fat, trimmed to 1/8" fat, choice, cooked, grilled	26.8	15.9	253	0.6
Beef, top loin filet, boneless, separable lean and fat, trimmed to 1/8" fat, select, cooked, grilled	28.3	11.6	219	0.4
Beef, top loin petite roast, boneless, separable lean and fat, trimmed to 1/8" fat, all grades, cooked, roasted	27	12.9	228	1
Beef, top loin petite roast, boneless, separable lean and fat, trimmed to 1/8" fat, choice, cooked, roasted	26.8	14.1	239	1.1
Beef, top loin petite roast, boneless, separable lean and fat, trimmed to 1/8" fat, select, cooked, roasted	27.1	11.2	213	0.9
Beef, top loin petite roast/filet, boneless, separable lean and fat, trimmed to 1/8" fat, all grades, raw	21.1	11.3	187	0.3
Beef, top loin petite roast/filet, boneless, separable lean and fat, trimmed to 1/8" fat, choice, raw	20.8	12.6	199	0.6
Beef, top loin petite roast/filet, boneless, separable lean and fat, trimmed to 1/8" fat, select, raw	21.6	9.3	170	0
Beef, Australian, imported, grass-fed, ground, 85% lean / 15% fat, raw	17.72	18.12	234	0
Beef, Australian, imported, grass-fed, loin, tenderloin steak/roast, boneless, separable lean only, raw	20.85	6.11	138	0
Beef, Australian, imported, Wagyu, loin, tenderloin steak/roast, boneless, separable lean only, Aust. marble score 4/5, raw	20.19	12.3	191	0
Beef, Australian, imported, grass-fed, external fat, raw	11.32	51.36	509	0.39
Beef, Australian, imported, grass-fed, seam fat, raw	9.58	57.73	562	1.06
Beef, Australian, imported, Wagyu, external fat, Aust. marble score 4/5, raw	6.54	63.27	596	0
Beef, Australian, imported, Wagyu, seam fat, Aust. marble score 4/5, raw	6	63.3	594	0
Beef, Australian, imported, Wagyu, external fat, Aust. marble score 9, raw	5.54	68.07	639	0.97

Food Name ---> per 100 g	Protein (g)	Fat (g)	Calories	Net Carb (g)
Beef, Australian, imported, Wagyu, seam fat, Aust. marble score 9, raw	5.16	67.33	627	0
Beef, Australian, imported, grass-fed, loin, tenderloin steak/roast, boneless, separable lean and fat, raw	20.53	7.63	151	0.01
Beef, Australian, imported, grass-fed, loin, top loin steak/roast, boneless, separable lean only, raw	21.79	4.87	131	0
Beef, Australian, imported, Wagyu, loin, tenderloin steak/roast, boneless, separable lean and fat, Aust. marble score 4/5, raw	19.71	14.09	206	0
Beef, Australian, imported, grass-fed, loin, top loin steak/roast, boneless, separable lean and fat, raw	19.9	13.17	199	0.11
Beef, Australian, imported, grass-fed, loin, top sirloin cap-off steak/roast, boneless, separable lean only, raw	21.9	3.87	122	0
Beef, Australian, imported, grass-fed, rib, ribeye steak/roast lip-on, boneless, separable lean only, raw	21.47	8.2	160	0
Beef, Australian, imported, grass-fed, round, bottom round steak/roast, boneless, separable lean only, raw	21.4	4.93	130	0
Beef, Australian, imported, grass-fed, round, top round cap-off steak/roast, boneless, separable lean only, raw	22.41	4.43	129	0
Beef, Australian, imported, Wagyu, loin, tenderloin steak/roast, boneless, separable lean only, Aust. marble score 9, raw	18.87	17.73	237	0.57
Beef, Australian, imported, Wagyu, loin, top loin steak/roast, boneless, separable lean only, Aust. marble score 4/5, raw	20.15	15.69	223	0.2
Beef, Australian, imported, Wagyu, loin, top loin steak/roast, boneless, separable lean only, Aust. marble score 9, raw	16.92	29.15	331	0.13
Beef, Australian, imported, Wagyu, rib, small end rib steak/roast, boneless, separable lean only, Aust. marble score 4/5, raw	20.35	16.93	234	0
Beef, Australian, imported, Wagyu, rib, small end rib steak/roast, boneless, separable lean only, Aust. marble score 9, raw	17.61	28.61	330	0.46
Beef, Australian, imported, grass-fed, loin, top sirloin cap-off steak/roast, boneless, separable lean and fat, raw	21.77	4.45	127	0.01
Beef, Australian, imported, grass-fed, rib, ribeye steak/roast lip-on, boneless, separable lean and fat, raw	19.8	15.21	217	0.11
Beef, Australian, imported, grass-fed, round, bottom round steak/roast, boneless, separable lean and fat, raw	21.13	6.16	140	0.01
Beef, Australian, imported, grass-fed, round, top round cap-off steak/roast, boneless, separable lean and fat, raw	22.24	4.4	129	0
Beef, Australian, imported, Wagyu, loin, top loin steak/roast, boneless, separable lean and fat, Aust. marble score 4/5, raw	17.67	24.2	289	0.17

Food Name ---> per 100 g	Protein (g)	Fat (g)	Calories	Net Carb (g)
Beef, Australian, imported, Wagyu, loin, top loin steak/roast, separable lean and fat, Aust. marble score 9, raw	14.58	36.98	392	0.22
Beef, Australian, imported, Wagyu, rib, small end rib steak/roast, boneless, separable lean and fat, Aust. marble score 4/5, raw	17.07	27.64	317	0
Beef, Australian, imported, Wagyu, rib, small end rib steak/roast, boneless, separable lean and fat, Aust. marble score 9, raw	14.54	38.3	405	0.42
Beef, Australian, imported, Wagyu, loin, tenderloin steak/roast, boneless, separable lean and fat, Aust. marble score 9, raw	18.5	19.11	248	0.58
Beef, round, top round steak, boneless, separable lean and fat, trimmed to 0" fat, all grades, raw	23.49	3.34	124	0
Beef, round, top round steak, boneless, separable lean and fat, trimmed to 0" fat, choice, raw	23.49	3.66	127	0
Beef, round, top round steak, boneless, separable lean and fat, trimmed to 0" fat, select, raw	23.49	2.85	120	0
Beef, round, top round roast, boneless, separable lean and fat, trimmed to 0" fat, all grades, raw	23.45	3.5	125	0
Beef, round, top round roast, boneless, separable lean and fat, trimmed to 0" fat, choice, raw	23.46	3.81	128	0
Beef, round, top round roast, boneless, separable lean and fat, trimmed to 0" fat, select, raw	23.44	3.04	121	0
Beef, round, eye of round roast, boneless, separable lean and fat, trimmed to 0" fat, all grades, raw	23.27	3.44	124	0
Beef, round, eye of round roast, boneless, separable lean and fat, trimmed to 0" fat, choice, raw	23.26	3.74	127	0
Beef, round, eye of round roast, boneless, separable lean and fat, trimmed to 0" fat, select, raw	23.28	3	120	0
Beef, round, eye of round steak, boneless, separable lean and fat, trimmed to 0" fat, all grades, raw	23.26	3.48	124	0
Beef, round, eye of round steak, boneless separable lean and fat, trimmed to 0" fat, choice, raw	23.24	3.83	127	0
Beef, round, eye of round steak, boneless, separable lean and fat, trimmed to 0" fat, select, raw	23.3	2.95	120	0
Beef, loin, tenderloin roast, boneless, separable lean and fat, trimmed to 0" fat, all grades, raw	21.67	6.93	149	0
Beef, loin, tenderloin roast, boneless, separable lean and fat, trimmed to 0" fat, choice, raw	21.5	7.4	153	0
Beef, loin, tenderloin roast, boneless, separable lean and fat, trimmed to 0" fat, select, raw	21.91	6.21	144	0

Food Name ---> per 100 g	Protein (g)	Fat (g)	Calories	Net Carb (g)
Beef, loin, top loin steak, boneless, lip off, separable lean and fat, trimmed to 0" fat, all grades, raw	22.43	8.17	163	0
Beef, loin, top loin steak, boneless, lip off, separable lean and fat, trimmed to 0" fat, choice, raw	22.19	9.16	171	0
Beef, loin, top loin steak, boneless, lip off, separable lean and fat, trimmed to 0" fat, select, raw	22.79	6.67	151	0
Beef, loin, tenderloin steak, boneless, separable lean and fat, trimmed to 0" fat, all grades, raw	21.72	6.67	147	0
Beef, loin, tenderloin steak, boneless, separable lean and fat, trimmed to 0" fat, choice, raw	21.57	7.1	150	0
Beef, loin, tenderloin steak, boneless, separable lean and fat, trimmed to 0" fat, select, raw	21.95	6.02	142	0
Beef, loin, tenderloin roast, boneless, separable lean and fat, trimmed to 0" fat, all grades, cooked, roasted	27.31	8.14	183	0
Beef, loin, tenderloin roast, boneless, separable lean and fat, trimmed to 0" fat, choice, cooked, roasted	27.26	8.82	188	0
Beef, loin, tenderloin roast, boneless, separable lean and fat, trimmed to 0" fat, select, cooked, roasted	27.38	7.12	174	0
Beef, round, top round roast, boneless, separable lean and fat, trimmed to 0" fat, all grades, cooked, roasted	29.9	4.49	160	0
Beef, round, top round roast, boneless, separable lean and fat, trimmed to 0" fat, choice, cooked, roasted	30.08	4.79	163	0
Beef, round, top round roast, boneless, separable lean and fat, trimmed to 0" fat, select, cooked, roasted	30.97	3.72	157	0
Beef, round, eye of round steak, boneless, separable lean and fat, trimmed to 0" fat, all grades, cooked, grilled	29.66	4.47	159	0
Beef, round, eye of round steak, boneless, separable lean and fat, trimmed to 0" fat, choice, cooked, grilled	29.79	4.83	163	0
Beef, round, eye of round steak, boneless, separable lean and fat, trimmed to 0" fat, select, cooked, grilled	29.47	3.98	154	0
Beef, round, top round steak, boneless, separable lean only, trimmed to 0" fat, all grades, raw	23.59	2.94	121	0
Beef, round, top round steak, boneless, separable lean only, trimmed to 0" fat, choice, raw	23.59	3.26	124	0
Beef, round, top round steak, boneless, separable lean only, trimmed to 0" fat, select, raw	23.59	2.45	116	0
Beef, round, top round roast, boneless, separable lean only, trimmed to 0" fat, all grades, raw	23.59	2.94	121	0

Food Name ---> per 100 g	Protein (g)	Fat (g)	Calories	Net Carb (g)
Beef, round, top round roast, boneless, separable lean only, trimmed to 0" fat, choice, raw	23.59	3.26	124	0
Beef, round, top round roast, boneless, separable lean only, trimmed to 0" fat, select, raw	23.59	2.45	116	0
Beef, round, eye of round roast, boneless, separable lean only, trimmed to 0" fat, all grades, raw	23.37	3.04	121	0
Beef, round, eye of round roast, boneless, separable lean only, trimmed to 0" fat, choice, raw	23.35	3.38	124	0
Beef, round, eye of round roast, boneless, separable lean only, trimmed to 0" fat, select, raw	23.41	2.52	116	0
Beef, round, eye of round steak, boneless, separable lean only, trimmed to 0" fat, all grades, raw	23.37	3.04	121	0
Beef, round, eye of round steak, boneless, separable lean only, trimmed to 0" fat, choice, raw	23.35	3.38	124	0
Beef, round, eye of round steak, boneless, separable lean only, trimmed to 0" fat, select, raw	23.41	2.52	116	0
Beef, loin, tenderloin roast, boneless, separable lean only, trimmed to 0" fat, all grades, raw	21.94	5.74	139	0
Beef, loin, tenderloin roast, boneless, separable lean only, trimmed to 0" fat, choice, raw	21.78	6.16	143	0
Beef, loin, tenderloin roast, boneless, separable lean only, trimmed to 0" fat, select, raw	22.16	5.1	135	0
Beef, loin, top loin steak, boneless, lip off, separable lean only, trimmed to 0" fat, all grades, raw	23.07	5.67	143	0
Beef, loin, top loin steak, boneless, lip off, separable lean only, trimmed to 0" fat, choice, raw	22.93	6.34	149	0
Beef, loin, top loin steak, boneless, lip off, separable lean only, trimmed to 0" fat, select, raw	23.3	4.66	135	0
Beef, loin, tenderloin steak, boneless, separable lean only, trimmed to 0" fat, all grades, raw	21.94	5.74	139	0
Beef, loin, tenderloin steak, boneless, separable lean only, trimmed to 0" fat, choice, raw	21.78	6.16	143	0
Beef, loin, tenderloin steak, boneless, separable lean only, trimmed to 0" fat, select, raw	22.16	5.1	135	0
Beef, loin, tenderloin roast, boneless, separable lean only, trimmed to 0" fat, all grades, cooked, roasted	27.51	7.49	177	0
Beef, loin, tenderloin roast, boneless, separable lean only, trimmed to 0" fat, choice, cooked, roasted	27.48	8.13	183	0

Food Name ---> per 100 g	Protein (g)	Fat (g)	Calories	Net Carb (g)
Beef, loin, tenderloin roast, separable lean only, boneless, trimmed to 0" fat, select, cooked, roasted	27.55	6.54	169	0
Beef, round, top round roast, boneless, separable lean only, trimmed to 0" fat, all grades, cooked, roasted	30.09	3.77	162	0
Beef, round, top round roast, boneless, separable lean only, trimmed to 0" fat, choice, cooked, roasted	30.24	4.11	158	0.06
Beef, round, top round roast, boneless, separable lean only, trimmed to 0" fat, select, cooked, roasted	29.81	3.37	150	0
Beef, round, eye of round steak, boneless, separable lean only, trimmed to 0" fat, all grades, cooked, grilled	29.85	3.9	155	0
Beef, round, eye of round steak, boneless, separable lean only, trimmed to 0" fat, choice, cooked, grilled	29.94	4.26	158	0
Beef, round, eye of round steak, boneless, separable lean only, trimmed to 0" fat, select, cooked, grilled	29.52	3.43	149	0
Beef, loin, top loin steak, boneless, lip-on, separable lean only, trimmed to 1/8" fat, select, raw	23.3	4.66	135	0
Beef, loin, top loin steak, boneless, lip-on, separable lean only, trimmed to 1/8" fat, choice, raw	22.93	6.34	149	0
Beef, loin, top loin steak, boneless, lip-on, separable lean only, trimmed to 1/8" fat, all grades, raw	23.07	5.67	143	0
Beef, loin, top loin steak, boneless, lip-on, separable lean and fat, trimmed to 1/8" fat, select, raw	21.54	11.65	191	0
Beef, loin, top loin steak, boneless, lip-on, separable lean and fat, trimmed to 1/8" fat, all grades, raw	21.29	12.68	199	0
Beef, loin, top loin steak, boneless, lip-on, separable lean and fat, trimmed to 1/8" fat, choice, cooked, grilled	25.69	19.19	275	0
Beef, loin, top loin steak, boneless, lip-on, separable lean and fat, trimmed to 1/8" fat, select, cooked, grilled	26.92	15.44	247	0
Beef, loin, top loin steak, boneless, lip-on, separable lean and fat, trimmed to 1/8" fat, all grades, cooked, grilled	26.18	17.69	264	0
Beef, loin, top loin steak, boneless, lip-on, separable lean only, trimmed to 1/8" fat, choice, cooked, grilled	28.66	10.34	208	0
Beef, loin, top loin steak, boneless, lip-on, separable lean only, trimmed to 1/8" fat, select, cooked, grilled	29.67	7.26	184	0
Beef, loin, top loin steak, boneless, lip-on, separable lean only, trimmed to 1/8" fat, all grades, cooked, grilled	29.06	9.11	198	0
Beef, loin, top loin steak, boneless, lip-on, separable lean and fat, trimmed to 1/8" fat, choice, raw	21.13	13.36	205	0

Food Name ---> per 100 g	Protein (g)	Fat (g)	Calories	Net Carb (g)
Beef, New Zealand, imported, bolar blade, separable lean only, cooked, fast roasted	33.53	6.57	193	0
Beef, New Zealand, imported, bolar blade, separable lean only, raw	22.09	4.49	129	0
Beef, New Zealand, imported, brisket navel end, separable lean only, cooked, braised	29.35	16.37	265	0
Beef, New Zealand, imported, brisket navel end, separable lean only, raw	19.74	12.75	194	0
Beef, New Zealand, imported, brisket point end, separable lean only, cooked, braised	34.51	7.05	202	0
Beef, New Zealand, imported, brisket point end, separable lean only, raw	20.92	4.62	125	0
Beef, New Zealand, imported, chuck eye roll, separable lean only, raw	20.46	5.41	131	0
Beef, New Zealand, imported, chuck eye roll, separable lean only, cooked, braised	32.08	8.89	208	0
Beef, New Zealand, imported, cube roll, separable lean only, cooked, fast roasted	30.09	13.22	239	0
Beef, New Zealand, imported, cube roll, separable lean only, raw	19.77	8.51	161	1.38
Beef, New Zealand, imported, eye round, separable lean only, cooked, slow roasted	29.68	4.98	164	0
Beef, New Zealand, imported, eye round, separable lean only, raw	20.15	3.35	116	1.35
Beef, New Zealand, imported, flank, separable lean only, cooked, braised	30.75	7.92	194	0
Beef, New Zealand, imported, flank, separable lean only, raw	20.53	6.67	142	0
Beef, New Zealand, imported, flat, separable lean only, cooked, braised	33.22	10.3	226	0
Beef, New Zealand, imported, flat, separable lean only, raw	21.3	7.69	154	0
Beef, New Zealand, imported, variety meats and by-products, heart, cooked, boiled	31.29	6	179	0
Beef, New Zealand, imported, variety meats and by-products, heart, raw	18.52	3.4	105	0
Beef, New Zealand, imported, hind shin, separable lean only, cooked, braised	31.23	4.64	167	0
Beef, New Zealand, imported, hind shin, separable lean only, raw	21.46	3.12	114	0
Beef, New Zealand, imported, inside, raw	22.16	4.36	128	0.1

Food Name ---> per 100 g	Protein (g)	Fat (g)	Calories	Net Carb (g)
Beef, New Zealand, imported, intermuscular fat, cooked	7.9	57.22	560	3.39
Beef, New Zealand, imported, intermuscular fat, raw	6.97	63.78	602	0.01
Beef, New Zealand, imported, variety meats and by-products, kidney, cooked, boiled	27.28	5.27	157	0
Beef, New Zealand, imported, knuckle, cooked, fast fried	27.51	7.58	178	0
Beef, New Zealand, imported, variety meats and by-products, kidney, raw	15.68	2.64	87	0
Beef, New Zealand, imported, variety meats and by-products liver, cooked, boiled	23.3	4.68	150	3.78
Beef, New Zealand, imported, variety meats and by-products, liver, raw	20.5	4.05	133	3.6
Beef, New Zealand, imported, manufacturing beef, cooked, boiled	24.21	3.26	126	0
Beef, New Zealand, imported, manufacturing beef, raw	21.23	3.68	119	0.23
Beef, New Zealand, imported, oyster blade, separable lean only, cooked, braised	29.87	8.46	196	0
Beef, New Zealand, imported, oyster blade, separable lean only, raw	21.83	7.56	155	0
Beef, New Zealand, imported, ribs prepared, cooked, fast roasted	27.23	9.74	197	0.09
Beef, New Zealand, imported, ribs prepared, raw	21.31	6.78	146	0
Beef, New Zealand, imported, rump centre, separable lean only, cooked, fast fried	30.17	7.48	188	0
Beef, New Zealand, imported, striploin, separable lean only, cooked, fast fried	28.53	11.4	217	0
Beef, New Zealand, imported, striploin, separable lean only, raw	20.93	7	150	0.74
Beef, New Zealand, imported, subcutaneous fat, cooked	6.5	78.3	731	0
Beef, New Zealand, imported, subcutaneous fat, raw	8.5	72.38	685	0
Beef, New Zealand, imported, sweetbread, cooked, boiled	12.53	29.79	318	0
Beef, New Zealand, imported, sweetbread, raw	11.51	28.6	303	0
Beef, New Zealand, imported, tenderloin, separable lean only, cooked, fast fried	29.37	9.01	200	0.27
Beef, New Zealand, imported, oyster blade, separable lean and fat, raw	21.27	10.31	178	0
Beef, New Zealand, imported, tenderloin, separable lean only, raw	21.19	6.1	140	0

Food Name ---> per 100 g	Protein (g)	Fat (g)	Calories	Net Carb (g)
Beef, New Zealand, imported, variety meats and by-products, tongue, cooked, boiled	18.31	20.34	271	3.68
Beef, New Zealand, imported, variety meats and by-products, tongue, raw	17.77	19.09	243	0
Beef, New Zealand, imported, variety meats and by-products, tripe cooked, boiled	19	2.98	103	0
Beef, New Zealand, imported, variety meats and by-products, tripe uncooked, raw	14.86	1.98	77	0
Beef, New Zealand, imported, bolar blade, separable lean and fat, cooked, fast roasted	31.3	11.37	228	0
Beef, New Zealand, imported, bolar blade, separable lean and fat, raw	21.29	8.22	159	0
Beef, New Zealand, imported, brisket navel end, separable lean and fat, cooked, braised	20.14	41.33	453	0
Beef, New Zealand, imported, brisket navel end, separable lean and fat, raw	15.81	31.27	345	0
Beef, New Zealand, imported, brisket point end, separable lean and fat, cooked, braised	31.94	13.6	250	0
Beef, New Zealand, imported, brisket point end, separable lean and fat, raw	20.05	9.23	163	0
Beef, New Zealand, imported, chuck eye roll, separable lean and fat, cooked, braised	29.92	14.74	252	0
Beef, New Zealand, imported, chuck eye roll, separable lean and fat, raw	19.38	11.45	181	0
Beef, New Zealand, imported, cube roll, separable lean and fat, cooked, fast roasted	27.79	19.45	286	0.03
Beef, New Zealand, imported, cube roll, separable lean and fat, raw	18.22	16.31	225	1.31
Beef, New Zealand, imported, eye round, separable lean and fat, cooked, slow roasted	29.49	5.57	168	0
Beef, New Zealand, imported, eye round, separable lean and fat, raw	19.88	4.92	129	1.32
Beef, New Zealand, imported, flank, separable lean and fat, cooked, braised	30.13	9.73	208	0
Beef, New Zealand, imported, flank, separable lean and fat, raw	20.12	8.9	161	0
Beef, New Zealand, imported, flat, separable lean and fat, cooked, braised	31.86	13.79	252	0
Beef, New Zealand, imported, flat, separable lean and fat, raw	20.57	10.55	177	0

Food Name ---> per 100 g	Protein (g)	Fat (g)	Calories	Net Carb (g)
Beef, New Zealand, imported, hind shin, separable lean and fat, cooked, braised	29.82	8.5	196	0.07
Beef, New Zealand, imported, hind shin, separable lean and fat, raw	20.61	7.2	147	0
Beef, New Zealand, imported, oyster blade, separable lean and fat, cooked, braised	29.79	8.68	197	0
Beef, New Zealand, imported, rump centre, separable lean and fat, cooked, fast fried	30.01	7.96	192	0
Beef, New Zealand, imported, rump centre, separable lean only, raw	21.74	6.05	141	0
Beef, New Zealand, imported, rump centre, separable lean and fat, raw	21.65	6.5	145	0
Beef, New Zealand, imported, striploin, separable lean and fat, cooked, fast fried	24.89	22.33	301	0.02
Beef, New Zealand, imported, striploin, separable lean and fat, raw	18.49	19.53	252	0.6
Beef, New Zealand, imported, tenderloin, separable lean and fat, cooked, fast fried	29.26	9.35	202	0.27
Beef, New Zealand, imported, tenderloin, separable lean and fat, raw	21.04	6.88	146	0
Beef, ground, 93% lean meat / 7% fat, raw	20.85	7	152	0
Beef, ground, 93% lean meat / 7% fat, patty, cooked, broiled	26.22	8.94	193	0
Beef, ground, 93% lean meat /7% fat, patty, cooked, pan-broiled	25.56	8.01	182	0.06
Beef, ground, 93% lean meat / 7% fat, loaf, cooked, baked	27.03	8.43	192	0
Beef, ground, 93% lean meat / 7% fat, crumbles, cooked, pan-browned	28.88	9.51	209	0
Beef, ground, 97% lean meat / 3% fat, raw	21.98	3	121	0
Beef, ground, 97% lean meat / 3% fat, patty, cooked, broiled	26.36	4.46	153	0
Beef, ground, 97% lean meat /3% fat, patty, cooked, pan-broiled	26.03	3.65	144	0
Beef, ground, 97% lean meat / 3% fat, loaf, cooked, baked	27.58	4.06	154	0
Beef, ground, 97% lean meat / 3% fat, crumbles, cooked, pan-browned	29.46	5.46	175	0
Beef, composite of trimmed retail cuts, separable lean and fat, trimmed to 0" fat, all grades, raw	20.95	9.3	169	0.05
Beef, composite of trimmed retail cuts, separable lean only, trimmed to 1/8" fat, all grades, raw	22.15	5.38	140	0

Food Name ---> per 100 g	Protein (g)	Fat (g)	Calories	Net Carb (g)
Beef, composite of trimmed retail cuts, separable lean only, trimmed to 1/8" fat, all grades, cooked	28.95	8.15	194	0
Beef, composite of trimmed retail cuts, separable lean only, trimmed to 0" fat, all grades, raw	22.15	5.54	139	0.08
Beef, composite of trimmed retail cuts, separable lean only, trimmed to 1/8" fat, choice, raw	22.01	6.05	147	0
Beef composite, separable lean only, trimmed to 1/8" fat, choice, cooked	28.73	9.16	203	0
Beef, composite of trimmed retail cuts, separable lean and fat, trimmed to 0" fat, choice, raw	21.34	10.08	176	0.06
Beef, composite of trimmed retail cuts, separable lean only, trimmed to 0" fat, choice, raw	21.55	7.24	151	0
Beef, composite of trimmed retail cuts, separable lean only, trimmed to 0" fat, select, raw	22.03	4.99	133	0.05
Beef, composite of trimmed retail cuts, separable lean and fat, trimmed to 0" fat, select, raw	21.2	8	157	0.04
Beef, composite of trimmed retail cuts, separable lean only, trimmed to 1/8" fat, select, cooked	27.51	6.37	167	0
Beef, composite of trimmed retail cuts, separable lean only, trimmed to 1/8" fat, select, raw	22.37	4.55	130	0
USDA Commodity, beef patties with VPP, frozen, cooked	15.64	16.94	247	6.49
USDA Commodity, beef, ground bulk/coarse ground, frozen, cooked	26.06	16.34	259	0
USDA Commodity, beef, patties (100%), frozen, cooked	22.98	16.37	249	0.91
USDA Commodity, beef patties with VPP, frozen, raw	15.21	16.48	225	2.54
USDA Commodity, beef, patties (100%), frozen, raw	14.63	15.69	204	0
USDA Commodity, beef, ground, bulk/coarse ground, frozen, raw	17.37	17.07	228	0
Beef, chuck, mock tender steak, separable lean only, trimmed to 0" fat, all grades, cooked, broiled	25.9	5.42	159	0
Beef, chuck, top blade, separable lean only, trimmed to 0" fat, all grades, cooked, broiled	26.13	10.16	203	0
Beef, chuck, clod roast, separable lean only, trimmed to 1/4" fat, all grades, raw	19.63	5.02	129	0
Beef, chuck, clod roast, separable lean only, trimmed to 0" fat, all grades, cooked, roasted	26.82	6.34	172	0
Beef, chuck, clod roast, separable lean only, trimmed to 1/4" fat, all grades, cooked, roasted	26.36	6.75	173	0

Food Name ---> per 100 g	Protein (g)	Fat (g)	Calories	Net Carb (g)
Beef, shoulder steak, boneless, separable lean only, trimmed to 0" fat, all grades, cooked, grilled	28.6	5.82	175	0
Beef, chuck, clod steak, separable lean only, trimmed to 1/4" fat, all grades, cooked, braised	29.34	7.04	189	0
Beef, chuck, mock tender steak, separable lean and fat, trimmed to 0" fat, USDA choice, cooked, broiled	25.73	5.72	161	0
Beef, chuck, mock tender steak, separable lean and fat, trimmed to 0" fat, USDA select, cooked, broiled	26.08	5.24	159	0
Beef, chuck, top blade, separable lean and fat, trimmed to 0" fat, choice, cooked, broiled	25.77	12.93	227	0
Beef, chuck, top blade, separable lean and fat, trimmed to 0" fat, select, cooked, broiled	25.67	9.99	200	0
Beef, chuck, clod roast, separable lean and fat, trimmed to 0" fat, choice, cooked, roasted	24.61	12.26	216	0
Beef, chuck, clod roast, separable lean and fat, trimmed to 0" fat, select, cooked, roasted	27.3	8.76	196	0
Beef, shoulder steak, boneless, separable lean and fat, trimmed to 0" fat, choice, cooked, grilled	28.22	7.25	186	0
Beef, shoulder steak, boneless, separable lean and fat, trimmed to 0" fat, select, cooked, grilled	28.41	6.14	177	0
Beef, plate, inside skirt steak, separable lean and fat, trimmed to 0" fat, all grades, cooked, broiled	26.13	12.05	220	0
Beef, plate, outside skirt steak, separable lean and fat, trimmed to 0" fat, all grades, cooked, broiled	23.51	17.13	255	0
Beef, loin, bottom sirloin butt, tri-tip steak, separable lean and fat, trimmed to 0" fat, all grades, cooked, broiled	29.97	15.18	265	0
Beef, chuck, mock tender steak, separable lean and fat, trimmed to 0" fat, all grades, cooked, broiled	25.87	5.52	160	0
Beef, chuck, top blade, separable lean and fat, trimmed to 0" fat, all grades, cooked, broiled	25.73	11.73	216	0
Beef, chuck, clod roast, separable lean and fat, trimmed to 0" fat, all grades, cooked, roasted	25.7	10.84	207	0
Beef, shoulder steak, boneless, separable lean and fat, trimmed to 0" fat, all grades, cooked, grilled	28.29	6.8	182	0
Beef, ground, 95% lean meat / 5% fat, raw	21.41	5	137	0
Beef, ground, 95% lean meat / 5% fat, patty, cooked, broiled	26.29	6.8	174	0
Beef, ground, 95% lean meat / 5% fat, patty, cooked, pan-broiled	25.8	5.94	164	0

Food Name ---> per 100 g	Protein (g)	Fat (g)	Calories	Net Carb (g)
Beef, ground, 95% lean meat / 5% fat, crumbles, cooked, pan-browned	29.17	7.58	193	0
Beef, ground, 95% lean meat / 5% fat, loaf, cooked, baked	27.31	6.37	174	0
Beef, ground, 90% lean meat / 10% fat, raw	20	10	176	0
Beef, ground, 90% lean meat / 10% fat, patty, cooked, broiled	26.11	11.75	217	0
Beef, ground, 90% lean meat / 10% fat, patty, cooked, pan-broiled	25.21	10.68	204	0
Beef, ground, 90% lean meat / 10% fat, crumbles, cooked, pan-browned	28.45	12.04	230	0
Beef, ground, 90% lean meat / 10% fat, loaf, cooked, baked	26.62	11.1	214	0
Beef, ground, 85% lean meat / 15% fat, raw	18.59	15	215	0
Beef, ground, 85% lean meat / 15% fat, patty, cooked, broiled	25.93	15.41	250	0
Beef, ground, 85% lean meat / 15% fat, patty, cooked, pan-broiled	24.62	14.02	232	0
Beef, ground, 85% lean meat / 15% fat, crumbles, cooked, pan-browned	27.73	15.3	256	0
Beef, ground, 85% lean meat / 15% fat, loaf, cooked, baked	25.93	14.36	240	0
Beef, ground, 80% lean meat / 20% fat, raw	17.17	20	254	0
Beef, ground, 80% lean meat / 20% fat, patty, cooked, broiled	25.75	17.78	270	0
Beef, ground, 80% lean meat / 20% fat, patty, cooked, pan-broiled	24.04	15.94	246	0
Beef, ground, 80% lean meat / 20% fat, crumbles, cooked, pan-browned	27	17.36	272	0
Beef, ground, 80% lean meat / 20% fat, loaf, cooked, baked	25.25	16.17	254	0
Beef, ground, 75% lean meat / 25% fat, raw	15.76	25	293	0
Beef, ground, 75% lean meat / 25% fat, patty, cooked, broiled	25.56	18.87	279	0
Beef, ground, 75% lean meat / 25% fat, patty, cooked, pan-broiled	23.45	16.44	248	0
Beef, ground, 75% lean meat / 25% fat, crumbles, cooked, pan-browned	26.28	18.21	277	0
Beef, ground, 75% lean meat / 25% fat, loaf, cooked, baked	24.56	16.5	254	0
Beef, rib, small end (ribs 10-12), separable lean only, trimmed to 1/8" fat, select, raw	22.53	4.2	134	0
Beef, tenderloin, steak, separable lean only, trimmed to 1/8" fat, select, raw	22.06	5.93	148	0

Food Name ---> per 100 g	Protein (g)	Fat (g)	Calories	Net Carb (g)
Beef, top sirloin, steak, separable lean only, trimmed to 1/8" fat, select, raw	22.27	3.54	127	0
Beef, short loin, top loin, steak, separable lean only, trimmed to 1/8" fat, select, raw	23.07	3.88	133	0
Beef, rib, small end (ribs 10-12), separable lean only, trimmed to 1/8" fat, select, cooked, broiled	30.87	6.22	188	0
Beef, tenderloin, steak, separable lean only, trimmed to 1/8" fat, select, cooked, broiled	29.07	7.76	194	0
Beef, top sirloin, steak, separable lean only, trimmed to 1/8" fat, select, cooked, broiled	29.34	4.96	170	0
Beef, short loin, top loin, steak, separable lean only, trimmed to 1/8" fat, select, cooked, grilled	29.44	5.73	177	0
Beef, round, bottom round , roast, separable lean only, trimmed to 1/8" fat, select, cooked, roasted	28.45	4.67	164	0
Beef, round, eye of round, roast, separable lean only, trimmed to 1/8" fat, select, cooked, roasted	29.59	4.11	163	0
Beef, round, top round, steak, separable lean only, trimmed to 1/8" fat, select, cooked, broiled	31.61	4.65	177	0
Beef, round, bottom round, steak, separable lean only, trimmed to 1/8" fat, select, cooked, braised	34.46	6.43	205	0
Beef, round, bottom round, roast, separable lean only, trimmed to 1/8" fat, all grades, raw	22.19	4.31	128	0
Beef, brisket, flat half, separable lean only, trimmed to 1/8" fat, all grades, cooked, braised	33.15	6	196	0
Beef, brisket, flat half, separable lean only, trimmed to 1/8" fat, all grades, raw	21.57	3.84	127	0
Beef, round, eye of round, roast, separable lean only, trimmed to 1/8" fat, all grades, raw	22.6	3	124	0
Beef, round, eye of round, roast, separable lean only, trimmed to 1/8" fat, all grades, cooked, roasted	29.73	4.71	169	0
Beef, rib, small end (ribs 10-12), separable lean only, trimmed to 1/8" fat, all grades, raw	22.33	5.04	141	0
Beef, tenderloin, steak, separable lean only, trimmed to 1/8" fat, all grades, cooked, broiled	29.04	8.39	200	0
Beef, tenderloin, steak, separable lean only, trimmed to 1/8" fat, all grades, raw	22.12	6.52	153	0
Beef, chuck, arm pot roast, separable lean only, trimmed to 1/8" fat, all grades, cooked, braised	34.66	7.36	214	0

Food Name ---> per 100 g	Protein (g)	Fat (g)	Calories	Net Carb (g)
Beef, chuck, arm pot roast, separable lean only, trimmed to 1/8" fat, all grades, raw	22.11	4.19	132	0
Beef, round, bottom round, roast, separable lean only, trimmed to 1/8" fat, all grades, cooked	28	5.72	163	0
Beef, round, bottom round, steak, separable lean only, trimmed to 1/8" fat, all grades, cooked, braised	34.34	7.73	216	0
Beef, short loin, top loin, steak, separable lean only, trimmed to 1/8" fat, all grades, cooked, broiled	29.3	7.09	189	0
Beef, short loin, top loin steak, separable lean only, trimmed to 1/8" fat, all grades, raw	22.93	5.15	138	0
Beef, round, top round, steak, separable lean only, trimmed to 1/8" fat, all grades, cooked, broiled	31.82	5.45	185	0
Beef, round, top round, steak, separable lean only, trimmed to 1/8" fat, all grades, raw	22.91	4.09	135	0
Beef, top sirloin, steak, separable lean only, trimmed to 1/8" fat, all grades, cooked, broiled	29.42	5.84	178	0
Beef, top sirloin, steak, separable lean only, trimmed to 1/8" fat, all grades, raw	22.09	4.08	131	0
Beef, chuck, arm pot roast, separable lean only, trimmed to 1/8" fat, choice, raw	21.96	5.05	139	0
Beef, brisket, flat half, separable lean only, trimmed to 1/8" fat, choice, raw	21.69	4.06	129	0
Beef, chuck, arm pot roast, separable lean only, trimmed to 1/8" fat, choice, cooked, braised	34.72	8.37	224	0
Beef, brisket, flat half, separable lean only, trimmed to 1/8" fat, choice, cooked, braised	33.13	6.79	203	0
Beef, round, eye of round, roast, separable lean only, trimmed to 1/8" fat, choice, raw	22.88	3.38	128	0
Beef, round, top round, steak, separable lean only, trimmed to 1/8" fat, choice, raw	22.69	4.78	140	0
Beef, round, bottom round, roast, separable lean only, trimmed to 1/8" fat, choice, raw	22.22	4.96	140	0
Beef, round, bottom round, roast, separable lean only, trimmed to 1/8" fat, choice, cooked, roasted	27.56	6.77	179	0
Beef, round, eye of round, roast, separable lean only, trimmed to 1/8" fat, choice, cooked, roasted	29.87	5.3	175	0
Beef, round, top round, steak, separable lean only, trimmed to 1/8" fat, choice, cooked, broiled	32.04	6.25	193	0

Food Name ---> per 100 g	Protein (g)	Fat (g)	Calories	Net Carb (g)
Beef, round, bottom round, steak, separable lean only, trimmed to 1/8" fat, choice, cooked, braised	34.22	9.02	228	0
Beef, rib, small end (ribs 10-12), separable lean only, trimmed to 1/8" fat, choice, raw	22.12	5.91	148	0
Beef, tenderloin, steak, separable lean only, trimmed to 1/8" fat, choice, raw	22.17	7.07	158	0
Beef, top sirloin, steak, separable lean only, trimmed to 1/8" fat, choice, raw	21.91	4.62	135	0
Beef, rib, small end (ribs 10-12), separable lean only, trimmed to 1/8"fat, choice, cooked, broiled	28.29	9.05	202	0
Beef, short loin, top loin, steak, separable lean only, trimmed to 1/8" fat, choice, raw	22.78	6.43	155	0
Beef, tenderloin, steak, separable lean only, trimmed to 1/8" fat, choice, cooked, broiled	29.01	9.1	206	0
Beef, top sirloin, steak, separable lean only, trimmed to 1/8" fat, choice, cooked, broiled	29.51	6.72	187	0
Beef, short loin, top loin, steak, separable lean only, trimmed to 1/8" fat, choice, cooked, broiled	29.16	8.45	201	0
Beef, chuck, arm pot roast, separable lean only, trimmed to 1/8" fat, select, raw	22.26	3.32	125	0
Beef, brisket, flat half, separable lean only, trimmed to 1/8" fat, select, raw	21.45	3.61	124	0
Beef, chuck, arm pot roast, separable lean only, trimmed to 1/8" fat, select, cooked, braised	34.6	6.35	205	0
Beef, brisket, flat half, separable lean only, trimmed to 1/8" fat, select, cooked, braised	33.18	5.21	189	0
Beef, round, eye of round, roast, separable lean only, trimmed to 1/8" fat, select, raw	22.31	2.62	119	0
Beef, round, top round, steak, separable lean only, trimmed to 1/8" fat, select, raw	23.13	3.37	129	0
Beef, round, bottom round, roast, separable lean only, trimmed to 1/8" fat, select, raw	22.18	3.66	128	0
Beef, rib, small end (ribs 10-12), separable lean only, trimmed to 1/8" fat, all grades, cooked, broiled	29.58	7.63	195	0
Beef, variety meats and by-products, tripe, cooked, simmered	11.71	4.05	94	1.99
Beef, bottom sirloin, tri-tip roast, separable lean only, trimmed to 0" fat, all grades, raw	21.26	5.63	142	0

Food Name ---> per 100 g	Protein (g)	Fat (g)	Calories	Net Carb (g)
Beef, bottom sirloin, tri-tip roast, separable lean only, trimmed to 0" fat, choice, cooked, roasted	26.34	9.73	193	0
Beef, bottom sirloin, tri-tip roast, separable lean only, trimmed to 0" fat, choice, raw	21.17	7.06	154	0
Beef, bottom sirloin, tri-tip roast, separable lean only, trimmed to 0" fat, select, cooked, roasted	27.17	6.95	179	0
Beef, bottom sirloin, tri-tip roast, separable lean only, trimmed to 0" fat, select, raw	21.34	4.21	129	0
Beef, round, tip round, roast, separable lean only, trimmed to 0" fat, all grades, raw	21.07	3.95	126	0
Beef, round, tip round, roast, separable lean only, trimmed to 0" fat, choice, raw	20.76	4.55	130	0
Beef, round, tip round, roast, separable lean only, trimmed to 0" fat, select, raw	21.38	3.35	122	0
Beef, flank, steak, separable lean only, trimmed to 0" fat, all grades, cooked, broiled	27.89	7.4	186	0
Beef, flank, steak, separable lean only, trimmed to 0" fat, select, cooked, broiled	27.96	6.48	178	0
Beef, flank, steak, separable lean only, trimmed to 0" fat, all grades, raw	21.57	5.47	141	0
Beef, flank, steak, separable lean only, trimmed to 0" fat, select, raw	21.43	5	137	0
Beef, brisket, flat half, separable lean and fat, trimmed to 1/8" fat, choice, raw	18.12	22.15	278	0.12
Beef, brisket, flat half, separable lean and fat, trimmed to 1/8" fat, select, raw	17.77	22.21	276	0
Beef, brisket, flat half, separable lean and fat, trimmed to 1/8" fat, choice, cooked, braised	28.66	19.47	298	0

Cereal Grains and Pasta

Food Name ---> per 100 g	Protein (g)	Fat (g)	Calories	Net Carb (g)
Amaranth grain, uncooked	13.56	7.02	371	58.55
Amaranth grain, cooked	3.8	1.58	102	16.59
Arrowroot flour	0.3	0.1	357	84.75
Barley, hulled	12.48	2.3	354	56.18
Barley, pearled, raw	9.91	1.16	352	62.12
Barley, pearled, cooked	2.26	0.44	123	24.42
Buckwheat	13.25	3.4	343	61.5
Buckwheat groats, roasted, dry	11.73	2.71	346	64.65
Buckwheat groats, roasted, cooked	3.38	0.62	92	17.24
Buckwheat flour, whole-groat	12.62	3.1	335	60.59
Bulgur, dry	12.29	1.33	342	63.37
Bulgur, cooked	3.08	0.24	83	14.08
Corn grain, yellow	9.42	4.74	365	66.96
Corn bran, crude	8.36	0.92	224	6.64
Corn flour, whole-grain, yellow	6.93	3.86	361	69.55
Corn flour, masa, enriched, white	8.46	3.69	363	70.19
Corn flour, yellow, degermed, unenriched	5.59	1.39	375	80.85
Corn flour, masa, unenriched, white	8.46	3.69	363	70.19
Cornmeal, whole-grain, yellow	8.12	3.59	362	69.59
Cornmeal, degermed, enriched, yellow	7.11	1.75	370	75.55
Cornmeal, yellow, self-rising, bolted, plain, enriched	8.28	3.4	334	63.58
Cornmeal, yellow, self-rising, bolted, with wheat flour added, enriched	8.41	2.85	348	67.13
Cornmeal, yellow, self-rising, degermed, enriched	8.41	1.72	355	67.69
Cornstarch	0.26	0.05	381	90.37
Couscous, dry	12.76	0.64	376	72.43
Couscous, cooked	3.79	0.16	112	21.82
Hominy, canned, white	1.48	0.88	72	11.76
Millet, raw	11.02	4.22	378	64.35

Food Name ---> per 100 g	Protein (g)	Fat (g)	Calories	Net Carb (g)
Millet, cooked	3.51	1	119	22.37
Oat bran, raw	17.3	7.03	246	50.82
Oat bran, cooked	3.21	0.86	40	8.84
Quinoa, uncooked	14.12	6.07	368	57.16
Rice, brown, long-grain, raw	7.54	3.2	367	72.65
Rice, brown, long-grain, cooked	2.74	0.97	123	23.98
Oats	16.89	6.9	389	55.67
Rice, brown, medium-grain, raw	7.5	2.68	362	72.77
Rice, brown, medium-grain, cooked	2.32	0.83	112	21.71
Rice, brown, parboiled, dry, UNCLE BEN'S	7.6	2.75	370	75.18
Rice, white, long-grain, regular, raw, enriched	7.13	0.66	365	78.65
Rice, white, long-grain, regular, enriched, cooked	2.69	0.28	130	27.77
Rice, white, long-grain, parboiled, enriched, dry	7.51	1.03	374	79.09
Rice, white, long-grain, parboiled, enriched, cooked	2.91	0.37	123	25.15
Rice, white, long-grain, precooked or instant, enriched, dry	7.82	0.94	380	80.42
Rice, white, long-grain, precooked or instant, enriched, prepared	2.18	0.5	124	26.16
Rice, white, medium-grain, raw, enriched	6.61	0.58	360	77.94
Rice, white, medium-grain, enriched, cooked	2.38	0.21	130	28.29
Rice, white, short-grain, enriched, uncooked	6.5	0.52	358	76.35
Rice, white, short-grain, enriched, cooked	2.36	0.19	130	28.73
Rice, white, glutinous, unenriched, uncooked	6.81	0.55	370	78.88
Rice, white, glutinous, unenriched, cooked	2.02	0.19	97	20.09
Rice, white, steamed, Chinese restaurant	3.2	0.27	151	32.98
Rice bran, crude	13.35	20.85	316	28.69
Rice flour, white, unenriched	5.95	1.42	366	77.73
Rye grain	10.34	1.63	338	60.76
Rye flour, dark	15.91	2.22	325	44.83
Rye flour, medium	10.88	1.52	349	63.63
Rye flour, light	9.82	1.33	357	68.68
Semolina, enriched	12.68	1.05	360	68.93
Sorghum grain	10.62	3.46	329	65.39

Food Name ---> per 100 g	Protein (g)	Fat (g)	Calories	Net Carb (g)
Tapioca, pearl, dry	0.19	0.02	358	87.79
Triticale	13.05	2.09	336	72.13
Triticale flour, whole-grain	13.18	1.81	338	58.54
Wheat, hard red spring	15.4	1.92	329	55.83
Wheat, hard red winter	12.61	1.54	327	58.98
Wheat, soft red winter	10.35	1.56	331	61.74
Wheat, hard white	11.31	1.71	342	63.7
Wheat, soft white	10.69	1.99	340	62.66
Wheat, durum	13.68	2.47	339	71.13
Wheat bran, crude	15.55	4.25	216	21.71
Wheat germ, crude	23.15	9.72	360	38.6
Wheat flour, whole-grain	13.21	2.5	340	61.27
Wheat flour, white, all-purpose, enriched, bleached	10.33	0.98	364	73.61
Wheat flour, white, all-purpose, self-rising, enriched	9.89	0.97	354	71.52
Wheat flour, white, bread, enriched	11.98	1.66	361	70.13
Wheat flour, white, cake, enriched	8.2	0.86	362	76.33
Wheat flour, white, tortilla mix, enriched	9.66	10.63	405	67.14
Wheat, sprouted	7.49	1.27	198	41.43
Wild rice, raw	14.73	1.08	357	68.7
Wild rice, cooked	3.99	0.34	101	19.54
Rice flour, brown	7.23	2.78	363	71.88
Pasta, gluten-free, corn, dry	7.46	2.08	357	68.26
Pasta, gluten-free, corn, cooked	2.63	0.73	126	23.11
Pasta, fresh-refrigerated, plain, as purchased	11.31	2.3	288	54.73
Pasta, fresh-refrigerated, plain, cooked	5.15	1.05	131	24.93
Pasta, fresh-refrigerated, spinach, as purchased	11.26	2.1	289	55.72
Pasta, fresh-refrigerated, spinach, cooked	5.06	0.94	130	25.04
Pasta, homemade, made with egg, cooked	5.28	1.74	130	23.54
Pasta, homemade, made without egg, cooked	4.37	0.98	124	25.12
Macaroni, vegetable, enriched, dry	13.14	1.04	367	70.58
Macaroni, vegetable, enriched, cooked	4.53	0.11	128	22.31

Food Name ---> per 100 g	Protein (g)	Fat (g)	Calories	Net Carb (g)
Noodles, egg, dry, enriched	14.16	4.44	384	67.97
Noodles, egg, enriched, cooked	4.54	2.07	138	23.96
Noodles, egg, spinach, enriched, dry	14.61	4.55	382	63.52
Noodles, egg, spinach, enriched, cooked	5.04	1.57	132	21.95
Noodles, chinese, chow mein	8.11	15.43	475	69.1
Noodles, japanese, soba, dry	14.38	0.71	336	74.62
Noodles, japanese, soba, cooked	5.06	0.1	99	21.44
Noodles, japanese, somen, dry	11.35	0.81	356	69.8
Noodles, japanese, somen, cooked	4	0.18	131	27.54
Noodles, flat, crunchy, Chinese restaurant	10.33	31.72	521	50
Pasta, dry, enriched	13.04	1.51	371	71.47
Pasta, cooked, enriched, without added salt	5.8	0.93	158	29.06
Pasta, whole-wheat, dry	13.87	2.93	352	64.17
Pasta, whole-wheat, cooked	5.99	1.71	149	26.17
Spaghetti, spinach, dry	13.35	1.57	372	64.21
Spaghetti, spinach, cooked	4.58	0.63	130	26.15
Wheat flours, bread, unenriched	11.98	1.66	361	70.13
Barley flour or meal	10.5	1.6	345	64.42
Barley malt flour	10.28	1.84	361	71.2
Oat flour, partially debranned	14.66	9.12	404	59.2
Rice noodles, dry	5.95	0.56	364	78.58
Rice noodles, cooked	1.79	0.2	108	23.01
Pasta, whole grain, 51% whole wheat, remaining unenriched semolina, dry	13.51	2.68	362	63
Pasta, whole grain, 51% whole wheat, remaining unenriched semolina, cooked	5.82	1.5	159	26.91
Quinoa, cooked	4.4	1.92	120	18.5
Wheat, KAMUT khorasan, uncooked	14.54	2.13	337	59.48
Wheat, KAMUT khorasan, cooked	5.71	0.83	132	23.3
Spelt, uncooked	14.57	2.43	338	59.49
Spelt, cooked	5.5	0.85	127	22.54
Teff, uncooked	13.3	2.38	367	65.13

Food Name ---> per 100 g	Protein (g)	Fat (g)	Calories	Net Carb (g)
Teff, cooked	3.87	0.65	101	17.06
Noodles, egg, cooked, enriched, with added salt	4.54	2.07	138	23.96
Corn grain, white	9.42	4.74	365	74.26
Corn flour, whole-grain, blue (harina de maiz morado)	8.75	5.09	364	65.49
Corn flour, whole-grain, white	6.93	3.86	361	69.55
Corn flour, yellow, masa, enriched	8.46	3.69	363	70.19
Cornmeal, whole-grain, white	8.12	3.59	362	69.59
Pasta, cooked, enriched, with added salt	5.8	0.93	157	28.79
Cornmeal, degermed, enriched, white	7.11	1.75	370	75.55
Cornmeal, white, self-rising, bolted, plain, enriched	8.28	3.4	334	63.58
Cornmeal, white, self-rising, bolted, with wheat flour added, enriched	8.41	2.85	348	67.13
Cornmeal, white, self-rising, degermed, enriched	8.41	1.72	355	67.69
Hominy, canned, yellow	1.48	0.88	72	11.76
Rice, white, long-grain, regular, cooked, enriched, with salt	2.69	0.28	130	27.77
Wheat flour, white, all-purpose, enriched, calcium-fortified	10.33	0.98	364	73.61
Noodles, egg, dry, unenriched	14.16	4.44	384	67.97
Noodles, egg, unenriched, cooked, without added salt	4.54	2.07	138	23.96
Pasta, dry, unenriched	13.04	1.51	371	71.47
Pasta, cooked, unenriched, without added salt	5.8	0.93	158	29.06
Cornmeal, degermed, unenriched, yellow	7.11	1.75	370	75.55
Rice, white, long-grain, regular, raw, unenriched	7.13	0.66	365	78.65
Rice, white, long-grain, regular, unenriched, cooked without salt	2.69	0.28	130	27.77
Rice, white, long-grain, parboiled, unenriched, dry	7.51	1.03	374	79.09
Rice, white, long-grain, parboiled, unenriched, cooked	2.91	0.37	123	25.15
Rice, white, medium-grain, raw, unenriched	6.61	0.58	360	79.34
Rice, white, medium-grain, cooked, unenriched	2.38	0.21	130	28.59
Rice, white, short-grain, raw, unenriched	6.5	0.52	358	79.15
Rice, white, short-grain, cooked, unenriched	2.36	0.19	130	28.73
Semolina, unenriched	12.68	1.05	360	68.93
Wheat flour, white, all-purpose, unenriched	10.33	0.98	364	73.61

Food Name ---> per 100 g	Protein (g)	Fat (g)	Calories	Net Carb (g)
Noodles, egg, cooked, unenriched, with added salt	4.54	2.07	138	23.96
Pasta, cooked, unenriched, with added salt	5.8	0.93	157	28.79
Cornmeal, degermed, unenriched, white	7.11	1.75	370	75.55
Spaghetti, protein-fortified, cooked, enriched (n x 6.25)	8.86	0.21	164	28.88
Rice, white, long-grain, regular, cooked, unenriched, with salt	2.69	0.28	130	27.77
Wheat flour, white, all-purpose, enriched, unbleached	10.33	0.98	364	73.61
Spaghetti, protein-fortified, dry, enriched (n x 6.25)	21.78	2.23	374	63.25
Wheat flour, white (industrial), 9% protein, bleached, enriched	8.89	1.43	367	77.32
Wheat flour, white (industrial), 9% protein, bleached, unenriched	8.89	1.43	367	74.92
Wheat flour, white (industrial), 10% protein, bleached, enriched	9.71	1.48	366	73.82
Wheat flour, white (industrial), 10% protein, bleached, unenriched	9.71	1.48	366	73.82
Wheat flour, white (industrial), 10% protein, unbleached, enriched	9.71	1.48	366	73.82
Wheat flour, white (industrial), 11.5% protein, bleached, enriched	11.5	1.45	363	71.41
Wheat flour, white (industrial), 11.5% protein, bleached, unenriched	11.5	1.45	363	71.41
Wheat flour, white (industrial), 11.5% protein, unbleached, enriched	11.5	1.45	363	71.41
Wheat flour, white (industrial), 13% protein, bleached, enriched	13.07	1.38	362	69.8
Wheat flour, white (industrial), 13% protein, bleached, unenriched	13.07	1.38	362	69.8
Wheat flour, white (industrial), 15% protein, bleached, enriched	15.33	1.41	362	67.48
Wheat flour, white (industrial), 15% protein, bleached, unenriched	15.33	1.41	362	67.48
Millet flour	10.75	4.25	382	71.62
Sorghum flour, whole-grain	8.43	3.34	359	70.04
Vital wheat gluten	75.16	1.85	370	13.19

Dairy and Egg Products

Food Name ---> per 100 g	Protein (g)	Fat (g)	Calories	Net Carb (g)
Butter, salted	0.85	81.11	717	0.06
Butter, whipped, with salt	0.49	78.3	718	2.87
Butter oil, anhydrous	0.28	99.48	876	0
Cheese, blue	21.4	28.74	353	2.34
Cheese, brick	23.24	29.68	371	2.79
Cheese, brie	20.75	27.68	334	0.45
Cheese, camembert	19.8	24.26	300	0.46
Cheese, caraway	25.18	29.2	376	3.06
Cheese, cheddar	22.87	33.31	404	3.09
Cheese, cheshire	23.37	30.6	387	4.78
Cheese, colby	23.76	32.11	394	2.57
Cheese, cottage, creamed, large or small curd	11.12	4.3	98	3.38
Cheese, cottage, creamed, with fruit	10.69	3.85	97	4.41
Cheese, cottage, nonfat, uncreamed, dry, large or small curd	10.34	0.29	72	6.66
Cheese, cottage, lowfat, 2% milkfat	10.45	2.27	81	4.76
Cheese, cottage, lowfat, 1% milkfat	12.39	1.02	72	2.72
Cheese, cream	6.15	34.44	350	5.52
Cheese, edam	24.99	27.8	357	1.43
Cheese, feta	14.21	21.28	264	4.09
Cheese, fontina	25.6	31.14	389	1.55
Cheese, gjetost	9.65	29.51	466	42.65
Cheese, gouda	24.94	27.44	356	2.22
Cheese, gruyere	29.81	32.34	413	0.36
Cheese, limburger	20.05	27.25	327	0.49
Cheese, monterey	24.48	30.28	373	0.68
Cheese, mozzarella, whole milk	22.17	22.35	300	2.19
Cheese, mozzarella, whole milk, low moisture	21.6	24.64	318	2.47
Cheese, mozzarella, part skim milk	24.26	15.92	254	2.77

Food Name ---> per 100 g	Protein (g)	Fat (g)	Calories	Net Carb (g)
Cheese, mozzarella, low moisture, part-skim	23.75	19.78	295	5.58
Cheese, muenster	23.41	30.04	368	1.12
Cheese, neufchatel	9.15	22.78	253	3.59
Cheese, parmesan, grated	28.42	27.84	420	13.91
Cheese, parmesan, hard	35.75	25.83	392	3.22
Cheese, port de salut	23.78	28.2	352	0.57
Cheese, provolone	25.58	26.62	351	2.14
Cheese, ricotta, whole milk	11.26	12.98	174	3.04
Cheese, ricotta, part skim milk	11.39	7.91	138	5.14
Cheese, romano	31.8	26.94	387	3.63
Cheese, roquefort	21.54	30.64	369	2
Cheese, swiss	26.96	30.99	393	1.44
Cheese, tilsit	24.41	25.98	340	1.88
Cheese, pasteurized process, American, fortified with vitamin D	18.13	30.71	366	4.78
Cheese, pasteurized process, pimento	22.13	31.2	375	1.63
Cheese, pasteurized process, swiss	24.73	25.01	334	2.1
Cheese food, cold pack, American	19.66	24.46	331	8.32
Cheese food, pasteurized process, American, vitamin D fortified	16.86	25.63	330	8.56
Cheese food, pasteurized process, swiss	21.92	24.14	323	4.5
Cheese spread, pasteurized process, American	16.41	21.23	290	8.73
Cream, fluid, half and half	3.13	10.39	123	4.73
Cream, fluid, light (coffee cream or table cream)	2.96	19.1	191	2.82
Cream, fluid, light whipping	2.17	30.91	292	2.96
Cream, fluid, heavy whipping	2.84	36.08	340	2.74
Cream, whipped, cream topping, pressurized	3.2	22.22	257	12.49
Cream, sour, reduced fat, cultured	2.94	12	135	4.26
Cream, sour, cultured	2.44	19.35	198	4.63
Eggnog	4.55	4.19	88	8.05
Sour dressing, non-butterfat, cultured, filled cream-type	3.25	16.57	178	4.68
Milk, filled, fluid, with blend of hydrogenated vegetable oils	3.33	3.46	63	4.74
Milk, filled, fluid, with lauric acid oil	3.33	3.4	63	4.74

Food Name ---> per 100 g	Protein (g)	Fat (g)	Calories	Net Carb (g)
Cheese, American, nonfat or fat free	21.05	0	126	10.53
Cream substitute, liquid, with hydrogenated vegetable oil and soy protein	1	9.97	136	11.38
Cream substitute, liquid, with lauric acid oil and sodium caseinate	1	9.97	136	11.38
Cream substitute, powdered	2.48	32.92	529	59.29
Dessert topping, powdered	4.9	39.92	577	52.54
Dessert topping, powdered, 1.5 ounce prepared with 1/2 cup milk	3.61	12.72	194	17.13
Dessert topping, pressurized	0.98	22.3	264	16.07
Dessert topping, semi solid, frozen	1.25	25.31	318	23.05
Sour cream, imitation, cultured	2.4	19.52	208	6.63
Milk substitutes, fluid, with lauric acid oil	1.75	3.41	61	6.16
Milk, whole, 3.25% milkfat, with added vitamin D	3.15	3.25	61	4.8
Milk, producer, fluid, 3.7% milkfat	3.28	3.66	64	4.65
Milk, reduced fat, fluid, 2% milkfat, with added vitamin A and vitamin D	3.3	1.98	50	4.8
Milk, reduced fat, fluid, 2% milkfat, with added nonfat milk solids and vitamin A and vitamin D	3.48	1.92	51	4.97
Milk, reduced fat, fluid, 2% milkfat, protein fortified, with added vitamin A and vitamin D	3.95	1.98	56	5.49
Milk, lowfat, fluid, 1% milkfat, with added vitamin A and vitamin D	3.37	0.97	42	4.99
Milk, lowfat, fluid, 1% milkfat, with added nonfat milk solids, vitamin A and vitamin D	3.48	0.97	43	4.97
Milk, lowfat, fluid, 1% milkfat, protein fortified, with added vitamin A and vitamin D	3.93	1.17	48	5.52
Milk, nonfat, fluid, with added vitamin A and vitamin D (fat free or skim)	3.37	0.08	34	4.96
Milk, nonfat, fluid, with added nonfat milk solids, vitamin A and vitamin D (fat free or skim)	3.57	0.25	37	5.02
Milk, nonfat, fluid, protein fortified, with added vitamin A and vitamin D (fat free and skim)	3.96	0.25	41	5.56
Milk, buttermilk, fluid, cultured, lowfat	3.31	0.88	40	4.79
Milk, low sodium, fluid	3.1	3.46	61	4.46
Milk, dry, whole, with added vitamin D	26.32	26.71	496	38.42

Food Name ---> per 100 g	Protein (g)	Fat (g)	Calories	Net Carb (g)
Milk, dry, nonfat, regular, without added vitamin A and vitamin D	36.16	0.77	362	51.98
Milk, dry, nonfat, instant, with added vitamin A and vitamin D	35.1	0.72	358	52.19
Milk, dry, nonfat, calcium reduced	35.5	0.2	354	51.8
Milk, buttermilk, dried	34.3	5.78	387	49
Milk, chocolate, fluid, commercial, whole, with added vitamin A and vitamin D	3.17	3.39	83	9.54
Milk, chocolate, fluid, commercial, reduced fat, with added vitamin A and vitamin D	2.99	1.9	76	11.43
Milk, chocolate, lowfat, with added vitamin A and vitamin D	3.46	1	62	9.76
Milk, chocolate beverage, hot cocoa, homemade	3.52	2.34	77	9.74
Milk, goat, fluid, with added vitamin D	3.56	4.14	69	4.45
Milk, human, mature, fluid	1.03	4.38	70	6.89
Milk, indian buffalo, fluid	3.75	6.89	97	5.18
Milk, sheep, fluid	5.98	7	108	5.36
Milk shakes, thick chocolate	3.05	2.7	119	20.85
Milk shakes, thick vanilla	3.86	3.03	112	17.75
Whey, acid, fluid	0.76	0.09	24	5.12
Whey, acid, dried	11.73	0.54	339	73.45
Whey, sweet, fluid	0.85	0.36	27	5.14
Whey, sweet, dried	12.93	1.07	353	74.46
Yogurt, plain, whole milk, 8 grams protein per 8 ounce	3.47	3.25	61	4.66
Yogurt, plain, low fat, 12 grams protein per 8 ounce	5.25	1.55	63	7.04
Yogurt, plain, skim milk, 13 grams protein per 8 ounce	5.73	0.18	56	7.68
Yogurt, vanilla, low fat, 11 grams protein per 8 ounce	4.93	1.25	85	13.8
Yogurt, fruit, low fat, 9 grams protein per 8 ounce	3.98	1.15	99	18.64
Yogurt, fruit, low fat, 10 grams protein per 8 ounce	4.37	1.08	102	19.05
Yogurt, fruit, low fat, 11 grams protein per 8 ounce	4.86	1.41	105	18.6
Egg, whole, raw, fresh	12.56	9.51	143	0.72
Egg, white, raw, fresh	10.9	0.17	52	0.73
Egg, yolk, raw, fresh	15.86	26.54	322	3.59
Egg, whole, cooked, fried	13.61	14.84	196	0.83

Food Name ---> per 100 g	Protein (g)	Fat (g)	Calories	Net Carb (g)
Egg, whole, cooked, hard-boiled	12.58	10.61	155	1.12
Egg, whole, cooked, poached	12.51	9.47	143	0.71
Egg, yolk, dried	33.63	59.13	669	0.66
Egg, duck, whole, fresh, raw	12.81	13.77	185	1.45
Egg, goose, whole, fresh, raw	13.87	13.27	185	1.35
Egg, quail, whole, fresh, raw	13.05	11.09	158	0.41
Egg, turkey, whole, fresh, raw	13.68	11.88	171	1.15
Egg substitute, powder	55.5	13	444	21.8
Butter, without salt	0.85	81.11	717	0.06
Cheese, parmesan, shredded	37.86	27.34	415	3.41
Milk, nonfat, fluid, without added vitamin A and vitamin D (fat free or skim)	3.37	0.08	34	4.96
Milk, reduced fat, fluid, 2% milkfat, with added nonfat milk solids, without added vitamin A	3.95	1.98	56	5.49
Milk, canned, evaporated, with added vitamin A	6.81	7.56	134	10.04
Milk, dry, nonfat, regular, with added vitamin A and vitamin D	36.16	0.77	362	51.98
Milk, dry, nonfat, instant, without added vitamin A and vitamin D	35.1	0.72	358	52.19
Cheese, goat, hard type	30.52	35.59	452	2.17
Cheese, goat, semisoft type	21.58	29.84	364	0.12
Cheese, goat, soft type	18.52	21.08	264	0
Egg, yolk, raw, frozen, salted, pasteurized	14.07	22.93	275	1.77
Cheese substitute, mozzarella	11.47	12.22	248	23.67
Cheese sauce, prepared from recipe	10.33	14.92	197	5.38
Cheese, mexican, queso anejo	21.44	29.98	373	4.63
Cheese, mexican, queso asadero	22.6	28.26	356	2.87
Cheese, mexican, queso chihuahua	21.56	29.68	374	5.56
Cheese, low fat, cheddar or colby	24.35	7	173	1.91
Cheese, low-sodium, cheddar or colby	24.35	32.62	398	1.91
Egg, whole, raw, frozen, pasteurized	12.33	9.95	147	1.01
Egg, white, raw, frozen, pasteurized	10.2	0	48	1.04
Egg, white, dried	81.1	0	382	7.8

Food Name ---> per 100 g	Protein (g)	Fat (g)	Calories	Net Carb (g)
Milk, reduced fat, fluid, 2% milkfat, without added vitamin A and vitamin D	3.3	1.98	50	4.8
Milk, fluid, 1% fat, without added vitamin A and vitamin D	3.37	0.97	42	4.99
Sour cream, reduced fat	7	14.1	181	7
Sour cream, light	3.5	10.6	136	7.1
Sour cream, fat free	3.1	0	74	15.6
USDA Commodity, cheese, cheddar, reduced fat	27.2	18.3	282	2
Yogurt, vanilla or lemon flavor, nonfat milk, sweetened with low-calorie sweetener	3.86	0.18	43	7.5
Parmesan cheese topping, fat free	40	5	370	40
Cheese, cream, fat free	15.69	1	105	7.66
Yogurt, chocolate, nonfat milk	3.53	0	112	22.33
KRAFT CHEEZ WHIZ Pasteurized Process Cheese Sauce	12	21	276	8.9
KRAFT CHEEZ WHIZ LIGHT Pasteurized Process Cheese Product	16.3	9.5	215	16
KRAFT FREE Singles American Nonfat Pasteurized Process Cheese Product	22.7	1	148	11.5
KRAFT VELVEETA Pasteurized Process Cheese Spread	16.3	22	303	9.8
KRAFT VELVEETA LIGHT Reduced Fat Pasteurized Process Cheese Product	19.6	10.6	222	11.8
KRAFT BREAKSTONE'S Reduced Fat Sour Cream	4.5	12	152	6.4
KRAFT BREAKSTONE'S FREE Fat Free Sour Cream	4.7	1.3	91	15.1
Cream, half and half, fat free	2.6	1.4	59	9
Reddi Wip Fat Free Whipped Topping	3	5	149	24.6
Milk, chocolate, fluid, commercial, reduced fat, with added calcium	2.99	1.9	78	11.43
Yogurt, fruit, lowfat, with low calorie sweetener	4.86	1.41	105	18.6
Cheese, parmesan, dry grated, reduced fat	20	20	265	1.37
Cream substitute, flavored, liquid	0.69	13.5	251	33.97
Cream substitute, flavored, powdered	0.68	21.47	482	74.22
Cheese, provolone, reduced fat	24.7	17.6	274	3.5
Cheese, Mexican, blend, reduced fat	24.69	19.4	282	3.41
Egg Mix, USDA Commodity	35.6	34.5	555	23.97

Food Name ---> per 100 g	Protein (g)	Fat (g)	Calories	Net Carb (g)
Milk, whole, 3.25% milkfat, without added vitamin A and vitamin D	3.15	3.27	61	4.78
Milk, dry, whole, without added vitamin D	26.32	26.71	496	38.42
Milk, canned, evaporated, without added vitamin A and vitamin D	6.81	7.56	135	10.04
Cheese product, pasteurized process, American, reduced fat, fortified with vitamin D	17.6	14.1	240	10.6
Yogurt, fruit, low fat, 9 grams protein per 8 ounce, fortified with vitamin D	3.98	1.15	99	18.64
Yogurt, fruit, low fat, 10 grams protein per 8 ounce, fortified with vitamin D	4.37	1.08	102	19.05
Yogurt, fruit variety, nonfat, fortified with vitamin D	4.4	0.2	95	19
Yogurt, fruit, lowfat, with low calorie sweetener, fortified with vitamin D	4.86	1.41	105	18.6
Yogurt, vanilla, low fat, 11 grams protein per 8 ounce, fortified with vitamin D	4.93	1.25	85	13.8
Yogurt, vanilla or lemon flavor, nonfat milk, sweetened with low-calorie sweetener, fortified with vitamin D	3.86	0.18	43	7.5
Yogurt, chocolate, nonfat milk, fortified with vitamin D	3.53	0	112	22.33
Protein supplement, milk based, Muscle Milk, powder	45.71	17.14	411	11.4
Protein supplement, milk based, Muscle Milk Light, powder	50	12	396	20
Dulce de Leche	6.84	7.35	315	55.35
Egg substitute, liquid or frozen, fat free	10	0	48	2
Cheese, dry white, queso seco	24.51	24.35	325	2.04
Cheese, fresh, queso fresco	18.09	23.82	299	2.98
Cheese, white, queso blanco	20.38	24.31	310	2.53
Milk, buttermilk, fluid, whole	3.21	3.31	62	4.88
Yogurt, vanilla flavor, lowfat milk, sweetened with low calorie sweetener	4.93	1.25	86	13.8
Yogurt, frozen, flavors not chocolate, nonfat milk, with low-calorie sweetener	4.4	0.8	104	17.7
Ice cream, soft serve, chocolate	4.1	13	222	21.5
Ice cream, bar or stick, chocolate covered	4.1	24.1	331	23.7
Ice cream sandwich	4.29	8.57	237	37.14
Ice cream cookie sandwich	3.7	7.4	240	38.4

Food Name ---> per 100 g	Protein (g)	Fat (g)	Calories	Net Carb (g)
Ice cream cone, chocolate covered, with nuts, flavors other than chocolate	5.21	21.88	354	33.38
Ice cream sandwich, made with light ice cream, vanilla	4.29	3.04	186	39.64
Ice cream sandwich, vanilla, light, no sugar added	5.71	2.86	200	35.76
Fat free ice cream, no sugar added, flavors other than chocolate	4.41	0	129	20.54
Milk dessert bar, frozen, made from lowfat milk	4.41	1.47	147	26.49
Nutritional supplement for people with diabetes, liquid	4.4	3.08	88	9.68
Cheese, Mexican blend	23.54	28.51	358	1.75
Cheese product, pasteurized process, American, vitamin D fortified	17.12	23.11	312	8.8
Cheese, pasteurized process, American, without added vitamin D	18.13	31.79	371	3.7
Cheese food, pasteurized process, American, without added vitamin D	16.86	25.63	330	8.56
Egg, whole, raw, frozen, salted, pasteurized	10.97	10.07	138	0.83
Yogurt, Greek, plain, nonfat	10.19	0.39	59	3.6
Egg, white, dried, stabilized, glucose reduced	84.08	0.32	357	4.51
Cheese spread, American or Cheddar cheese base, reduced fat	13.41	8.88	176	10.71
Cheese, cheddar, reduced fat	27.35	20.41	309	4.06
Ice cream, light, soft serve, chocolate	3.36	3.69	141	23.15
Ice cream bar, stick or nugget, with crunch coating	2.11	25.26	358	36.02
Cheese, cheddar, nonfat or fat free	32.14	0	157	7.14
Cheese, Swiss, nonfat or fat free	28.4	0	127	3.4
Cheese, mexican, queso cotija	20	30	366	3.97
Cheese, cheddar, sharp, sliced	24.25	33.82	410	2.13
Cheese, mozzarella, low moisture, part-skim, shredded	23.63	19.72	304	8.06
Yogurt, Greek, nonfat, vanilla, CHOBANI	9.07	0.22	71	7.79
Yogurt, Greek, strawberry, DANNON OIKOS	8.25	2.92	106	10.67
Yogurt, Greek, nonfat, vanilla, DANNON OIKOS	8.12	0.14	85	12.22
Yogurt, Greek, nonfat, strawberry, DANNON OIKOS	8.03	0.22	84	12.13
Yogurt, Greek, nonfat, strawberry, CHOBANI	8.03	0.12	80	10.92
Yogurt, Greek, strawberry, lowfat	8.17	2.57	103	10.89
Yogurt, Greek, strawberry, nonfat	8.05	0.15	82	11.47

Food Name ---> per 100 g	Protein (g)	Fat (g)	Calories	Net Carb (g)
Yogurt, Greek, vanilla, nonfat	8.64	0.18	78	9.87
Yogurt, Greek, plain, lowfat	9.95	1.92	73	3.94
Kefir, lowfat, plain, LIFEWAY	3.79	0.93	41	4.48
Kefir, lowfat, strawberry, LIFEWAY	3.39	0.9	62	10.2
Milk, evaporated, 2% fat, with added vitamin A and vitamin D	6.67	2	107	15.74
Milk, chocolate, fat free, with added vitamin A and vitamin D	3.39	0	67	13.46
Yogurt, Greek, plain, whole milk	9	5	97	3.98
Yogurt, Greek, fruit, whole milk	7.33	3	106	12.29
Yogurt, vanilla, non-fat	2.94	0	78	17.04
Yogurt, Greek, vanilla, lowfat	8.64	2.5	95	9.54
Yogurt, frozen, flavors other than chocolate, lowfat	8	2.5	139	21
Ice cream bar, covered with chocolate and nuts	5.62	25.84	303	10.79
Ice cream sundae cone	3	14	254	27.89
Light ice cream, Creamsicle	1.54	3.08	165	32.75
Cream, half and half, lowfat	3.33	5	72	3.33
Milk, chocolate, lowfat, reduced sugar	3.43	1.04	54	7.68
Ice cream, lowfat, no sugar added, cone, added peanuts and chocolate sauce	5.33	9.33	265	30.71
Imitation cheese, american or cheddar, low cholesterol	25	32	390	1
Whipped topping, frozen, low fat	3	13.1	224	23.6
Cream substitute, powdered, light	1.9	15.7	431	73.4
Cream substitute, liquid, light	0.8	3.5	71	9.1
Cheese, monterey, low fat	28.2	21.6	313	0.7
Milk, buttermilk, fluid, cultured, reduced fat	4.1	2	56	5.3
Cheese, pasteurized process, cheddar or American, fat-free	22.5	0.8	148	13.4
Cheese, cottage, lowfat, 1% milkfat, lactose reduced	12.4	1	74	2.6
Cheese product, pasteurized process, cheddar, reduced fat	17.6	14.1	240	10.6
Milk, fluid, nonfat, calcium fortified (fat free or skim)	3.4	0.18	35	4.85
Cheese, muenster, low fat	24.7	17.6	271	3.5
Cheese, mozzarella, nonfat	31.7	0	141	1.7
Beverage, milkshake mix, dry, not chocolate	23.5	2.6	329	51.3
Beverage, instant breakfast powder, chocolate, not reconstituted	19.9	1.4	353	65.8

Food Name ---> per 100 g	Protein (g)	Fat (g)	Calories	Net Carb (g)
Beverage, instant breakfast powder, chocolate, sugar-free, not reconstituted	35.8	5.1	358	39
Yogurt, fruit variety, nonfat	4.4	0.2	95	19
Whipped cream substitute, dietetic, made from powdered mix	0.9	6	100	10.6
Cheese, cottage, with vegetables	10.9	4.2	95	2.9
Cheese, cream, low fat	7.85	15.28	201	8.13
Cheese, pasteurized process, American, low fat	24.6	7	180	3.5
Cheese spread, cream cheese base	7.1	28.6	295	3.5
Cheese, american cheddar, imitation	16.7	14	239	11.6
Eggs, scrambled, frozen mixture	13.1	5.6	131	7.5
Cheese, parmesan, low sodium	41.6	29.99	451	3.7
Cheese, cottage, lowfat, 1% milkfat, no sodium added	12.4	1	72	2.7
Cheese, pasteurized process, swiss, low fat	25.5	5.1	165	4.3
Cheese, cottage, lowfat, 1% milkfat, with vegetables	10.9	1	67	3
Cheese, pasteurized process, cheddar or American, low sodium	22.2	31.19	376	1.6
Cheese, swiss, low sodium	28.4	27.4	374	3.4
Milk, imitation, non-soy	1.6	2	46	5.3
Cheese, swiss, low fat	28.4	5.1	179	3.4
Cheese, mozzarella, low sodium	27.5	17.1	280	3.1
Cheese food, pasteurized process, American, imitation, without added vitamin D	4.08	19.5	257	16.18

Fats and Oils

Food Name ---> per 100 g	Protein (g)	Fat (g)	Calories	Net Carb (g)
Fat, beef tallow	0	100	902	0
Lard	0	100	902	0
Salad dressing, russian dressing	0.69	26.18	355	31.2
Salad dressing, sesame seed dressing, regular	3.1	45.2	443	7.6
Salad dressing, thousand island, commercial, regular	1.09	35.06	379	13.84
Salad dressing, mayonnaise type, regular, with salt	0.65	21.6	250	14.78
Salad dressing, french dressing, reduced fat	0.58	11.52	222	29.72
Salad dressing, italian dressing, commercial, reduced fat	0.39	6.68	102	9.99
Salad dressing, russian dressing, low calorie	0.5	4	141	27.3
Salad dressing, thousand island dressing, reduced fat	0.83	11.32	195	22.86
Salad dressing, mayonnaise, regular	0.96	74.85	680	0.57
Salad dressing, mayonnaise, soybean and safflower oil, with salt	1.1	79.4	717	2.7
Salad dressing, mayonnaise, imitation, soybean	0.3	19.2	232	16
Salad dressing, mayonnaise, imitation, milk cream	2.1	5.1	97	11.1
Salad dressing, mayonnaise, imitation, soybean without cholesterol	0.1	47.7	482	15.8
Sandwich spread, with chopped pickle, regular, unspecified oils	0.9	34	389	22
Shortening, household, soybean (partially hydrogenated)-cottonseed (partially hydrogenated)	0	100	884	0
Oil, soybean, salad or cooking, (partially hydrogenated)	0	100	884	0
Oil, rice bran	0	100	884	0
Oil, wheat germ	0	100	884	0
Oil, peanut, salad or cooking	0	100	884	0
Oil, soybean, salad or cooking	0	100	884	0
Oil, coconut	0	99.06	892	0
Oil, olive, salad or cooking	0	100	884	0
Oil, palm	0	100	884	0
Oil, sesame, salad or cooking	0	100	884	0
Salad dressing, french, home recipe	0.1	70.2	631	3.4

Food Name ---> per 100 g	Protein (g)	Fat (g)	Calories	Net Carb (g)
Salad dressing, home recipe, vinegar and oil	0	50.1	449	2.5
Salad dressing, french dressing, commercial, regular, without salt	0.77	44.81	459	15.58
Salad dressing, french dressing, reduced fat, without salt	0.58	13.46	233	28.18
Salad dressing, italian dressing, commercial, regular, without salt	0.38	28.37	292	10.43
Salad dressing, italian dressing, reduced fat, without salt	0.47	6.38	76	4.57
Salad dressing, mayonnaise, soybean oil, without salt	1.1	79.4	717	2.7
Salad dressing, french, cottonseed, oil, home recipe	0.1	70.2	631	3.4
Salad dressing, french dressing, fat-free	0.2	0.27	132	29.94
Oil, cocoa butter	0	100	884	0
Oil, cottonseed, salad or cooking	0	100	884	0
Oil, sunflower, linoleic, (approx. 65%)	0	100	884	0
Oil, safflower, salad or cooking, linoleic, (over 70%)	0	100	884	0
Oil, safflower, salad or cooking, high oleic (primary safflower oil of commerce)	0	100	884	0
Vegetable oil, palm kernel	0	100	862	0
Oil, poppyseed	0	100	884	0
Oil, tomatoseed	0	100	884	0
Oil, teaseed	0	100	884	0
Oil, grapeseed	0	100	884	0
Oil, corn, industrial and retail, all purpose salad or cooking	0	100	900	0
Fat, mutton tallow	0	100	902	0
Oil, walnut	0	100	884	0
Oil, almond	0	100	884	0
Oil, apricot kernel	0	100	884	0
Oil, soybean lecithin	0	100	763	0
Oil, hazelnut	0	100	884	0
Oil, babassu	0	100	884	0
Oil, sheanut	0	100	884	0
Salad dressing, blue or roquefort cheese dressing, commercial, regular	1.37	51.1	484	4.37
Oil, cupu assu	0	100	884	0
Fat, chicken	0	99.8	900	0

Food Name ---> per 100 g	Protein (g)	Fat (g)	Calories	Net Carb (g)
Oil, soybean, salad or cooking, (partially hydrogenated) and cottonseed	0	100	884	0
Shortening, household, lard and vegetable oil	0	100	900	0
Oil, sunflower, linoleic, (partially hydrogenated)	0	100	884	0
Shortening bread, soybean (hydrogenated) and cottonseed	0	100	884	0
Shortening cake mix, soybean (hydrogenated) and cottonseed (hydrogenated)	0	100	884	0
Shortening industrial, lard and vegetable oil	0	100	900	0
Shortening frying (heavy duty), beef tallow and cottonseed	0	100	900	0
Shortening confectionery, coconut (hydrogenated) and or palm kernel (hydrogenated)	0	100	884	0
Shortening industrial, soybean (hydrogenated) and cottonseed	0	100	884	0
Shortening frying (heavy duty), palm (hydrogenated)	0	100	884	0
Shortening household soybean (hydrogenated) and palm	0	100	884	0
Shortening frying (heavy duty), soybean (hydrogenated), linoleic (less than 1%)	0	100	884	0
Shortening, confectionery, fractionated palm	0	100	884	0
Oil, nutmeg butter	0	100	884	0
Oil, ucuhuba butter	0	100	884	0
Fat, duck	0	99.8	882	0
Fat, turkey	0	99.8	900	0
Fat, goose	0	99.8	900	0
Oil, avocado	0	100	884	0
Oil, canola	0	100	884	0
Oil, mustard	0	100	884	0
Oil, sunflower, high oleic (70% and over)	0	100	884	0
Margarine-like, margarine-butter blend, soybean oil and butter	0.31	80.32	727	0.77
Shortening, special purpose for cakes and frostings, soybean (hydrogenated)	0	100	884	0
Shortening, special purpose for baking, soybean (hydrogenated) palm and cottonseed	0	100	884	0
Oil, oat	0	100	884	0
Fish oil, cod liver	0	100	902	0

Food Name ---> per 100 g	Protein (g)	Fat (g)	Calories	Net Carb (g)
Fish oil, herring	0	100	902	0
Fish oil, menhaden	0	100	902	0
Fish oil, menhaden, fully hydrogenated	0	100	902	0
Fish oil, salmon	0	100	902	0
Fish oil, sardine	0	100	902	0
Shortening, multipurpose, soybean (hydrogenated) and palm (hydrogenated)	0	100	884	0
Margarine-like, vegetable oil-butter spread, tub, with salt	1	40	362	1
Butter, light, stick, with salt	3.3	55.1	499	0
Butter, light, stick, without salt	3.3	55.1	499	0
Meat drippings (lard, beef tallow, mutton tallow)	0	98.59	889	0
Animal fat, bacon grease	0	99.5	897	0
Oil, industrial, soy (partially hydrogenated), palm, principal uses icings and fillings	0	100	884	0
Margarine, industrial, non-dairy, cottonseed, soy oil (partially hydrogenated), for flaky pastries	1.9	80.2	714	0
Shortening, industrial, soy (partially hydrogenated) and corn for frying	0	100	884	0
Shortening, industrial, soy (partially hydrogenated) for baking and confections	0	100	884	0
Margarine, industrial, soy and partially hydrogenated soy oil, use for baking, sauces and candy	0.18	80	714	0.71
USDA Commodity Food, oil, vegetable, soybean, refined	0	100	884	0
USDA Commodity Food, oil, vegetable, low saturated fat	0	100	884	0
Margarine, margarine-like vegetable oil spread, 67-70% fat, tub	0.07	68.29	606	0.59
Margarine, 80% fat, tub, CANOLA HARVEST Soft Spread (canola, palm and palm kernel oils)	0.41	80.32	730	1.39
Oil, cooking and salad, ENOVA, 80% diglycerides	0	100	884	0
Salad dressing, honey mustard dressing, reduced calorie	0.98	10	207	27.46
Margarine-like spread, BENECOL Light Spread	0	38.71	357	5.71
Salad dressing, spray-style dressing, assorted flavors	0.16	10.75	165	16.3
Salad Dressing, mayonnaise, light, SMART BALANCE, Omega Plus light	1.53	34.18	333	9.19
Oil, industrial, canola, high oleic	0	100	900	0

Food Name ---> per 100 g	Protein (g)	Fat (g)	Calories	Net Carb (g)
Oil, industrial, soy, low linolenic	0	100	900	0
Oil, industrial, soy, ultra low linolenic	0	100	884	0
Oil, industrial, soy, fully hydrogenated	0	100	884	0
Oil, industrial, cottonseed, fully hydrogenated	0	100	884	0
Salad dressing, honey mustard, regular	0.87	40.83	464	22.93
Salad dressing, poppyseed, creamy	0.92	33.33	399	23.43
Salad dressing, caesar, fat-free	1.47	0.23	131	30.53
Dressing, honey mustard, fat-free	1.07	1.47	169	37.23
Oil, flaxseed, contains added sliced flaxseed	0.37	99.01	878	0.39
Mayonnaise, reduced fat, with olive oil	0.37	40	361	0
Salad dressing, mayonnaise-type, light	0.65	10	158	16.4
Creamy dressing, made with sour cream and/or buttermilk and oil, reduced calorie	1.5	14	160	7
Salad dressing, peppercorn dressing, commercial, regular	1.2	61.4	564	3.5
Mayonnaise, reduced-calorie or diet, cholesterol-free	0.9	33.3	333	6.7
Salad dressing, italian dressing, reduced calorie	0.3	20	200	6.5
Vegetable oil-butter spread, reduced calorie	0	53	465	0
Salad dressing, blue or roquefort cheese dressing, light	2.1	2.7	86	13.2
Creamy dressing, made with sour cream and/or buttermilk and oil, reduced calorie, fat-free	1.4	2.7	107	20
Creamy dressing, made with sour cream and/or buttermilk and oil, reduced calorie, cholesterol-free	1	8	140	16
Salad dressing, french dressing, reduced calorie	0.4	13	227	27
Mayonnaise, made with tofu	5.95	31.79	322	1.96
Salad dressing, blue or roquefort cheese dressing, fat-free	1.52	1.01	115	23.8
Salad Dressing, mayonnaise-like, fat-free	0.2	2.7	84	13.6
Salad Dressing, coleslaw dressing, reduced fat	0	20	329	39.6
Oil, flaxseed, cold pressed	0.11	99.98	884	0
Margarine-like, vegetable oil spread, stick or tub, sweetened	0	52	534	16.7
Oil, corn and canola	0	100	884	0
Margarine-like, butter-margarine blend, 80% fat, stick, without salt	0.9	80.7	718	0.6

Food Name ---> per 100 g	Protein (g)	Fat (g)	Calories	Net Carb (g)
Margarine-like, vegetable oil-butter spread, reduced calorie, tub, with salt	1	50	450	1
Salad dressing, caesar dressing, regular	2.17	57.85	542	2.8
Salad dressing, coleslaw	0.9	33.4	390	23.7
Salad dressing, green goddess, regular	1.9	43.33	427	7.26
Salad dressing, sweet and sour	0.1	0	15	3.7
Salad dressing, blue or roquefort cheese, low calorie	5.1	7.2	99	2.9
Salad dressing, caesar, low calorie	0.3	4.4	110	18.5
Butter replacement, without fat, powder	2	1	373	89
Salad dressing, buttermilk, lite	1.25	12.42	202	20.23
Salad dressing, mayonnaise and mayonnaise-type, low calorie	0.9	19	263	23.9
Salad dressing, bacon and tomato	1.8	35	326	1.8
Mayonnaise, low sodium, low calorie or diet	0.3	19.2	231	16
Mayonnaise dressing, no cholesterol	0	77.8	688	0.3
Oil, corn, peanut, and olive	0	100	884	0

Finfish and Shellfish Products

Food Name ---> per 100 g	Protein (g)	Fat (g)	Calories	Net Carb (g)
Fish, anchovy, european, raw	20.35	4.84	131	0
Fish, anchovy, european, canned in oil, drained solids	28.89	9.71	210	0
Fish, bass, fresh water, mixed species, raw	18.86	3.69	114	0
Fish, bass, striped, raw	17.73	2.33	97	0
Fish, bluefish, raw	20.04	4.24	124	0
Fish, burbot, raw	19.31	0.81	90	0
Fish, butterfish, raw	17.28	8.02	146	0
Fish, carp, raw	17.83	5.6	127	0
Fish, carp, cooked, dry heat	22.86	7.17	162	0
Fish, catfish, channel, wild, raw	16.38	2.82	95	0
Fish, catfish, channel, cooked, breaded and fried	18.09	13.33	229	7.34
Fish, caviar, black and red, granular	24.6	17.9	264	4
Fish, cisco, raw	18.99	1.91	98	0
Fish, cisco, smoked	16.36	11.9	177	0
Fish, cod, Atlantic, raw	17.81	0.67	82	0
Fish, cod, Atlantic, cooked, dry heat	22.83	0.86	105	0
Fish, cod, Atlantic, canned, solids and liquid	22.76	0.86	105	0
Fish, cod, Atlantic, dried and salted	62.82	2.37	290	0
Fish, cod, Pacific, raw (may have been previously frozen)	15.27	0.41	69	0
Fish, croaker, Atlantic, raw	17.78	3.17	104	0
Fish, croaker, Atlantic, cooked, breaded and fried	18.2	12.67	221	7.14
Fish, cusk, raw	18.99	0.69	87	0
Fish, mahimahi, raw	18.5	0.7	85	0
Fish, drum, freshwater, raw	17.54	4.93	119	0
Fish, eel, mixed species, raw	18.44	11.66	184	0
Fish, eel, mixed species, cooked, dry heat	23.65	14.95	236	0
Fish, fish sticks, frozen, prepared	11.01	16.23	277	20.16
Fish, flatfish (flounder and sole species), raw	12.41	1.93	70	0
Fish, flatfish (flounder and sole species), cooked, dry heat	15.24	2.37	86	0
Fish, gefiltefish, commercial, sweet recipe	9.07	1.73	84	7.41
Fish, grouper, mixed species, raw	19.38	1.02	92	0

Food Name ---> per 100 g	Protein (g)	Fat (g)	Calories	Net Carb (g)
Fish, grouper, mixed species, cooked, dry heat	24.84	1.3	118	0
Fish, haddock, raw	16.32	0.45	74	0
Fish, haddock, cooked, dry heat	19.99	0.55	90	0
Fish, haddock, smoked	25.23	0.96	116	0
Fish, halibut, Atlantic and Pacific, raw	18.56	1.33	91	0
Fish, halibut, Atlantic and Pacific, cooked, dry heat	22.54	1.61	111	0
Fish, halibut, Greenland, raw	14.37	13.84	186	0
Fish, herring, Atlantic, raw	17.96	9.04	158	0
Fish, herring, Atlantic, cooked, dry heat	23.03	11.59	203	0
Fish, herring, Atlantic, pickled	14.19	18	262	9.64
Fish, herring, Atlantic, kippered	24.58	12.37	217	0
Fish, herring, Pacific, raw	16.39	13.88	195	0
Fish, ling, raw	18.99	0.64	87	0
Fish, lingcod, raw	17.66	1.06	85	0
Fish, mackerel, Atlantic, raw	18.6	13.89	205	0
Fish, mackerel, Atlantic, cooked, dry heat	23.85	17.81	262	0
Fish, mackerel, jack, canned, drained solids	23.19	6.3	156	0
Fish, mackerel, king, raw	20.28	2	105	0
Fish, mackerel, Pacific and jack, mixed species, raw	20.07	7.89	158	0
Fish, mackerel, spanish, raw	19.29	6.3	139	0
Fish, mackerel, spanish, cooked, dry heat	23.59	6.32	158	0
Fish, milkfish, raw	20.53	6.73	148	0
Fish, monkfish, raw	14.48	1.52	76	0
Fish, mullet, striped, raw	19.35	3.79	117	0
Fish, mullet, striped, cooked, dry heat	24.81	4.86	150	0
Fish, ocean perch, Atlantic, raw	15.31	1.54	79	0
Fish, ocean perch, Atlantic, cooked, dry heat	18.51	1.87	96	0
Fish, pout, ocean, raw	16.64	0.91	79	0
Fish, perch, mixed species, raw	19.39	0.92	91	0
Fish, perch, mixed species, cooked, dry heat	24.86	1.18	117	0
Fish, pike, northern, raw	19.26	0.69	88	0

Food Name ---> per 100 g	Protein (g)	Fat (g)	Calories	Net Carb (g)
Fish, pike, northern, cooked, dry heat	24.69	0.88	113	0
Fish, pike, walleye, raw	19.14	1.22	93	0
Fish, pollock, Atlantic, raw	19.44	0.98	92	0
Fish, pollock, Alaska, raw (may have been previously frozen)	12.19	0.41	56	0
Fish, pollock, Alaska, cooked, dry heat (may have been previously frozen)	23.48	1.18	111	0
Fish, pompano, florida, raw	18.48	9.47	164	0
Fish, pompano, florida, cooked, dry heat	23.69	12.14	211	0
Fish, rockfish, Pacific, mixed species, raw	18.36	1.34	90	0
Fish, rockfish, Pacific, mixed species, cooked, dry heat	22.23	1.62	109	0
Fish, roe, mixed species, raw	22.32	6.42	143	1.5
Fish, roughy, orange, raw	16.41	0.7	76	0
Fish, sablefish, raw	13.41	15.3	195	0
Fish, sablefish, smoked	17.65	20.14	257	0
Fish, salmon, Atlantic, wild, raw	19.84	6.34	142	0
Fish, salmon, chinook, smoked	18.28	4.32	117	0
Fish, salmon, chinook, raw	19.93	10.43	179	0
Fish, salmon, chum, raw	20.14	3.77	120	0
Fish, salmon, chum, canned, drained solids with bone	21.43	5.5	141	0
Fish, salmon, coho, wild, raw	21.62	5.93	146	0
Fish, salmon, coho, wild, cooked, moist heat	27.36	7.5	184	0
Fish, salmon, pink, raw	20.5	4.4	127	0
Fish, salmon, pink, canned, total can contents	19.68	4.97	129	0
Fish, salmon, sockeye, raw	22.25	4.69	131	0
Fish, salmon, sockeye, cooked, dry heat	26.48	5.57	156	0
Fish, salmon, sockeye, canned, drained solids	23.59	7.39	167	0
Fish, sardine, Atlantic, canned in oil, drained solids with bone	24.62	11.45	208	0
Fish, sardine, Pacific, canned in tomato sauce, drained solids with bone	20.86	10.45	185	0.44
Fish, scup, raw	18.88	2.73	105	0
Fish, sea bass, mixed species, raw	18.43	2	97	0
Fish, sea bass, mixed species, cooked, dry heat	23.63	2.56	124	0

Food Name ---> per 100 g	Protein (g)	Fat (g)	Calories	Net Carb (g)
Fish, seatrout, mixed species, raw	16.74	3.61	104	0
Fish, shad, american, raw	16.93	13.77	197	0
Fish, shark, mixed species, raw	20.98	4.51	130	0
Fish, shark, mixed species, cooked, batter-dipped and fried	18.62	13.82	228	6.39
Fish, sheepshead, raw	20.21	2.41	108	0
Fish, sheepshead, cooked, dry heat	26.02	1.63	126	0
Fish, smelt, rainbow, raw	17.63	2.42	97	0
Fish, smelt, rainbow, cooked, dry heat	22.6	3.1	124	0
Fish, snapper, mixed species, raw	20.51	1.34	100	0
Fish, snapper, mixed species, cooked, dry heat	26.3	1.72	128	0
Fish, spot, raw	18.51	4.9	123	0
Fish, sturgeon, mixed species, raw	16.14	4.04	105	0
Fish, sturgeon, mixed species, cooked, dry heat	20.7	5.18	135	0
Fish, sturgeon, mixed species, smoked	31.2	4.4	173	0
Fish, sucker, white, raw	16.76	2.32	92	0
Fish, sunfish, pumpkin seed, raw	19.4	0.7	89	0
Fish, surimi	15.18	0.9	99	6.85
Fish, swordfish, raw	19.66	6.65	144	0
Fish, swordfish, cooked, dry heat	23.45	7.93	172	0
Fish, tilefish, raw	17.5	2.31	96	0
Fish, tilefish, cooked, dry heat	24.49	4.69	147	0
Fish, trout, mixed species, raw	20.77	6.61	148	0
Fish, trout, rainbow, wild, raw	20.48	3.46	119	0
Fish, trout, rainbow, wild, cooked, dry heat	22.92	5.82	150	0
Fish, tuna, fresh, bluefin, raw	23.33	4.9	144	0
Fish, tuna, fresh, bluefin, cooked, dry heat	29.91	6.28	184	0
Fish, tuna, light, canned in oil, drained solids	29.13	8.21	198	0
Fish, tuna, light, canned in water, drained solids	19.44	0.96	86	0
Fish, tuna, fresh, skipjack, raw	22	1.01	103	0
Fish, tuna, white, canned in oil, drained solids	26.53	8.08	186	0
Fish, tuna, white, canned in water, drained solids	23.62	2.97	128	0

Food Name ---> per 100 g	Protein (g)	Fat (g)	Calories	Net Carb (g)
Fish, tuna, fresh, yellowfin, raw	24.4	0.49	109	0
Fish, tuna salad	16.04	9.26	187	9.41
Fish, turbot, european, raw	16.05	2.95	95	0
Fish, whitefish, mixed species, raw	19.09	5.86	134	0
Fish, whitefish, mixed species, smoked	23.4	0.93	108	0
Fish, whiting, mixed species, raw	18.31	1.31	90	0
Fish, whiting, mixed species, cooked, dry heat	23.48	1.69	116	0
Fish, wolffish, Atlantic, raw	17.5	2.39	96	0
Fish, yellowtail, mixed species, raw	23.14	5.24	146	0
Crustaceans, crab, alaska king, raw	18.29	0.6	84	0
Crustaceans, crab, alaska king, cooked, moist heat	19.35	1.54	97	0
Crustaceans, crab, alaska king, imitation, made from surimi	7.62	0.46	95	14.5
Crustaceans, crab, blue, raw	18.06	1.08	87	0.04
Crustaceans, crab, blue, cooked, moist heat	17.88	0.74	83	0
Crustaceans, crab, blue, canned	17.88	0.74	83	0
Crustaceans, crab, blue, crab cakes, home recipe	20.21	7.52	155	0.48
Crustaceans, crab, dungeness, raw	17.41	0.97	86	0.74
Crustaceans, crab, queen, raw	18.5	1.18	90	0
Crustaceans, crayfish, mixed species, wild, raw	15.97	0.95	77	0
Crustaceans, crayfish, mixed species, wild, cooked, moist heat	16.77	1.2	82	0
Crustaceans, lobster, northern, raw	16.52	0.75	77	0
Crustaceans, lobster, northern, cooked, moist heat	19	0.86	89	0
Crustaceans, shrimp, mixed species, raw (may have been previously frozen)	13.61	1.01	71	0.91
Crustaceans, shrimp, mixed species, cooked, breaded and fried	21.39	12.28	242	11.07
Crustaceans, shrimp, mixed species, cooked, moist heat (may have been previously frozen)	22.78	1.7	119	1.52
Crustaceans, shrimp, mixed species, canned	20.42	1.36	100	0
Crustaceans, shrimp, mixed species, imitation, made from surimi	12.39	1.47	101	9.13
Crustaceans, spiny lobster, mixed species, raw	20.6	1.51	112	2.43
Mollusks, abalone, mixed species, raw	17.1	0.76	105	6.01

Food Name ---> per 100 g	Protein (g)	Fat (g)	Calories	Net Carb (g)
Mollusks, abalone, mixed species, cooked, fried	19.63	6.78	189	11.05
Mollusks, clam, mixed species, raw	14.67	0.96	86	3.57
Mollusks, clam, mixed species, cooked, breaded and fried	14.24	11.15	202	10.33
Mollusks, clam, mixed species, cooked, moist heat	25.55	1.95	148	5.13
Mollusks, clam, mixed species, canned, drained solids	24.25	1.59	142	5.9
Mollusks, clam, mixed species, canned, liquid	0.4	0.02	2	0.1
Mollusks, cuttlefish, mixed species, raw	16.24	0.7	79	0.82
Mollusks, mussel, blue, raw	11.9	2.24	86	3.69
Mollusks, mussel, blue, cooked, moist heat	23.8	4.48	172	7.39
Mollusks, octopus, common, raw	14.91	1.04	82	2.2
Mollusks, oyster, eastern, wild, raw	5.71	1.71	51	2.72
Mollusks, oyster, eastern, cooked, breaded and fried	8.77	12.58	199	11.62
Mollusks, oyster, eastern, wild, cooked, moist heat	11.42	3.42	102	5.45
Mollusks, oyster, eastern, canned	7.06	2.47	68	3.91
Mollusks, oyster, Pacific, raw	9.45	2.3	81	4.95
Mollusks, scallop, mixed species, raw	12.06	0.49	69	3.18
Mollusks, scallop, mixed species, cooked, breaded and fried	18.07	10.94	216	10.13
Mollusks, scallop, mixed species, imitation, made from surimi	12.77	0.41	99	10.62
Mollusks, squid, mixed species, raw	15.58	1.38	92	3.08
Mollusks, squid, mixed species, cooked, fried	17.94	7.48	175	7.79
Mollusks, whelk, unspecified, raw	23.84	0.4	137	7.76
Mollusks, whelk, unspecified, cooked, moist heat	47.68	0.8	275	15.52
Fish, salmon, chinook, smoked, (lox), regular	18.28	4.32	117	0
Fish, salmon, chum, canned, without salt, drained solids with bone	21.43	5.5	141	0
Fish, salmon, pink, canned, without salt, solids with bone and liquid	19.78	6.05	139	0
Fish, salmon, sockeye, canned, without salt, drained solids with bone	20.47	7.31	153	0
Fish, tuna, light, canned in oil, without salt, drained solids	29.13	8.21	198	0
Fish, tuna, light, canned in water, without salt, drained solids	25.51	0.82	116	0
Fish, tuna, white, canned in oil, without salt, drained solids	26.53	8.08	186	0

Food Name ---> per 100 g	Protein (g)	Fat (g)	Calories	Net Carb (g)
Fish, tuna, white, canned in water, without salt, drained solids	23.62	2.97	128	0
Fish, bass, freshwater, mixed species, cooked, dry heat	24.18	4.73	146	0
Fish, bass, striped, cooked, dry heat	22.73	2.99	124	0
Fish, bluefish, cooked, dry heat	25.69	5.44	159	0
Fish, burbot, cooked, dry heat	24.76	1.04	115	0
Fish, butterfish, cooked, dry heat	22.15	10.28	187	0
Fish, cod, Pacific, cooked, dry heat (may have been previously frozen)	18.73	0.5	85	0
Fish, cusk, cooked, dry heat	24.35	0.88	112	0
Fish, mahimahi, cooked, dry heat	23.72	0.9	109	0
Fish, drum, freshwater, cooked, dry heat	22.49	6.32	153	0
Fish, halibut, greenland, cooked, dry heat	18.42	17.74	239	0
Fish, herring, Pacific, cooked, dry heat	21.01	17.79	250	0
Fish, ling, cooked, dry heat	24.35	0.82	111	0
Fish, lingcod, cooked, dry heat	22.64	1.36	109	0
Fish, mackerel, king, cooked, dry heat	26	2.56	134	0
Fish, mackerel, Pacific and jack, mixed species, cooked, dry heat	25.73	10.12	201	0
Fish, milkfish, cooked, dry heat	26.32	8.63	190	0
Fish, monkfish; cooked, dry heat	18.56	1.95	97	0
Fish, pike, walleye, cooked, dry heat	24.54	1.56	119	0
Fish, pollock, Atlantic, cooked, dry heat	24.92	1.26	118	0
Fish, pout, ocean, cooked, dry heat	21.33	1.17	102	0
Fish, roe, mixed species, cooked, dry heat	28.62	8.23	204	1.92
Fish, sablefish, cooked, dry heat	17.19	19.62	250	0
Fish, salmon, Atlantic, wild, cooked, dry heat	25.44	8.13	182	0
Fish, salmon, chinook, cooked, dry heat	25.72	13.38	231	0
Fish, salmon, chum, cooked, dry heat	25.82	4.83	154	0
Fish, salmon, pink, cooked, dry heat	24.58	5.28	153	0
Fish, scup, cooked, dry heat	24.21	3.5	135	0
Fish, seatrout, mixed species, cooked, dry heat	21.46	4.63	133	0
Fish, shad, american, cooked, dry heat	21.71	17.65	252	0

Food Name ---> per 100 g	Protein (g)	Fat (g)	Calories	Net Carb (g)
Fish, spot, cooked, dry heat	23.73	6.28	158	0
Fish, sucker, white, cooked, dry heat	21.49	2.97	119	0
Fish, sunfish, pumpkin seed, cooked, dry heat	24.87	0.9	114	0
Fish, trout, mixed species, cooked, dry heat	26.63	8.47	190	0
Fish, tuna, skipjack, fresh, cooked, dry heat	28.21	1.29	132	0
Fish, tuna, yellowfin, fresh, cooked, dry heat	29.15	0.59	130	0
Fish, turbot, european, cooked, dry heat	20.58	3.78	122	0
Fish, whitefish, mixed species, cooked, dry heat	24.47	7.51	172	0
Fish, wolffish, Atlantic, cooked, dry heat	22.44	3.06	123	0
Fish, yellowtail, mixed species, cooked, dry heat	29.67	6.72	187	0
Crustaceans, crab, dungeness, cooked, moist heat	22.32	1.24	110	0.95
Crustaceans, crab, queen, cooked, moist heat	23.72	1.51	115	0
Crustaceans, spiny lobster, mixed species, cooked, moist heat	26.41	1.94	143	3.12
Mollusks, cuttlefish, mixed species, cooked, moist heat	32.48	1.4	158	1.64
Mollusks, octopus, common, cooked, moist heat	29.82	2.08	164	4.4
Mollusks, oyster, Pacific, cooked, moist heat	18.9	4.6	163	9.9
Fish, roughy, orange, cooked, dry heat	22.64	0.9	105	0
Fish, catfish, channel, wild, cooked, dry heat	18.47	2.85	105	0
Fish, catfish, channel, farmed, raw	15.23	5.94	119	0
Fish, catfish, channel, farmed, cooked, dry heat	18.44	7.19	144	0
Fish, salmon, Atlantic, farmed, raw	20.42	13.42	208	0
Fish, salmon, Atlantic, farmed, cooked, dry heat	22.1	12.35	206	0
Fish, salmon, coho, farmed, raw	21.27	7.67	160	0
Fish, salmon, coho, farmed, cooked, dry heat	24.3	8.23	178	0
Fish, trout, rainbow, farmed, raw	19.94	6.18	141	0
Fish, trout, rainbow, farmed, cooked, dry heat	23.8	7.38	168	0
Crustaceans, crayfish, mixed species, farmed, raw	14.85	0.97	72	0
Crustaceans, crayfish, mixed species, farmed, cooked, moist heat	17.52	1.3	87	0
Mollusks, oyster, eastern, wild, cooked, dry heat	8.87	2.65	79	4.23
Mollusks, oyster, eastern, farmed, raw	5.22	1.55	59	5.53
Mollusks, oyster, eastern, farmed, cooked, dry heat	7	2.12	79	7.28

Food Name ---> per 100 g	Protein (g)	Fat (g)	Calories	Net Carb (g)
Fish, salmon, coho, wild, cooked, dry heat	23.45	4.3	139	0
Mollusks, conch, baked or broiled	26.3	1.2	130	1.7
USDA Commodity, salmon nuggets, breaded, frozen, heated	12.69	11.72	212	13.96
USDA Commodity, salmon nuggets, cooked as purchased, unheated	11.97	10.43	189	11.85
Salmon, sockeye, canned, total can contents	20.63	7.17	153	0
Fish, salmon, pink, canned, drained solids	23.1	5.02	138	0
Fish, tilapia, raw	20.08	1.7	96	0
Fish, tilapia, cooked, dry heat	26.15	2.65	128	0
Salmon, sockeye, canned, drained solids, without skin and bones	26.33	5.87	158	0
Fish, Salmon, pink, canned, drained solids, without skin and bones	24.62	4.21	136	0
Fish, pollock, Alaska, raw (not previously frozen)	17.17	0.19	70	0
Fish, pollock, Alaska, cooked (not previously frozen)	19.42	0.26	80	0
Fish, cod, Pacific, raw (not previously frozen)	17.54	0.2	72	0
Fish, cod, Pacific, cooked (not previously frozen)	20.42	0.25	84	0
Crustaceans, shrimp, raw (not previously frozen)	20.1	0.51	85	0
Crustaceans, shrimp, cooked (not previously frozen)	23.98	0.28	99	0.2
Fish, trout, brook, raw, New York State	21.23	2.73	110	0
Jellyfish, dried, salted	5.5	1.4	36	0
Frog legs, raw	16.4	0.3	73	0
Fish, mackerel, salted	18.5	25.1	305	0
Mollusks, scallop, (bay and sea), cooked, steamed	20.54	0.84	111	5.41
Mollusks, snail, raw	16.1	1.4	90	2

Fruits and Fruits Juices

Food Name ---> per 100 g	Protein (g)	Fat (g)	Calories	Net Carb (g)
Acerola, (west indian cherry), raw	0.4	0.3	32	6.59
Acerola juice, raw	0.4	0.3	23	4.5
Apples, raw, with skin	0.26	0.17	52	11.41
Apples, raw, without skin	0.27	0.13	48	11.46
Apples, raw, without skin, cooked, boiled	0.26	0.36	53	11.24
Apples, raw, without skin, cooked, microwave	0.28	0.42	56	11.61
Apples, canned, sweetened, sliced, drained, unheated	0.18	0.49	67	15
Apples, canned, sweetened, sliced, drained, heated	0.18	0.43	67	14.84
Apples, dehydrated (low moisture), sulfured, uncooked	1.32	0.58	346	81.13
Apples, dehydrated (low moisture), sulfured, stewed	0.28	0.12	74	17.31
Apples, dried, sulfured, uncooked	0.93	0.32	243	57.19
Apples, dried, sulfured, stewed, without added sugar	0.22	0.07	57	13.32
Apples, dried, sulfured, stewed, with added sugar	0.2	0.07	83	18.83
Apples, frozen, unsweetened, unheated	0.28	0.32	48	11.01
Apples, frozen, unsweetened, heated	0.29	0.33	47	10.7
Apple juice, canned or bottled, unsweetened, without added ascorbic acid	0.1	0.13	46	11.1
Apple juice, frozen concentrate, unsweetened, undiluted, without added ascorbic acid	0.51	0.37	166	40.6
Apple juice, frozen concentrate, unsweetened, diluted with 3 volume water without added ascorbic acid	0.14	0.1	47	11.44
Applesauce, canned, unsweetened, without added ascorbic acid (includes USDA commodity)	0.17	0.1	42	10.17
Applesauce, canned, sweetened, without salt (includes USDA commodity)	0.16	0.17	68	16.29
Apricots, raw	1.4	0.39	48	9.12
Apricots, canned, water pack, with skin, solids and liquids	0.71	0.16	27	4.79
Apricots, canned, water pack, without skin, solids and liquids	0.69	0.03	22	4.38
Apricots, canned, juice pack, with skin, solids and liquids	0.63	0.04	48	10.74

Food Name ---> per 100 g	Protein (g)	Fat (g)	Calories	Net Carb (g)
Apricots, canned, extra light syrup pack, with skin, solids and liquids	0.6	0.1	49	10.9
Apricots, canned, light syrup pack, with skin, solids and liquids	0.53	0.05	63	14.89
Apricots, canned, heavy syrup pack, with skin, solids and liquids	0.53	0.08	83	19.87
Apricots, canned, heavy syrup pack, without skin, solids and liquids	0.51	0.09	83	19.85
Apricots, canned, extra heavy syrup pack, without skin, solids and liquids	0.55	0.04	96	23.25
Apricots, dehydrated (low-moisture), sulfured, uncooked	4.9	0.62	320	82.89
Apricots, dehydrated (low-moisture), sulfured, stewed	1.93	0.24	126	32.62
Apricots, dried, sulfured, uncooked	3.39	0.51	241	55.34
Apricots, dried, sulfured, stewed, without added sugar	1.2	0.18	85	19.55
Apricots, dried, sulfured, stewed, with added sugar	1.17	0.15	113	25.16
Apricots, frozen, sweetened	0.7	0.1	98	22.9
Apricot nectar, canned, without added ascorbic acid	0.37	0.09	56	13.79
Avocados, raw, all commercial varieties	2	14.66	160	1.83
Avocados, raw, California	1.96	15.41	167	1.84
Avocados, raw, Florida	2.23	10.06	120	2.22
Bananas, raw	1.09	0.33	89	20.24
Bananas, dehydrated, or banana powder	3.89	1.81	346	78.38
Blackberries, raw	1.39	0.49	43	4.31
Blackberry juice, canned	0.3	0.6	38	7.7
Cherries, tart, dried, sweetened	1.25	0.73	333	77.95
Blackberries, canned, heavy syrup, solids and liquids	1.31	0.14	92	19.7
Blackberries, frozen, unsweetened	1.18	0.43	64	10.67
Blueberries, raw	0.74	0.33	57	12.09
Blueberries, canned, heavy syrup, solids and liquids	0.65	0.33	88	20.46
Blueberries, wild, frozen	0	0.16	57	9.45
Blueberries, frozen, unsweetened	0.42	0.64	51	9.47
Blueberries, frozen, sweetened	0.4	0.13	85	19.75
Boysenberries, canned, heavy syrup	0.99	0.12	88	19.71
Boysenberries, frozen, unsweetened	1.1	0.26	50	6.89

Food Name ---> per 100 g	Protein (g)	Fat (g)	Calories	Net Carb (g)
Breadfruit, raw	1.07	0.23	103	22.22
Carambola, (starfruit), raw	1.04	0.33	31	3.93
Carissa, (natal-plum), raw	0.5	1.3	62	13.63
Cherimoya, raw	1.57	0.68	75	14.71
Cherries, sour, red, raw	1	0.3	50	10.58
Cherries, sour, red, canned, water pack, solids and liquids (includes USDA commodity red tart cherries, canned)	0.77	0.1	36	7.84
Cherries, sour, red, canned, light syrup pack, solids and liquids	0.74	0.1	75	18.5
Cherries, sour, red, canned, heavy syrup pack, solids and liquids	0.73	0.1	91	22.17
Cherries, sour, red, canned, extra heavy syrup pack, solids and liquids	0.71	0.09	114	28.43
Cherries, sour, red, frozen, unsweetened	0.92	0.44	46	9.42
Cherries, sweet, raw	1.06	0.2	63	13.91
Cherries, sweet, canned, water pack, solids and liquids	0.77	0.13	46	10.26
Cherries, sweet, canned, juice pack, solids and liquids	0.91	0.02	54	12.31
Cherries, sweet, canned, light syrup pack, solids and liquids	0.61	0.15	67	15.79
Cherries, sweet, canned, pitted, heavy syrup pack, solids and liquids	0.6	0.15	83	19.87
Cherries, sweet, canned, extra heavy syrup pack, solids and liquids	0.59	0.15	102	24.73
Cherries, sweet, frozen, sweetened	1.15	0.13	89	20.26
Crabapples, raw	0.4	0.3	76	19.95
Cranberries, raw	0.46	0.13	46	8.37
Cranberries, dried, sweetened	0.17	1.09	308	77.5
Cranberry sauce, canned, sweetened	0.9	0.15	159	39.3
Cranberry-orange relish, canned	0.3	0.1	178	46.2
Currants, european black, raw	1.4	0.41	63	15.38
Currants, red and white, raw	1.4	0.2	56	9.5
Currants, zante, dried	4.08	0.27	283	67.28
Custard-apple, (bullock's-heart), raw	1.7	0.6	101	22.8
Dates, deglet noor	2.45	0.39	282	67.03
Elderberries, raw	0.66	0.5	73	11.4

Food Name ---> per 100 g	Protein (g)	Fat (g)	Calories	Net Carb (g)
Figs, raw	0.75	0.3	74	16.28
Figs, canned, water pack, solids and liquids	0.4	0.1	53	11.79
Figs, canned, light syrup pack, solids and liquids	0.39	0.1	69	16.15
Figs, canned, heavy syrup pack, solids and liquids	0.38	0.1	88	20.7
Figs, canned, extra heavy syrup pack, solids and liquids	0.38	0.1	107	27.86
Figs, dried, uncooked	3.3	0.93	249	54.07
Figs, dried, stewed	1.42	0.4	107	23.37
Fruit cocktail, (peach and pineapple and pear and grape and cherry), canned, water pack, solids and liquids	0.42	0.05	32	7.51
Fruit cocktail, (peach and pineapple and pear and grape and cherry), canned, juice pack, solids and liquids	0.46	0.01	46	10.86
Fruit cocktail, (peach and pineapple and pear and grape and cherry), canned, extra light syrup, solids and liquids	0.4	0.07	45	10.53
Fruit cocktail, (peach and pineapple and pear and grape and cherry), canned, light syrup, solids and liquids	0.4	0.07	57	13.93
Fruit cocktail, (peach and pineapple and pear and grape and cherry), canned, heavy syrup, solids and liquids	0.39	0.07	73	17.91
Fruit cocktail, (peach and pineapple and pear and grape and cherry), canned, extra heavy syrup, solids and liquids	0.39	0.07	88	21.79
Fruit salad, (peach and pear and apricot and pineapple and cherry), canned, water pack, solids and liquids	0.35	0.07	30	6.87
Fruit salad, (peach and pear and apricot and pineapple and cherry), canned, juice pack, solids and liquids	0.51	0.03	50	12.05
Fruit salad, (peach and pear and apricot and pineapple and cherry), canned, light syrup, solids and liquids	0.34	0.07	58	14.14
Fruit salad, (peach and pear and apricot and pineapple and cherry), canned, heavy syrup, solids and liquids	0.34	0.07	73	18.11
Fruit salad, (peach and pear and apricot and pineapple and cherry), canned, extra heavy syrup, solids and liquids	0.33	0.06	88	21.77
Gooseberries, raw	0.88	0.58	44	5.88
Gooseberries, canned, light syrup pack, solids and liquids	0.65	0.2	73	16.35
Goji berries, dried	14.26	0.39	349	64.06
Grapefruit, raw, pink and red and white, all areas	0.63	0.1	32	6.98
Grapefruit, raw, pink and red, all areas	0.77	0.14	42	9.06
Grapefruit, raw, pink and red, California and Arizona	0.5	0.1	37	9.69

Food Name ---> per 100 g	Protein (g)	Fat (g)	Calories	Net Carb (g)
Grapefruit, raw, pink and red, Florida	0.55	0.1	30	6.4
Grapefruit, raw, white, all areas	0.69	0.1	33	7.31
Grapefruit, raw, white, California	0.88	0.1	37	9.09
Grapefruit, raw, white, Florida	0.63	0.1	32	8.19
Grapefruit, sections, canned, water pack, solids and liquids	0.58	0.1	36	8.75
Grapefruit, sections, canned, juice pack, solids and liquids	0.7	0.09	37	8.81
Grapefruit, sections, canned, light syrup pack, solids and liquids	0.56	0.1	60	15.04
Grapefruit juice, white, canned or bottled, unsweetened	0.58	0.1	34	7.13
Grapefruit juice, white, canned, sweetened	0.58	0.09	46	11.03
Grapefruit juice, white, frozen concentrate, unsweetened, undiluted	1.97	0.48	146	34.16
Grapefruit juice, white, frozen concentrate, unsweetened, diluted with 3 volume water	0.55	0.13	41	9.63
Grapefruit juice, pink or red, with added calcium	0.5	0.1	38	8.69
Grapefruit juice, white, raw	0.5	0.1	39	9.1
Grapes, muscadine, raw	0.81	0.47	57	10.03
Grape juice, canned or bottled, unsweetened, with added ascorbic acid	0.37	0.13	60	14.57
Grapes, american type (slip skin), raw	0.63	0.35	67	16.25
Grapes, red or green (European type, such as Thompson seedless), raw	0.72	0.16	69	17.2
Grapes, canned, thompson seedless, water pack, solids and liquids	0.5	0.11	40	9.7
Grapes, canned, thompson seedless, heavy syrup pack, solids and liquids	0.48	0.1	76	19.05
Grape juice, canned or bottled, unsweetened, without added ascorbic acid	0.37	0.13	60	14.57
Groundcherries, (cape-gooseberries or poha), raw	1.9	0.7	53	11.2
Guavas, common, raw	2.55	0.95	68	8.92
Guavas, strawberry, raw	0.58	0.6	69	11.96
Guava sauce, cooked	0.32	0.14	36	5.88
Jackfruit, raw	1.72	0.64	95	21.75
Java-plum, (jambolan), raw	0.72	0.23	60	15.56

Food Name ---> per 100 g	Protein (g)	Fat (g)	Calories	Net Carb (g)
Jujube, raw	1.2	0.2	79	20.23
Jujube, Chinese, fresh, dried	4.72	0.5	281	66.52
Kiwifruit, green, raw	1.14	0.52	61	11.66
Kumquats, raw	1.88	0.86	71	9.4
Lemons, raw, without peel	1.1	0.3	29	6.52
Lemon juice, raw	0.35	0.24	22	6.6
Lemon juice from concentrate, canned or bottled	0.45	0.07	17	4.92
Lemon juice, frozen, unsweetened, single strength	0.46	0.32	22	6.1
Lemon peel, raw	1.5	0.3	47	5.4
Limes, raw	0.7	0.2	30	7.74
Lime juice, raw	0.42	0.07	25	8.02
Lime juice, canned or bottled, unsweetened	0.25	0.23	21	6.29
Blueberries, dried, sweetened	2.5	2.5	317	72.5
Litchis, raw	0.83	0.44	66	15.23
Litchis, dried	3.8	1.2	277	66.1
Loganberries, frozen	1.52	0.31	55	7.72
Longans, raw	1.31	0.1	60	14.04
Longans, dried	4.9	0.4	286	74
Loquats, raw	0.43	0.2	47	10.44
Mammy-apple, (mamey), raw	0.5	0.5	51	9.5
Mangos, raw	0.82	0.38	60	13.38
Mangosteen, canned, syrup pack	0.41	0.58	73	16.11
Mango, dried, sweetened	2.45	1.18	319	76.18
Melons, cantaloupe, raw	0.84	0.19	34	7.26
Melons, casaba, raw	1.11	0.1	28	5.68
Melons, honeydew, raw	0.54	0.14	36	8.29
Melon balls, frozen	0.84	0.25	33	7.24
Mulberries, raw	1.44	0.39	43	8.1
Nectarines, raw	1.06	0.32	44	8.85
Oheloberries, raw	0.38	0.22	28	6.84
Olives, ripe, canned (small-extra large)	0.84	10.68	115	3.06

Food Name ---> per 100 g	Protein (g)	Fat (g)	Calories	Net Carb (g)
Olives, ripe, canned (jumbo-super colossal)	0.97	6.87	81	3.11
Olives, pickled, canned or bottled, green	1.03	15.32	145	0.54
Oranges, raw, all commercial varieties	0.94	0.12	47	9.35
Oranges, raw, California, valencias	1.04	0.3	49	9.39
Oranges, raw, navels	0.91	0.15	49	10.34
Oranges, raw, Florida	0.7	0.21	46	9.14
Oranges, raw, with peel	1.3	0.3	63	11
Orange juice, raw	0.7	0.2	45	10.2
Orange juice, canned, unsweetened	0.68	0.15	47	10.71
Orange juice, chilled, includes from concentrate	0.68	0.12	49	11.24
Orange juice, chilled, includes from concentrate, with added calcium and vitamin D	0.68	0.12	47	10.97
Orange juice, chilled, includes from concentrate, with added calcium	0.68	0.12	47	10.97
Orange juice, frozen concentrate, unsweetened, diluted with 3 volume water, with added calcium	0.6	0.06	37	8.27
Orange juice, frozen concentrate, unsweetened, undiluted, with added calcium	2.4	0.25	147	32.86
Orange juice, frozen concentrate, unsweetened, undiluted	2.4	0.25	148	34.19
Orange juice, frozen concentrate, unsweetened, diluted with 3 volume water	0.6	0.06	37	8.6
Orange peel, raw	1.5	0.2	97	14.4
Orange-grapefruit juice, canned or bottled, unsweetened	0.6	0.1	43	10.18
Tangerines, (mandarin oranges), raw	0.81	0.31	53	11.54
Tangerines, (mandarin oranges), canned, juice pack	0.62	0.03	37	8.87
Tangerines, (mandarin oranges), canned, light syrup pack	0.45	0.1	61	15.49
Tangerine juice, raw	0.5	0.2	43	9.9
Tangerine juice, canned, sweetened	0.5	0.2	50	11.8
Papayas, raw	0.47	0.26	43	9.12
Papaya, canned, heavy syrup, drained	0.14	0.55	206	54.33
Papaya nectar, canned	0.17	0.15	57	13.91
Passion-fruit, (granadilla), purple, raw	2.2	0.7	97	12.98
Passion-fruit juice, purple, raw	0.39	0.05	51	13.4

Food Name ---> per 100 g	Protein (g)	Fat (g)	Calories	Net Carb (g)
Passion-fruit juice, yellow, raw	0.67	0.18	60	14.25
Peaches, yellow, raw	0.91	0.25	39	8.04
Peaches, canned, water pack, solids and liquids	0.44	0.06	24	4.81
Peaches, canned, juice pack, solids and liquids	0.63	0.03	44	10.27
Peaches, canned, extra light syrup, solids and liquids	0.4	0.1	42	10.1
Peaches, canned, light syrup pack, solids and liquids	0.45	0.03	54	13.25
Peaches, canned, heavy syrup pack, solids and liquids	0.45	0.1	74	18.64
Peaches, canned, extra heavy syrup pack, solids and liquids	0.47	0.03	96	25.06
Peaches, spiced, canned, heavy syrup pack, solids and liquids	0.41	0.1	75	18.78
Peaches, dehydrated (low-moisture), sulfured, uncooked	4.89	1.03	325	83.18
Peaches, dehydrated (low-moisture), sulfured, stewed	2.01	0.42	133	34.14
Peaches, dried, sulfured, uncooked	3.61	0.76	239	53.13
Peaches, dried, sulfured, stewed, without added sugar	1.16	0.25	77	16.99
Peaches, dried, sulfured, stewed, with added sugar	1.06	0.22	103	24.2
Peaches, frozen, sliced, sweetened	0.63	0.13	94	22.18
Peach nectar, canned, without added ascorbic acid	0.27	0.02	54	13.32
Pears, raw	0.36	0.14	57	12.13
Pears, canned, water pack, solids and liquids	0.19	0.03	29	6.21
Pears, canned, juice pack, solids and liquids	0.34	0.07	50	11.34
Pears, canned, extra light syrup pack, solids and liquids	0.3	0.1	47	10.6
Pears, canned, light syrup pack, solids and liquids	0.19	0.03	57	13.57
Pears, canned, heavy syrup pack, solids and liquids	0.2	0.13	74	17.57
Pears, canned, extra heavy syrup pack, solids and liquids	0.19	0.13	97	23.65
Pears, dried, sulfured, uncooked	1.87	0.63	262	62.2
Pears, dried, sulfured, stewed, without added sugar	0.91	0.31	127	27.41
Pears, dried, sulfured, stewed, with added sugar	0.86	0.29	140	31.34
Pear nectar, canned, without added ascorbic acid	0.11	0.01	60	15.16
Persimmons, japanese, raw	0.58	0.19	70	14.99
Persimmons, japanese, dried	1.38	0.59	274	58.93
Persimmons, native, raw	0.8	0.4	127	33.5
Pineapple, raw, all varieties	0.54	0.12	50	11.72

Food Name ---> per 100 g	Protein (g)	Fat (g)	Calories	Net Carb (g)
Pineapple, canned, water pack, solids and liquids	0.43	0.09	32	7.5
Pineapple, canned, juice pack, solids and liquids	0.42	0.08	60	14.9
Pineapple, canned, light syrup pack, solids and liquids	0.36	0.12	52	12.65
Pineapple, canned, heavy syrup pack, solids and liquids	0.35	0.11	78	19.4
Pineapple, canned, extra heavy syrup pack, solids and liquids	0.34	0.11	83	20.7
Pineapple, frozen, chunks, sweetened	0.4	0.1	86	21.1
Pineapple juice, canned or bottled, unsweetened, without added ascorbic acid	0.36	0.12	53	12.67
Pineapple juice, frozen concentrate, unsweetened, undiluted	1.3	0.1	179	43.6
Pineapple juice, frozen concentrate, unsweetened, diluted with 3 volume water	0.4	0.03	51	12.47
Pitanga, (surinam-cherry), raw	0.8	0.4	33	7.49
Plantains, raw	1.3	0.37	122	29.59
Plantains, cooked	0.79	0.18	116	28.85
Plums, raw	0.7	0.28	46	10.02
Plums, canned, purple, water pack, solids and liquids	0.39	0.01	41	10.13
Plums, canned, purple, juice pack, solids and liquids	0.51	0.02	58	14.25
Plums, canned, purple, light syrup pack, solids and liquids	0.37	0.1	63	15.38
Plums, canned, purple, heavy syrup pack, solids and liquids	0.36	0.1	89	22.34
Plums, canned, purple, extra heavy syrup pack, solids and liquids	0.36	0.1	101	25.31
Pomegranates, raw	1.67	1.17	83	14.7
Prickly pears, raw	0.73	0.51	41	5.97
Prunes, canned, heavy syrup pack, solids and liquids	0.87	0.2	105	24
Prunes, dehydrated (low-moisture), uncooked	3.7	0.73	339	89.07
Prunes, dehydrated (low-moisture), stewed	1.23	0.24	113	29.7
Plums, dried (prunes), uncooked	2.18	0.38	240	56.78
Plums, dried (prunes), stewed, without added sugar	0.96	0.16	107	24.98
Plums, dried (prunes), stewed, with added sugar	1.09	0.22	124	29.08
Prune juice, canned	0.61	0.03	71	16.45
Pummelo, raw	0.76	0.04	38	8.62
Quinces, raw	0.4	0.1	57	13.4

Food Name ---> per 100 g	Protein (g)	Fat (g)	Calories	Net Carb (g)
Raisins, golden seedless	3.39	0.46	302	75.52
Raisins, seedless	3.07	0.46	299	75.48
Raisins, seeded	2.52	0.54	296	71.67
Rambutan, canned, syrup pack	0.65	0.21	82	19.97
Raspberries, raw	1.2	0.65	52	5.44
Raspberries, canned, red, heavy syrup pack, solids and liquids	0.83	0.12	91	20.06
Raspberries, frozen, red, sweetened	0.7	0.16	103	21.76
Rhubarb, raw	0.9	0.2	21	2.74
Rhubarb, frozen, uncooked	0.55	0.11	21	3.3
Rhubarb, frozen, cooked, with sugar	0.39	0.05	116	29.2
Roselle, raw	0.96	0.64	49	11.31
Rose-apples, raw	0.6	0.3	25	5.7
Sapodilla, raw	0.44	1.1	83	14.66
Sapote, mamey, raw	1.45	0.46	124	26.7
Soursop, raw	1	0.3	66	13.54
Strawberries, raw	0.67	0.3	32	5.68
Strawberries, canned, heavy syrup pack, solids and liquids	0.56	0.26	92	21.83
Strawberries, frozen, unsweetened	0.43	0.11	35	7.03
Strawberries, frozen, sweetened, whole	0.52	0.14	78	19.1
Strawberries, frozen, sweetened, sliced	0.53	0.13	96	24.02
Sugar-apples, (sweetsop), raw	2.06	0.29	94	19.24
Tamarinds, raw	2.8	0.6	239	57.4
Fruit salad, (pineapple and papaya and banana and guava), tropical, canned, heavy syrup, solids and liquids	0.41	0.1	86	21.06
Watermelon, raw	0.61	0.15	30	7.15
Maraschino cherries, canned, drained	0.22	0.21	165	38.77
Feijoa, raw	0.71	0.42	61	8.81
Pears, asian, raw	0.5	0.23	42	7.05
Fruit cocktail, canned, heavy syrup, drained	0.47	0.1	70	17.1
Blueberries, canned, light syrup, drained	1.04	0.4	88	20.06
Blueberries, wild, canned, heavy syrup, drained	0.56	0.34	107	23.42
Pineapple, canned, juice pack, drained	0.51	0.11	60	14.26

Food Name ---> per 100 g	Protein (g)	Fat (g)	Calories	Net Carb (g)
Apricots, canned, heavy syrup, drained	0.64	0.11	83	18.61
Cherries, sour, canned, water pack, drained	0.69	0.21	42	9.25
Cherries, sweet, canned, pitted, heavy syrup, drained	0.73	0.21	83	18.77
Peaches, canned, heavy syrup, drained	0.52	0.18	72	17.23
Pears, canned, heavy syrup, drained	0.24	0.18	74	16.38
Plums, canned, heavy syrup, drained	0.44	0.14	89	21.62
Tangerines, (mandarin oranges), canned, juice pack, drained	0.75	0.04	38	8.21
Apple juice, canned or bottled, unsweetened, with added ascorbic acid	0.1	0.13	46	11.1
Applesauce, canned, unsweetened, with added ascorbic acid	0.17	0.1	42	10.17
Applesauce, canned, sweetened, with salt	0.18	0.18	76	18.71
Apricot nectar, canned, with added ascorbic acid	0.37	0.09	56	13.79
Grapefruit juice, pink, raw	0.5	0.1	39	9.2
Peach nectar, canned, with added ascorbic acid	0.27	0.02	54	13.32
Pear nectar, canned, with added ascorbic acid	0.11	0.01	60	15.16
Pineapple juice, canned or bottled, unsweetened, with added ascorbic acid	0.36	0.12	53	12.67
Apple juice, frozen concentrate, unsweetened, undiluted, with added ascorbic acid	0.51	0.37	166	41
Apple juice, frozen concentrate, unsweetened, diluted with 3 volume water, with added ascorbic acid	0.14	0.1	47	11.44
Pears, raw, bartlett	0.39	0.16	63	11.91
Pears, raw, red anjou	0.33	0.14	62	11.94
Pears, raw, bosc	0.36	0.09	67	13
Pears, raw, green anjou	0.44	0.1	66	12.69
Grapefruit juice, white, bottled, unsweetened, OCEAN SPRAY	0.58	0.1	34	7.13
Jackfruit, canned, syrup pack	0.36	0.14	92	23.04
Dates, medjool	1.81	0.15	277	68.27
Durian, raw or frozen	1.47	5.33	147	23.29
Prune puree	2.1	0.2	257	61.8
Candied fruit	0.34	0.07	322	81.14
Abiyuch, raw	1.5	0.1	69	12.3
Rowal, raw	2.3	2	111	17.7

Food Name ---> per 100 g	Protein (g)	Fat (g)	Calories	Net Carb (g)
Pineapple, raw, traditional varieties	0.55	0.13	45	11.82
Pineapple, raw, extra sweet variety	0.53	0.11	51	12.1
USDA Commodity, mixed fruit (peaches, pears, grapes), canned, light syrup, drained	0.46	0.1	57	13.05
USDA Commodity, mixed fruit (peaches, pears, grapes), canned, light syrup, solids and liquids	0.41	0.08	55	13.1
Clementines, raw	0.85	0.15	47	10.32
Guanabana nectar, canned	0.11	0.17	59	14.83
Guava nectar, canned, with added ascorbic acid	0.09	0.06	63	15.25
Mango nectar, canned	0.11	0.06	51	12.82
Tamarind nectar, canned	0.09	0.12	57	14.23
USDA Commodity peaches, canned, light syrup, drained	0.56	0.15	61	14.95
USDA Commodity pears, canned, juice pack, drained	0.34	0.19	51	10.71
USDA Commodity pears, canned, light syrup, drained	0.28	0.15	62	14.61
Pomegranate juice, bottled	0.15	0.29	54	13.03
Juice, apple and grape blend, with added ascorbic acid	0.16	0.12	50	12.26
Juice, apple, grape and pear blend, with added ascorbic acid and calcium	0.17	0.12	52	12.76
Plantains, green, fried	1.5	11.81	309	45.67
Plantains, yellow, fried, Latino restaurant	1.42	7.51	236	37.57
Nance, canned, syrup, drained	0.56	1.28	95	15.79
Nance, frozen, unsweetened	0.66	1.16	73	9.47
Naranjilla (lulo) pulp, frozen, unsweetened	0.44	0.22	25	4.8
Horned melon (Kiwano)	1.78	1.26	44	7.56
Orange Pineapple Juice Blend	0.41	0.08	51	12
Apples, raw, red delicious, with skin	0.27	0.2	59	11.76
Apples, raw, golden delicious, with skin	0.28	0.15	57	11.2
Apples, raw, granny smith, with skin	0.44	0.19	58	10.81
Apples, raw, gala, with skin	0.25	0.12	57	11.38
Apples, raw, fuji, with skin	0.2	0.18	63	13.12
Orange juice, chilled, includes from concentrate, with added calcium and vitamins A, D, E	0.68	0.12	49	11.24

Food Name ---> per 100 g	Protein (g)	Fat (g)	Calories	Net Carb (g)
Pineapple juice, canned, not from concentrate, unsweetened, with added vitamins A, C and E	0.36	0.14	50	11.98
Grape juice, canned or bottled, unsweetened, with added ascorbic acid and calcium	0.37	0.13	62	14.57
Apple juice, canned or bottled, unsweetened, with added ascorbic acid, calcium, and potassium	0.12	0.17	48	11.19
Raspberries, frozen, unsweetened	1.2	0.65	52	5.44
Guava nectar, with sucralose, canned	0.3	0.07	48	12.1
Kiwifruit, ZESPRI SunGold, raw	1.02	0.28	63	14.39
Cranberry juice blend, 100% juice, bottled, with added vitamin C and calcium	0.27	0.12	45	10.81
Lemon juice from concentrate, bottled, CONCORD	0.4	0.07	24	5.37
Lemon juice from concentrate, bottled, REAL LEMON	0.47	0.07	17	4.96
Cranberry sauce, whole, canned, OCEAN SPRAY	0.75	0.05	158	39.2
Cranberry sauce, jellied, canned, OCEAN SPRAY	1.05	0.04	160	39.61
Ruby Red grapefruit juice blend (grapefruit, grape, apple), OCEAN SPRAY, bottled, with added vitamin C	0.5	0.1	44	10.33
Fruit juice smoothie, ODWALLA, strawberry banana	0.5	0.32	48	10.45
Fruit juice smoothie, NAKED JUICE, strawberry banana	0.48	0.27	50	11.06
Cranberry juice, unsweetened	0.39	0.13	46	12.1

Fast food

Food Name ---> per serving	Weight (g)	Measure	Calories	Net Carb (g)
ARBY'S, roast beef sandw., classic	149	1 sand..	361	31.19
BURGER KING, Cheeseburger	133	1 item	380	30.23
BURGER KING, Chicken Strips	36	1strip	105	6.88
BURGER KING, CROISSAN'WICH with Egg and Cheese	110	1 item	311	26.47
BURGER KING, CROISSAN'WICH with Sausage and Cheese	131	1 item	493	29.23
BURGER KING, CROISSAN'WICH with Sausage, Egg and Cheese	171	1 sand..	527	24.09
BURGER KING, Double Cheeseburger	162	1 sand..	457	28.24
BURGER KING, DOUBLE WHOPPER, no cheese	374	1 item	942	46.19
BURGER KING, DOUBLE WHOPPER, with cheese	399	1 item	1061	47.54
BURGER KING, french fries	74	1 small serv	207	26.54
BURGER KING, french toast sticks	21	1 stick	73	8.35
BURGER KING, Hamburger	99	1 sand..	258	25.49
BURGER KING, Hash Brown Rounds	5.6	1 piece	17	1.54
BURGER KING, Onion Rings	91	1 small	379	37.16
BURGER KING, Original Chicken Sandw.	199	1 sand..	569	47.38
BURGER KING, Premium Fish Sandw.	220	1 sand..	572	56.72
BURGER KING, Vanilla Shake	24.8	1fl oz	42	4.72
BURGER KING, WHOPPER, no cheese	291	1 item	678	48.78
BURGER KING, WHOPPER, with cheese	316	1 item	790	49.57
CHICK-FIL-A, Chick-n-Strips	50	1strip	114	4.7
CHICK-FIL-A, chicken sandw.	187	1 sand..	466	36.46
CHICK-FIL-A, hash browns	5.5	1 piece	17	1.48
DIGIORNO Pizza, cheese topping, cheese stuffed crust, frozen, baked	164	1slice 1/4 of pie	458	45.87

Food Name ---> per serving	Weight (g)	Measure	Calories	Net Carb (g)
DIGIORNO Pizza, cheese topping, rising crust, frozen, baked	183	1slice 1/4 of pie	468	53.76
DIGIORNO Pizza, cheese topping, thin crispy crust, frozen, baked	161	1slice 1/4 of pie	398	37.82
DIGIORNO Pizza, pepperoni topping, cheese stuffed crust, frozen, baked	179	1slice 1/4 of pie	499	48.93
DIGIORNO Pizza, pepperoni topping, rising crust, frozen, baked	207	1slice 1/4 of pie	549	59.68
DIGIORNO Pizza, pepperoni topping, thin crispy crust, frozen, baked	145	1slice 1/4 of pie	410	37.47
DIGIORNO Pizza, supreme topping, rising crust, frozen, baked	227	1slice 1/4 of pie	579	58.2
DIGIORNO Pizza, supreme topping, thin crispy crust, frozen, baked	155	1slice 1/4 of pie	395	39.18
DOMINO'S 14" Cheese Pizza, Classic Hand-Tossed Crust	108	1slice	278	33.5
DOMINO'S 14" Cheese Pizza, Crunchy Thin Crust	70	1slice	209	17.93
DOMINO'S 14" Cheese Pizza, Ultimate Deep Dish Crust	118	1slice	313	36.71
DOMINO'S 14" EXTRAVAGANZZA FEAST Pizza, Classic Hand-Tossed Crust	151	1slice	368	35.84
DOMINO'S 14" Pepperoni Pizza, Classic Hand-Tossed Crust	113	1slice	308	33.6
DOMINO'S 14" Pepperoni Pizza, Crunchy Thin Crust	79	1slice	259	17.93
DOMINO'S 14" Pepperoni Pizza, Ultimate Deep Dish Crust	123	1slice	348	36.22
DOMINO'S 14" Sausage Pizza, Classic Hand-Tossed Crust	114	1slice	311	33.6
DOMINO'S 14" Sausage Pizza, Crunchy Thin Crust	78	1slice	249	17.73
DOMINO'S 14" Sausage Pizza, Ultimate Deep Dish Crust	129	1slice	357	36.81
Fast food, biscuit	55	1biscuit	204	22.15
Fast Food, Pizza Chain, 14" pizza, cheese topping, regular crust	107	1slice	285	33.16

Food Name ---> per serving	Weight (g)	Measure	Calories	Net Carb (g)
Fast Food, Pizza Chain, 14" pizza, cheese topping, stuffed crust	117	1slice 1/8 pizza	321	33.1
Fast Food, Pizza Chain, 14" pizza, cheese topping, thick crust	115	1slice	312	35.65
Fast Food, Pizza Chain, 14" pizza, cheese topping, thin crust	76	1slice	230	21.81
Fast Food, Pizza Chain, 14" pizza, meat and vegetable topping, regular crust	136	1slice	332	31.52
Fast Food, Pizza Chain, 14" pizza, pepperoni topping, regular crust	111	1slice	313	32.9
Fast Food, Pizza Chain, 14" pizza, pepperoni topping, thick crust	118	1slice	339	34.97
Fast Food, Pizza Chain, 14" pizza, pepperoni topping, thin crust	79	1slice	261	21.11
Fast Food, Pizza Chain, 14" pizza, sausage topping, regular crust	116	1slice	325	32.82
Fast Food, Pizza Chain, 14" pizza, sausage topping, thick crust	127	1slice	358	35.66
Fast Food, Pizza Chain, 14" pizza, sausage topping, thin crust	88	1slice	282	21.56
Fast foods, bagel, with breakfast steak, egg, cheese, and condiments	254	1 item	716	57.89
Fast foods, bagel, with egg, sausage patty, cheese, and condiments	219	1 item	646	49.18
Fast foods, biscuit, with crispy chicken fillet	132	1 item	396	38.54
Fast foods, biscuit, with egg and bacon	150	1biscuit	458	27.79
Fast foods, biscuit, with egg and ham	182	1biscuit	424	29.09
Fast Foods, biscuit, with egg and sausage	162	1 item	505	33.8
Fast foods, biscuit, with egg, cheese, and bacon	145	1 item	436	35.14
Fast foods, biscuit, with ham	162	1biscuit	554	61.67
Fast foods, biscuit, with sausage	111	1 item	412	32.89
Fast foods, breadstick, soft, prepared with garlic and parmesan cheese	43	1breadstick	147	18.13
Fast foods, breakfast burrito, with egg, cheese, and sausage	109	1burrito	302	23.74
Fast foods, burrito, with beans	217	2.0 pieces	447	71.44

Food Name ---> per serving	Weight (g)	Measure	Calories	Net Carb (g)
Fast foods, burrito, with beans and beef	241	1 item	460	39.84
Fast foods, burrito, with beans and cheese	185	1each burrito	379	49.98
Fast foods, burrito, with beans, cheese, and beef	241	1burrito	434	47.42
Fast foods, cheeseburger, double, regular patty and bun, with condiments	155	1 sand..	437	26.25
Fast foods, cheeseburger; double, large patty; with condiments	280	1 item	762	37.6
Fast Foods, cheeseburger; double, large patty; with condiments, vegetables and mayonnaise	355	1 item	898	40.2
Fast foods, cheeseburger; double, regular patty; double decker bun with condiments and special sauce	219	1 item	572	44.05
Fast foods, cheeseburger; double, regular patty; with condiments	155	1 sand..	437	26.45
Fast foods, cheeseburger; single, large patty; plain	182	1 sand..	564	40.71
Fast foods, cheeseburger; single, large patty; with condiments	199	1 item	535	36.84
Fast foods, cheeseburger; single, large patty; with condiments, vegetables and mayonnaise	215	1 sand..	576	35.72
Fast foods, cheeseburger; single, regular patty, with condiments	127	1 item	343	29.93
Fast foods, cheeseburger; single, regular patty, with condiments and vegetables	115	1 sand..	292	27.12
Fast foods, cheeseburger; single, regular patty; plain	91	1 sand..	280	23.71
Fast foods, chicken fillet sandw., plain with pickles	187	1 sand..	468	36.46
Fast foods, chicken tenders	30	1strip	81	4.77
Fast foods, chicken, breaded and fried, boneless pieces, plain	96	6.0 pieces	295	13.43
Fast foods, coleslaw	191	1cup	292	24.84
Fast Foods, crispy chicken filet sandw., with lettuce and mayonnaise	152	1 sand..	420	39.55
Fast foods, crispy chicken in tortilla, with lettuce, cheese, and ranch sauce	133	1 item	366	29.18

Food Name ---> per serving	Weight (g)	Measure	Calories	Net Carb (g)
Fast foods, crispy chicken, bacon, and tomato club sandw., with cheese, lettuce, and mayonnaise	271	1 sand..	696	57.97
Fast foods, croissant, with egg, cheese, and bacon	128	1 item	370	27.5
Fast foods, croissant, with egg, cheese, and ham	155	1 item	405	28.02
Fast foods, croissant, with egg, cheese, and sausage	171	1 sand..	527	24.09
Fast foods, egg, scrambled	96	2.0 eggs	204	2
Fast foods, english muffin, with cheese and sausage	108	1 item	365	26.8
Fast foods, english muffin, with egg, cheese, and canadian bacon	126	1 sand..	287	26.8
Fast foods, english muffin, with egg, cheese, and sausage	165	1 item	472	28.48
Fast foods, fish sandw., with tartar sauce	220	1 sand..	565	56.52
Fast foods, fish sandw., with tartar sauce and cheese	134	1 sand..	374	34.26
Fast foods, french toast sticks	65	3.0 pieces	221	25.89
Fast Foods, Fried Chicken, Breast, meat and skin and breading	203	1breast, with skin	467	12.04
Fast Foods, Fried Chicken, Breast, meat only, skin and breading removed	142	1breast without skin	217	0
Fast Foods, Fried Chicken, Drumstick, meat and skin with breading	75	1drumstick , with skin	200	5.29
Fast Foods, Fried Chicken, Drumstick, meat only, skin and breading removed	40	1drum stick,	69	0
Fast Foods, Fried Chicken, Thigh, meat and skin and breading	136	1thigh with skin	373	11.7
Fast Foods, Fried Chicken, Thigh, meat only, skin and breading removed	84	1thigh without skin	150	0.2
Fast Foods, Fried Chicken, Wing, meat and skin and breading	58	1wing, with skin	180	6.39
Fast Foods, Fried Chicken, Wing, meat only, skin and breading removed	37	1wing without skin	80	0.79

Food Name ---> per serving	Weight (g)	Measure	Calories	Net Carb (g)
Fast foods, griddle cake sandw., egg, cheese, and bacon	174	1 item 6.1 oz	473	44.17
Fast foods, griddle cake sandw., egg, cheese, and sausage	199	1 item	579	42.66
Fast foods, griddle cake sandw., sausage	135	1 item	429	40.79
Fast Foods, grilled chicken filet sandw., with lettuce, tomato and spread	230	1 sand..	419	36.49
Fast foods, grilled chicken in tortilla, with lettuce, cheese, and ranch sauce	123	1 item	273	21.57
Fast foods, grilled chicken, bacon and tomato club sandw., with cheese, lettuce, and mayonnaise	268	1 sand..	590	50.05
Fast foods, hamburger, large, single patty, with condiments	171	1 item	438	35.96
Fast foods, hamburger; double, large patty; with condiments, vegetables and mayonnaise	374	1 item	942	46.19
Fast foods, hamburger; single, large patty; with condiments, vegetables and mayonnaise	247	1 item	558	39.11
Fast foods, hamburger; single, regular patty; double decker bun with condiments and special sauce	205	1 item	531	43.61
Fast foods, hamburger; single, regular patty; plain	78	1 sand..	232	23.27
Fast foods, hamburger; single, regular patty; with condiments	97	1 sand..	255	26.98
Fast foods, hush puppies	22	1 piece	65	8.25
Fast foods, miniature cinnamon rolls	25	1each	101	12.75
Fast foods, nachos, with cheese	80	1serv	274	25.33
Fast foods, nachos, with cheese, beans, ground beef, and tomatoes	222	1serv	486	39.29
Fast foods, onion rings, breaded and fried	117	1package (18 onion rings)	481	47.79
Fast foods, potato, french fried in vegetable oil	71	1serv small	222	26.72
Fast foods, potato, mashed	242	1cup	215	32.35
Fast foods, potatoes, hash browns, round pieces or patty	5.5	1round piece	15	1.49

Food Name ---> per serving	Weight (g)	Measure	Calories	Net Carb (g)
Fast foods, quesadilla, with chicken	180	1each quesadilla	529	40.17
Fast foods, roast beef sandw., plain	149	1 sand..	364	31.19
Fast foods, shrimp, breaded and fried	39	3.0 pieces shrimp	120	10.62
Fast foods, strawberry banana smoothie made with ice and low-fat yogurt	347	12.0 fl oz	226	49.12
Fast foods, submarine sandw., bacon, lettuce, and tomato on white bread	148	6.0 inch sub	303	37.06
Fast foods, submarine sand., cold cut on white bread, lettuce and tomato	196	6.0 inch sub	417	37.64
Fast foods, submarine sandw., ham on white bread with lettuce and tomato	184	6.0 inch sub	278	39.75
Fast foods, submarine sandw., meatball marinara on white bread	209	6.0 inch sub	458	49.96
Fast foods, submarine sandw., oven roasted chicken on white bread with lettuce and tomato	198	6.0 inch sub	311	39.87
Fast foods, submarine sandw., roast beef on white bread with lettuce and tomato	190	6.0 inch sub	296	37.35
Fast foods, submarine sandw., steak and cheese on white bread with cheese, lettuce and tomato	201	6.0 inch sub	368	40.79
Fast foods, submarine sandw., sweet onion chicken teriyaki on white bread with lettuce, tomato and sweet onion sauce	228	6.0 inch sub	353	48.69
Fast foods, submarine sandw., tuna on white bread with lettuce and tomato	237	6.0 inch sub	517	36.1
Fast foods, submarine sandw., turkey breast on white bread with lettuce and tomato	184	6.0 inch sub	270	38.85
Fast foods, submarine sandw., turkey, roast beef and ham on white bread with lettuce and tomato	413	12.0 inch sub	603	78.29
Fast foods, sundae, caramel	155	1sundae	304	49.31
Fast foods, sundae, hot fudge	158	1sundae	284	47.67
Fast foods, sundae, strawberry	153	1sundae	268	44.65
Fast foods, taco with beef, cheese and lettuce, hard shell	69	1each taco	156	11
Fast foods, taco with beef, cheese and lettuce, soft	102	1each taco	210	17.63

Food Name ---> per serving	Weight (g)	Measure	Calories	Net Carb (g)
Fast foods, taco with chicken, lettuce and cheese, soft	98	1each taco	185	18.1
Fast foods, vanilla, light, soft-serve ice cream, with cone	120	1 item	196	31.53
KFC, biscuit	49	1biscuit	175	20.34
KFC, Coleslaw	112	1package	161	15.33
KFC, Crispy Chicken Strips	47	1strip	129	5.72
KFC, Fried Chicken, EXTRA CRISPY, Breast, meat and skin with breading	212	1breast, with skin	568	17.96
KFC, Fried Chicken, EXTRA CRISPY, Breast, meat only, skin and breading removed	140	1breast, without skin	214	0.35
KFC, Fried Chicken, EXTRA CRISPY, Drumstick, meat and skin with breading	81	1drumstick, with skin	222	6.45
KFC, Fried Chicken, EXTRA CRISPY, Drumstick, meat only, skin and breading removed	41	1drumstick	70	0
KFC, Fried Chicken, EXTRA CRISPY, Thigh, meat and skin with breading	152	1thigh, with skin	470	15.66
KFC, Fried Chicken, EXTRA CRISPY, Thigh, meat only, skin and breading removed	91	1thigh, without skin	163	0
KFC, Fried Chicken, EXTRA CRISPY, Wing, meat and skin with breading	68	1wing, with skin	229	7.93
KFC, Fried Chicken, EXTRA CRISPY, Wing, meat only, skin and breading removed	44	1wing, without skin	104	1.31
KFC, Fried Chicken, ORIGINAL RECIPE, Breast, meat and skin with breading	212	1breast, with skin	490	13.31
KFC, Fried Chicken, ORIGINAL RECIPE, Breast, meat only, skin and breading removed	152	1breast without skin	226	0
KFC, Fried Chicken, ORIGINAL RECIPE, Drumstick, meat and skin with breading	75	1drumstick, with skin	179	4.04
KFC, Fried Chicken, ORIGINAL RECIPE, Drumstick, meat only, skin and breading removed	40	1drumstick, bone and skin removed	70	0.04

Food Name ---> per serving	Weight (g)	Measure	Calories	Net Carb (g)
KFC, Fried Chicken, ORIGINAL RECIPE, Thigh, meat and skin with breading	135	1thigh, with skin	363	11.42
KFC, Fried Chicken, ORIGINAL RECIPE, Thigh, meat only, skin and breading removed	86	1thigh without skin	150	0.01
KFC, Fried Chicken, ORIGINAL RECIPE, Wing, meat and skin with breading	60	1wing, with skin	178	5.96
KFC, Fried Chicken, ORIGINAL RECIPE, Wing, meat only, skin and breading removed	39	1wing wing without skin	84	0.69
KFC, Popcorn Chicken	6.4	1 piece	22	1.26
Light Ice Cream, soft serve, blended with cookie pieces	337	12.0 fl oz cup	570	85.8
Light Ice Cream, soft serve, blended with milk chocolate candies	348	12.0 fl oz cup	633	92.63
LITTLE CAESARS 14" Cheese Pizza, Large Deep Dish Crust	102	1slice	268	29.4
LITTLE CAESARS 14" Cheese Pizza, Thin Crust	48	1slice	148	10.17
LITTLE CAESARS 14" Original Round Cheese Pizza, Regular Crust	89	1slice	236	26.54
LITTLE CAESARS 14" Original Round Meat and Vegetable Pizza, Regular Crust	115	1slice	279	24.17
LITTLE CAESARS 14" Original Round Pepperoni Pizza, Regular Crust	90	1slice	246	26.41
LITTLE CAESARS 14" Pepperoni Pizza, Large Deep Dish Crust	104	1slice	276	28.59
McDONALD'S Bacon Ranch Salad with Crispy Chicken	319	1 item 11.3 oz	389	16.2
McDONALD'S, Bacon Egg & Cheese Biscuit	142	1 item 4.9 oz	432	30.31
McDONALD'S, Bacon Ranch Salad with Grilled Chicken	305	1 item 10.8 oz	247	8.1
McDONALD'S, Bacon Ranch Salad without chicken	223	1 item 7.8 oz	136	6.07
McDONALD'S, Bacon, Egg & Cheese McGRIDDLES	165	1 item 5.8 oz	449	41.91

Food Name ---> per serving	Weight (g)	Measure	Calories	Net Carb (g)
McDONALD'S, BIG BREAKFAST	269	1 item 9.5 oz	767	44.08
McDONALD'S, BIG MAC	219	1 item 7.6 oz	563	40.48
McDONALD'S, BIG MAC (without Big Mac Sauce)	200	1 item	468	38.62
McDONALD'S, Cheeseburger	119	1 item 4 oz	313	31.79
McDONALD'S, Chicken McNUGGETS	64	4.0 pieces	193	9.66
McDONALD'S, Deluxe Breakfast, with syrup and margarine	420	1 item 14.8 oz	1197	119.62
McDONALD'S, Double Cheeseburger	155	1 sand..	437	27.92
McDONALD'S, DOUBLE QUARTER POUNDER with Cheese	280	1 item	734	37.6
McDONALD'S, Egg McMUFFIN	126	1 sand..	287	25.9
McDONALD'S, FILET-O-FISH	134	1 sand..	378	33.46
McDONALD'S, FILET-O-FISH (without tartar sauce)	124	1 item	301	37.34
McDONALD'S, french fries	71	1 small serv	229	27.43
McDONALD'S, Fruit 'n Yogurt Parfait	149	1 item 5.2 oz	156	29.37
McDONALD'S, Fruit 'n Yogurt Parfait (without granola)	142	1 item	128	23.79
McDONALD'S, Hamburger	95	1 sand..	251	27.57
McDONALD'S, Hash Brown	53	1serv 1 patty	144	13.64
McDONALD'S, Hot Caramel Sundae	182	1 item (6.4 oz)	342	60.72
McDONALD'S, Hot Fudge Sundae	179	1 item (6.3 oz)	333	53.09
McDONALD'S, Hotcakes (plain)	149	3.0 hotcakes 5.3 oz	340	54.92
McDONALD'S, Hotcakes (with 2 pats margarine & syrup)	221	1 item	601	99.84
McDONALD'S, Hotcakes and Sausage	192	1 item	564	69
McDONALD'S, McCHICKEN Sandw.	131	1 sand..	358	34.94

Food Name ---> per serving	Weight (g)	Measure	Calories	Net Carb (g)
McDONALD'S, McCHICKEN Sandw. (without mayonnaise)	138	1 item	331	40.81
McDONALD'S, McFLURRY with M & M'S CANDIES	348	1regular (12 fl oz)	616	92.63
McDONALD'S, McFLURRY with OREO cookies	337	1regular (12 fl oz)	556	85.8
McDONALD'S, QUARTER POUNDER	171	1 item	417	35.21
McDONALD'S, QUARTER POUNDER with Cheese	199	1 item 7.1 oz	513	36.9
McDONALD'S, RANCH SNACK WRAP, Crispy	133	1wrap	366	29.18
McDONALD'S, RANCH SNACK WRAP, Grilled	123	1wrap	273	21.57
McDONALD'S, Sausage Biscuit	117	1 item 4.1 oz	440	30.42
McDONALD'S, Sausage Biscuit with Egg	163	1 item 5.7 oz	507	30.13
McDONALD'S, Sausage Burrito	109	1burrito	302	23.74
McDONALD'S, Sausage McGRIDDLES	135	1 item	421	40.79
McDONALD'S, Sausage McMUFFIN	115	1 item 4 oz	383	26.6
McDONALD'S, Sausage McMUFFIN with Egg	165	1 item 5.8 oz	452	27.01
McDONALD'S, Sausage, Egg & Cheese McGRIDDLES	199	1 item 7 oz	563	42.66
McDONALD'S, Side Salad	87	1 item 3.1 oz	17	2.34
McDONALD'S, Southern Style Chicken Biscuit	132	1biscuit regular size biscuit	401	38.54
McDONALD'S, Strawberry Sundae	178	1 item (6.3 oz)	281	50
McDONALD'S, Vanilla Reduced Fat Ice Cream Cone	90	1 item (3.2 oz)	146	23.62
PAPA JOHN'S 14" Cheese Pizza, Original Crust	117	1slice	304	36.11
PAPA JOHN'S 14" Cheese Pizza, Thin Crust	87	1slice	257	20.85
PAPA JOHN'S 14" Pepperoni Pizza, Original Crust	123	1slice	338	35.45

Food Name ---> per serving	Weight (g)	Measure	Calories	Net Carb (g)
PAPA JOHN'S 14" The Works Pizza, Original Crust	153	1slice	367	37.04
PIZZA HUT 12" Cheese Pizza, Hand-Tossed Crust	96	1slice	260	28.27
PIZZA HUT 12" Cheese Pizza, Pan Crust	100	1slice	280	28.23
PIZZA HUT 12" Cheese Pizza, THIN 'N CRISPY Crust	69	1slice	209	18.66
PIZZA HUT 12" Pepperoni Pizza, Hand-Tossed Crust	96	1slice	269	28.69
PIZZA HUT 12" Pepperoni Pizza, Pan Crust	96	1slice	286	27.57
PIZZA HUT 12" Super Supreme Pizza, Hand-Tossed Crust	127	1slice	309	30.04
PIZZA HUT 14" Cheese Pizza, Hand-Tossed Crust	105	1slice	289	32.59
PIZZA HUT 14" Cheese Pizza, Pan Crust	112	1slice	309	34.39
PIZZA HUT 14" Cheese Pizza, Stuffed Crust	117	1slice	321	33.1
PIZZA HUT 14" Cheese Pizza, THIN 'N CRISPY Crust	79	1slice	242	25.13
PIZZA HUT 14" Pepperoni Pizza, Hand-Tossed Crust	110	1slice	320	32.42
PIZZA HUT 14" Pepperoni Pizza, Pan Crust	113	1slice	329	33.62
PIZZA HUT 14" Pepperoni Pizza, THIN 'N CRISPY Crust	80	1slice	266	24.43
PIZZA HUT 14" Sausage Pizza, Hand-Tossed Crust	119	1slice	342	32.27
PIZZA HUT 14" Sausage Pizza, Pan Crust	125	1slice	359	34.45
PIZZA HUT 14" Sausage Pizza, THIN 'N CRISPY Crust	92	1slice	297	24.2
PIZZA HUT 14" Super Supreme Pizza, Hand-Tossed Crust	123	1slice	305	29.19
PIZZA HUT, breadstick, parmesan garlic	43	1breadstick	147	18.13
Pizza, cheese topping, regular crust, frozen, cooked	81	1serv	217	21.71
Pizza, cheese topping, rising crust, frozen, cooked	139	1serv	361	42.24
Pizza, cheese topping, thin crust, frozen, cooked	69	1slice	181	17.77

Food Name ---> per serving	Weight (g)	Measure	Calories	Net Carb (g)
Pizza, meat and vegetable topping, regular crust, frozen, cooked	143	1serv	395	32.85
Pizza, meat and vegetable topping, rising crust, frozen, cooked	170	1serv	461	45.03
Pizza, meat topping, thick crust, frozen, cooked	103	1slice	282	29.28
Pizza, pepperoni topping, regular crust, frozen, cooked	127	0.25 pizza	348	28.86
POPEYES, biscuit	60	1biscuit	241	22.27
POPEYES, Coleslaw	120	1packag	193	14.94
POPEYES, Fried Chicken, Mild, Breast, meat and skin with breading	194	1breast, with skin	532	18.27
POPEYES, Fried Chicken, Mild, Breast, meat only, skin and breading removed	132	1breast without skin	207	0
POPEYES, Fried Chicken, Mild, Drumstick, meat and skin with breading	76	1drumst	223	7.48
POPEYES, Fried Chicken, Mild, Drumstick, meat only, skin and breading removed	44	1drumstick	75	0.02
POPEYES, Fried Chicken, Mild, Thigh, meat and skin with breading	138	1thigh with skin	428	14.76
POPEYES, Fried Chicken, Mild, Thigh, meat only, skin and breading removed	83	1thigh thigh without skin	156	0.71
POPEYES, Fried Chicken, Mild, Wing, meat and skin with breading	57	1wing, with skin	193	7.41
POPEYES, Fried Chicken, Mild, Wing, meat only, skin and breading removed	16	1wing	34	0.46
POPEYES, Mild Chicken Strips, analyzed 2006	54	1strip	146	10.03
POPEYES, Spicy Chicken Strips, analyzed 2006	53	1strip	134	9.22
School Lunch, chicken nuggets, whole grain breaded	88	5.0 pieces	238	18.22
School Lunch, chicken patty, whole grain breaded	86	1patty	212	8.75
School Lunch, pizza, BIG DADDY'S LS 16" 51% Whole Grain Rolled Edge Cheese Pizza, frozen	155	1slice 1/8 per pizza	377	37.81

Food Name ---> per serving	Weight (g)	Measure	Calories	Net Carb (g)
School Lunch, pizza, BIG DADDY'S LS 16" 51% Whole Grain Rolled Edge Turkey Pepperoni Pizza, frozen	156	1slice 1/8 per pizza	387	36.27
School Lunch, pizza, cheese topping, thick crust, whole grain, frozen, cooked	124	1slice per 1/10 pizza	315	31.22
School Lunch, pizza, cheese topping, thin crust, whole grain, frozen, cooked	130	1 piece 4"x6"	321	35.5
School Lunch, pizza, pepperoni topping, thick crust, whole grain, frozen, cooked	124	1slice per 1/10 pizza	321	29.79
School Lunch, pizza, pepperoni topping, thin crust, whole grain, frozen, cooked	127	1 piece 4"x6"	323	34.17
School Lunch, pizza, sausage topping, thick crust, whole grain, frozen, cooked	129	1/10 pizza	332	34.25
School Lunch, pizza, sausage topping, thin crust, whole grain, frozen, cooked	133	1 piece 4" x 6"	332	37.68
School Lunch, pizza, TONY'S Breakfast Pizza Sausage, frozen	91	1 piece 3.2 oz	218	22.76
School Lunch, pizza, TONY'S SMARTPIZZA Whole Grain 4x6 Cheese Pizza 50/50 Cheese, frozen	130	1 piece 4" x 6"	303	33.15
School Lunch, pizza, TONY'S SMARTPIZZA Whole Grain 4x6 Pepperoni Pizza 50/50 Cheese, frozen	127	1 piece 4"x6"	302	31.43
SUBWAY, B.L.T. sub on white bread with bacon, lettuce and tomato	148	6.0 inch sub	303	37.06
SUBWAY, black forest ham sub on white bread with lettuce and tomato	184	6.0 inch sub	278	39.75
SUBWAY, cold cut sub on white bread with lettuce and tomato	196	6.0 inch sub	419	37.64
SUBWAY, meatball marinara sub on white bread (no toppings)	209	6.0 inch sub	458	49.96
SUBWAY, oven roasted chicken sub on white bread with lettuce and tomato	198	6.0 inch sub	311	39.87
SUBWAY, roast beef sub on white bread with lettuce and tomato	190	6.0 inch sub	294	37.35
SUBWAY, steak & cheese sub on white bread with American cheese, lettuce and tomato	201	6.0 inch sub	368	40.79
SUBWAY, SUBWAY CLUB sub on white bread with lettuce and tomato	207	6.0 inch sub	302	39.25

Food Name ---> per serving	Weight (g)	Measure	Calories	Net Carb (g)
SUBWAY, sweet onion chicken teriyaki sub on white bread with lettuce, tomato and sweet sauce	228	6.0 inch sub	353	48.69
SUBWAY, tuna sub on white bread with lettuce and tomato	237	6.0 inch sub	524	36.1
SUBWAY, turkey breast sub on white bread with lettuce and tomato	184	6.0 inch sub	270	38.85
TACO BELL, Bean Burrito	185	1each burrito	387	49.98
TACO BELL, BURRITO SUPREME with beef	241	1burrito	441	47.42
TACO BELL, BURRITO SUPREME with chicken	248	1 item	444	44.86
TACO BELL, BURRITO SUPREME with steak	248	1 item	454	44.39
TACO BELL, Nachos	80	1serv	280	25.33
TACO BELL, Nachos Supreme	222	1serv	495	39.29
TACO BELL, Original Taco with beef, cheese and lettuce	69	1each taco	158	11
TACO BELL, Soft Taco with beef, cheese and lettuce	102	1each taco	210	17.63
TACO BELL, Soft Taco with chicken, cheese and lettuce	98	1each taco	185	18.1
TACO BELL, Soft Taco with steak	127	1 item	286	19.87
TACO BELL, Taco Salad	533	1 item	906	64.48
WEND'YS, Crispy Chicken Sandw.	126	1 sand..	350	33.21
WENDY'S, Chicken Nuggets	68	5.0 pieces	222	9.73
WENDY'S, CLASSIC DOUBLE, with cheese	310	1 item	747	32.9
WENDY'S, CLASSIC SINGLE Hamburger, no cheese	218	1 item	464	33.87
WENDY'S, CLASSIC SINGLE Hamburger, with cheese	236	1 item	522	30.21
WENDY'S, DAVE'S Hot 'N Juicy 1/4 LB, single	215	1 sand..	576	35.72
WENDY'S, Double Stack, with cheese	146	1 sand..	416	22.41
WENDY'S, french fries	71	1kid's meal Serv	214	25.41
WENDY'S, Frosty Dairy Dessert	113	1junior 6 oz. cup	149	22.99

Food Name ---> per serving	Weight (g)	Measure	Calories	Net Carb (g)
WENDY'S, Homestyle Chicken Fillet Sandw.	230	1 item	492	46.56
WENDY'S, Jr. Hamburger, with cheese	129	1 item	330	30.41
WENDY'S, Jr. Hamburger, without cheese	117	1 item	284	31.29
WENDY'S, Ultimate Chicken Grill Sandw.	225	1 item	403	39.98
Yogurt parfait, lowfat, with fruit and granola	149	1 item	125	22.03

Lamb, Veal, and Game Products

Food Name ---> per 100 g	Protein (g)	Fat (g)	Calorie	Net Carb (g)
Veal, Australian, rib, rib roast, separable lean only, raw	21.7	4.63	134	1.4
Lamb, domestic, composite of trimmed retail cuts, separable lean and fat, trimmed to 1/4" fat, choice, raw	16.88	21.59	267	0
Lamb, domestic, composite of trimmed retail cuts, separable lean and fat, trimmed to 1/4" fat, choice, cooked	24.52	20.94	294	0
Lamb, domestic, composite of trimmed retail cuts, separable lean only, trimmed to 1/4" fat, choice, raw	20.29	5.25	134	0
Lamb, domestic, composite of trimmed retail cuts, separable lean only, trimmed to 1/4" fat, choice, cooked	28.22	9.52	206	0
Lamb, domestic, composite of trimmed retail cuts, separable fat, trimmed to 1/4" fat, choice, raw	6.65	70.61	665	0
Lamb, domestic, composite of trimmed retail cuts, separable fat, trimmed to 1/4" fat, choice, cooked	12.16	59.18	586	0
Lamb, domestic, foreshank, separable lean and fat, trimmed to 1/4" fat, choice, raw	18.91	13.38	201	0
Lamb, domestic, foreshank, separable lean and fat, trimmed to 1/4" fat, choice, cooked, braised	28.37	13.46	243	0
Lamb, domestic, foreshank, separable lean only, trimmed to 1/4" fat, choice, raw	21.08	3.29	120	0
Lamb, domestic, foreshank, separable lean only, trimmed to 1/4" fat, choice, cooked, braised	31.01	6.02	187	0
Lamb, domestic, leg, whole (shank and sirloin), separable lean and fat, trimmed to 1/4" fat, choice, raw	17.91	17.07	230	0
Lamb, domestic, leg, whole (shank and sirloin), separable lean and fat, trimmed to 1/4" fat, choice, cooked, roasted	25.55	16.48	258	0
Lamb, domestic, leg, whole (shank and sirloin), separable lean only, trimmed to 1/4" fat, choice, raw	20.56	4.51	128	0
Lamb, domestic, leg, whole (shank and sirloin), separable lean only, trimmed to 1/4" fat, choice, cooked, roasted	28.3	7.74	191	0
Lamb, domestic, leg, shank half, separable lean and fat, trimmed to 1/4" fat, choice, raw	18.58	13.49	201	0
Lamb, domestic, leg, shank half, separable lean and fat, trimmed to 1/4" fat, choice, cooked, roasted	26.41	12.45	225	0
Lamb, domestic, leg, shank half, separable lean only, trimmed to 1/4" fat, choice, raw	20.52	4.19	125	0

Food Name ---> per 100 g	Protein (g)	Fat (g)	Calorie	Net Carb (g)
Lamb, domestic, leg, shank half, separable lean only, trimmed to 1/4" fat, choice, cooked, roasted	28.17	6.67	180	0
Lamb, domestic, leg, sirloin half, separable lean and fat, trimmed to 1/4" fat, choice, raw	16.94	22.11	272	0
Lamb, domestic, leg, sirloin half, separable lean and fat, trimmed to 1/4" fat, choice, cooked, roasted	24.63	20.67	292	0
Lamb, domestic, leg, sirloin half, separable lean only, trimmed to 1/4" fat, choice, raw	20.55	5.08	134	0
Lamb, domestic, leg, sirloin half, separable lean only, trimmed to 1/4" fat, choice, cooked, roasted	28.35	9.17	204	0
Lamb, domestic, loin, separable lean and fat, trimmed to 1/4" fat, choice, raw	16.32	26.63	310	0
Lamb, domestic, loin, separable lean and fat, trimmed to 1/4" fat, choice, cooked, broiled	25.17	23.08	316	0
Lamb, domestic, loin, separable lean and fat, trimmed to 1/4" fat, choice, cooked, roasted	22.55	23.59	309	0
Lamb, domestic, loin, separable lean only, trimmed to 1/4" fat, choice, raw	20.88	5.94	143	0
Lamb, domestic, loin, separable lean only, trimmed to 1/4" fat, choice, cooked, broiled	29.99	9.73	216	0
Lamb, domestic, loin, separable lean only, trimmed to 1/4" fat, choice, cooked, roasted	26.59	9.76	202	0
Lamb, domestic, rib, separable lean and fat, trimmed to 1/4" fat, choice, raw	14.52	34.39	372	0
Lamb, domestic, rib, separable lean and fat, trimmed to 1/4" fat, choice, cooked, broiled	22.13	29.59	361	0
Lamb, domestic, rib, separable lean and fat, trimmed to 1/4" fat, choice, cooked, roasted	21.12	29.82	359	0
Lamb, domestic, rib, separable lean only, trimmed to 1/4" fat, choice, raw	19.98	9.23	169	0
Lamb, domestic, rib, separable lean only, trimmed to 1/4" fat, choice, cooked, broiled	27.74	12.95	235	0
Lamb, domestic, rib, separable lean only, trimmed to 1/4" fat, choice, cooked, roasted	26.16	13.31	232	0
Lamb, domestic, shoulder, whole (arm and blade), separable lean and fat, trimmed to 1/4" fat, choice, raw	16.58	21.45	264	0
Lamb, domestic, shoulder, whole (arm and blade), separable lean and fat, trimmed to 1/4" fat, choice, cooked, braised	28.68	24.55	344	0

Food Name ---> per 100 g	Protein (g)	Fat (g)	Calorie	Net Carb (g)
Lamb, domestic, shoulder, whole (arm and blade), separable lean and fat, trimmed to 1/4" fat, choice, cooked, broiled	24.42	19.26	278	0
Lamb, domestic, shoulder, whole (arm and blade), separable lean and fat, trimmed to 1/4" fat, choice, cooked, roasted	22.51	19.97	276	0
Lamb, domestic, shoulder, whole (arm and blade), separable lean only, trimmed to 1/4" fat, choice, raw	19.55	6.76	144	0
Lamb, domestic, shoulder, whole (arm and blade), separable lean only, trimmed to 1/4" fat, choice, cooked, braised	32.81	15.89	283	0
Lamb, domestic, shoulder, whole (arm and blade), separable lean only, trimmed to 1/4" fat, choice, cooked, broiled	27.12	10.5	210	0
Lamb, domestic, shoulder, whole (arm and blade), separable lean only, trimmed to 1/4" fat, choice, cooked, roasted	24.94	10.77	204	0
Lamb, domestic, shoulder, arm, separable lean and fat, trimmed to 1/4" fat, choice, raw	16.79	20.9	260	0
Lamb, domestic, shoulder, arm, separable lean and fat, trimmed to 1/4" fat, choice, cooked, braised	30.39	24	346	0
Lamb, domestic, shoulder, arm, separable lean and fat, trimmed to 1/4" fat, choice, cooked, broiled	24.44	19.55	281	0
Lamb, domestic, shoulder, arm, separable lean and fat, trimmed to 1/4" fat, choice, cooked, roasted	22.53	20.24	279	0
Lamb, domestic, shoulder, arm, separable lean only, trimmed to 1/4" fat, choice, raw	19.99	5.2	132	0
Lamb, domestic, shoulder, arm, separable lean only, trimmed to 1/4" fat, choice, cooked, braised	35.54	14.08	279	0
Lamb, domestic, shoulder, arm, separable lean only, trimmed to 1/4" fat, choice, cooked, broiled	27.71	9.02	200	0
Lamb, domestic, shoulder, arm, separable lean only, trimmed to 1/4" fat, choice, cooked, roasted	25.46	9.26	192	0
Lamb, domestic, shoulder, blade, separable lean and fat, trimmed to 1/4" fat, choice, raw	16.63	20.86	259	0
Lamb, domestic, shoulder, blade, separable lean and fat, trimmed to 1/4" fat, choice, cooked, braised	28.51	24.73	345	0
Lamb, domestic, shoulder, blade, separable lean and fat, trimmed to 1/4" fat, choice, cooked, broiled	23.08	19.94	278	0
Lamb, domestic, shoulder, blade, separable lean and fat, trimmed to 1/4" fat, choice, cooked, roasted	22.25	20.61	281	0
Lamb, domestic, shoulder, blade, separable lean only, trimmed to 1/4" fat, choice, raw	19.29	7.63	151	0

Food Name ---> per 100 g	Protein (g)	Fat (g)	Calorie	Net Carb (g)
Lamb, domestic, shoulder, blade, separable lean only, trimmed to 1/4" fat, choice, cooked, braised	32.35	16.64	288	0
Lamb, domestic, shoulder, blade, separable lean only, trimmed to 1/4" fat, choice, cooked, broiled	25.48	11.32	211	0
Lamb, domestic, shoulder, blade, separable lean only, trimmed to 1/4" fat, choice, cooked, roasted	24.61	11.57	209	0
Lamb, domestic, cubed for stew or kabob (leg and shoulder), separable lean only, trimmed to 1/4" fat, raw	20.21	5.28	134	0
Lamb, domestic, cubed for stew or kabob (leg and shoulder), separable lean only, trimmed to 1/4" fat, cooked, braised	33.69	8.8	223	0
Lamb, domestic, cubed for stew or kabob (leg and shoulder), separable lean only, trimmed to 1/4" fat, cooked, broiled	28.08	7.33	186	0
Lamb, New Zealand, imported, frozen, composite of trimmed retail cuts, separable lean and fat, raw	16.74	22.74	277	0
Lamb, New Zealand, imported, frozen, composite of trimmed retail cuts, separable lean and fat, cooked	24.42	22.26	305	0
Lamb, New Zealand, imported, frozen, composite of trimmed retail cuts, separable lean only, raw	20.75	4.41	128	0
Lamb, New Zealand, imported, frozen, composite of trimmed retail cuts, separable lean only, cooked	29.59	8.86	206	0
Lamb, New Zealand, imported, frozen, composite of trimmed retail cuts, separable fat, raw	6.92	67.63	640	0
Lamb, New Zealand, imported, frozen, composite of trimmed retail cuts, separable fat, cooked	9.72	60.39	586	0
Lamb, New Zealand, imported, fore-shank, separable lean and fat, raw	20.09	11.38	183	0.09
Lamb, New Zealand, imported, fore-shank, separable lean and fat, cooked, braised	30.35	14.99	256	0.03
Lamb, New Zealand, imported, fore-shank, separable lean only, raw	22.05	3.77	122	0
Lamb, New Zealand, imported, fore-shank, separable lean only, cooked, braised	33.31	8.4	209	0
Lamb, New Zealand, imported, leg chop/steak, bone-in, separable lean and fat, raw	18.64	14.52	206	0.13
Lamb, New Zealand, imported, frozen, leg, whole (shank and sirloin), separable lean and fat, cooked, roasted	24.81	15.56	246	0
Lamb, New Zealand, imported, leg chop/steak, bone-in, separable lean only, raw	21.1	4.64	126	0

Food Name ---> per 100 g	Protein (g)	Fat (g)	Calorie	Net Carb (g)
Lamb, New Zealand, imported, frozen, leg, whole (shank and sirloin), separable lean only, cooked, roasted	27.68	7.01	181	0
Lamb, New Zealand, imported, loin chop, separable lean and fat, raw	15.4	26.19	298	0.22
Lamb, New Zealand, imported, frozen, loin, separable lean and fat, cooked, broiled	23.43	23.88	315	0
Lamb, New Zealand, imported, loin chop, separable lean only, raw	19.98	6.88	142	0
Lamb, New Zealand, imported, frozen, loin, separable lean only, cooked, broiled	29.31	8.24	199	0
Lamb, New Zealand, imported, rack - partly frenched, separable lean and fat, raw	18.12	18.52	240	0.13
Lamb, New Zealand, imported, rack - partly frenched, separable lean and fat, cooked, fast roasted	22.06	18.29	253	0.04
Lamb, New Zealand, imported, rack - partly frenched, separable lean only, raw	20.65	8.61	160	0
Lamb, New Zealand, imported, rack - partly frenched, separable lean only, cooked, fast roasted	24.43	10.63	193	0
Lamb, New Zealand, imported, square-cut shoulder, separable lean and fat, raw	16.16	22.89	272	0.24
Lamb, New Zealand, imported, frozen, shoulder, whole (arm and blade), separable lean and fat, cooked, braised	28.21	26.27	357	0
Lamb, New Zealand, imported, square-cut shoulder, separable lean only, raw	19.72	8.3	154	0
Lamb, New Zealand, imported, frozen, shoulder, whole (arm and blade), separable lean only, cooked, braised	34.06	15.5	285	0
Veal, composite of trimmed retail cuts, separable lean and fat, raw	19.35	6.77	144	0
Veal, composite of trimmed retail cuts, separable lean and fat, cooked	30.1	11.39	231	0
Veal, composite of trimmed retail cuts, separable lean only, raw	20.2	2.87	112	0
Veal, composite of trimmed retail cuts, separable lean only, cooked	31.9	6.58	196	0
Veal, composite of trimmed retail cuts, separable fat, raw	6.02	67.83	638	0
Veal, composite of trimmed retail cuts, separable fat, cooked	9.42	66.74	642	0
Veal, leg (top round), separable lean and fat, raw	20.98	3.08	117	0
Veal, leg (top round), separable lean and fat, cooked, braised	36.16	6.33	211	0

Food Name ---> per 100 g	Protein (g)	Fat (g)	Calorie	Net Carb (g)
Veal, leg (top round), separable lean and fat, cooked, pan-fried, breaded	27.29	9.18	238	9.61
Veal, leg (top round), separable lean and fat, cooked, pan-fried, not breaded	31.75	8.35	211	0
Veal, leg (top round), separable lean and fat, cooked, roasted	27.7	4.65	160	0
Veal, leg (top round), separable lean only, raw	21.28	1.76	107	0
Veal, leg (top round), separable lean only, cooked, braised	36.71	5.09	203	0
Veal, leg (top round), separable lean only, cooked, pan-fried, breaded	28.41	6.27	216	9.64
Veal, leg (top round), separable lean only, cooked, pan-fried, not breaded	33.17	4.62	183	0
Veal, leg (top round), separable lean only, cooked, roasted	28.07	3.39	150	0
Veal, loin, separable lean and fat, raw	20.07	10.07	177	0.07
Veal, loin, separable lean and fat, cooked, braised	30.19	17.21	284	0
Veal, loin, separable lean and fat, cooked, roasted	24.8	12.32	217	0
Veal, loin, separable lean only, raw	21.85	2.9	114	0
Veal, loin, separable lean only, cooked, braised	33.57	9.15	226	0
Veal, loin, separable lean only, cooked, roasted	26.32	6.94	175	0
Veal, rib, separable lean and fat, raw	18.86	9.01	162	0
Veal, rib, separable lean and fat, cooked, braised	32.43	12.53	251	0
Veal, rib, separable lean and fat, cooked, roasted	23.96	13.96	228	0
Veal, rib, separable lean only, raw	19.97	3.89	120	0
Veal, rib, separable lean only, cooked, braised	34.44	7.81	218	0
Veal, rib, separable lean only, cooked, roasted	25.76	7.44	177	0
Veal, shoulder, whole (arm and blade), separable lean and fat, raw	19.27	5.28	130	0
Veal, shoulder, whole (arm and blade), separable lean and fat, cooked, braised	32.06	10.14	228	0
Veal, shoulder, whole (arm and blade), separable lean and fat, cooked, roasted	25.32	8.42	184	0
Veal, shoulder, whole (arm and blade), separable lean only, raw	19.79	3	112	0
Veal, shoulder, whole (arm and blade), separable lean only, cooked, braised	33.68	6.1	199	0
Veal, shoulder, whole (arm and blade), separable lean only, cooked, roasted	25.81	6.62	170	0

Food Name ---> per 100 g	Protein (g)	Fat (g)	Calorie	Net Carb (g)
Veal, shoulder, arm, separable lean and fat, raw	19.34	5.44	132	0
Veal, shoulder, arm, separable lean and fat, cooked, braised	33.63	10.24	236	0
Veal, shoulder, arm, separable lean and fat, cooked, roasted	25.46	8.25	183	0
Veal, shoulder, arm, separable lean only, raw	20.04	2.16	105	0
Veal, shoulder, arm, separable lean only, cooked, braised	35.73	5.33	201	0
Veal, shoulder, arm, separable lean only, cooked, roasted	26.13	5.81	164	0
Veal, shoulder, blade chop, separable lean and fat, raw	18.72	7.61	148	0.03
Veal, shoulder, blade, separable lean and fat, cooked, braised	31.26	10.09	225	0
Veal, shoulder, blade, separable lean and fat, cooked, roasted	25.15	8.67	186	0
Veal, shoulder, blade chop, separable lean only, raw	19.6	2.88	110	0
Veal, shoulder, blade, separable lean only, cooked, braised	32.66	6.48	198	0
Veal, shoulder, blade, separable lean only, cooked, roasted	25.64	6.88	171	0
Veal, sirloin, separable lean and fat, raw	19.07	7.81	152	0
Veal, sirloin, separable lean and fat, cooked, braised	31.26	13.14	252	0
Veal, sirloin, separable lean and fat, cooked, roasted	25.14	10.45	202	0
Veal, sirloin, separable lean only, raw	20.2	2.59	110	0
Veal, sirloin, separable lean only, cooked, braised	33.96	6.51	204	0
Veal, sirloin, separable lean only, cooked, roasted	26.32	6.22	168	0
Veal, cubed for stew (leg and shoulder), separable lean only, raw	20.27	2.5	109	0
Veal, cubed for stew (leg and shoulder), separable lean only, cooked, braised	34.94	4.31	188	0
Veal, ground, raw	18.58	13.06	197	0
Veal, ground, cooked, broiled	24.38	7.56	172	0
Game meat, antelope, raw	22.38	2.03	114	0
Game meat, antelope, cooked, roasted	29.45	2.67	150	0
Game meat, bear, raw	20.1	8.3	161	0
Game meat, bear, cooked, simmered	32.42	13.39	259	0
Bison, ground, grass-fed, cooked	25.45	8.62	179	0
Bison, ground, grass-fed, raw	20.23	7.21	146	0.05
Game meat, beaver, raw	24.05	4.8	146	0
Game meat, beaver, cooked, roasted	34.85	6.96	212	0
Game meat, beefalo, composite of cuts, raw	23.3	4.8	143	0

Food Name ---> per 100 g	Protein (g)	Fat (g)	Calorie	Net Carb (g)
Game meat, beefalo, composite of cuts, cooked, roasted	30.66	6.32	188	0
Veal, Australian, separable fat, raw	9.91	52.17	509	0
Veal, Australian, rib, rib roast, separable lean and fat, raw	19.6	13.1	201	1.15
Game meat, bison, separable lean only, raw	21.62	1.84	109	0
Game meat, bison, separable lean only, cooked, roasted	28.44	2.42	143	0
Game meat, boar, wild, raw	21.51	3.33	122	0
Game meat, boar, wild, cooked, roasted	28.3	4.38	160	0
Game meat, buffalo, water, raw	20.39	1.37	99	0
Game meat, buffalo, water, cooked, roasted	26.83	1.8	131	0
Game meat, caribou, raw	22.63	3.36	127	0
Game meat, caribou, cooked, roasted	29.77	4.42	167	0
Game meat, deer, raw	22.96	2.42	120	0
Game meat, deer, cooked, roasted	30.21	3.19	158	0
Game meat, elk, raw	22.95	1.45	111	0
Game meat, elk, cooked, roasted	30.19	1.9	146	0
Goat, raw	20.6	2.31	109	0
Game meat, goat, cooked, roasted	27.1	3.03	143	0
Game meat, horse, raw	21.39	4.6	133	0
Game meat, horse, cooked, roasted	28.14	6.05	175	0
Game meat, moose, raw	22.24	0.74	102	0
Game meat, moose, cooked, roasted	29.27	0.97	134	0
Game meat, muskrat, raw	20.76	8.1	162	0
Game meat, muskrat, cooked, roasted	30.09	11.74	234	0
Game meat, opossum, cooked, roasted	30.2	10.2	221	0
Game meat, rabbit, domesticated, composite of cuts, raw	20.05	5.55	136	0
Game meat, rabbit, domesticated, composite of cuts, cooked, roasted	29.06	8.05	197	0
Game meat, rabbit, domesticated, composite of cuts, cooked, stewed	30.38	8.41	206	0
Game meat, rabbit, wild, raw	21.79	2.32	114	0
Game meat, rabbit, wild, cooked, stewed	33.02	3.51	173	0
Game meat, raccoon, cooked, roasted	29.2	14.5	255	0

Food Name ---> per 100 g	Protein (g)	Fat (g)	Calorie	Net Carb (g)
Game meat, squirrel, raw	21.23	3.21	120	0
Game meat, squirrel, cooked, roasted	30.77	4.69	173	0
Lamb, variety meats and by-products, brain, raw	10.4	8.58	122	0
Lamb, variety meats and by-products, brain, cooked, braised	12.55	10.17	145	0
Lamb, variety meats and by-products, brain, cooked, pan-fried	16.97	22.19	273	0
Veal, variety meats and by-products, brain, raw	10.32	8.21	118	0
Veal, variety meats and by-products, brain, cooked, braised	11.48	9.63	136	0
Veal, variety meats and by-products, brain, cooked, pan-fried	14.48	16.75	213	0
Lamb, variety meats and by-products, heart, raw	16.47	5.68	122	0.21
Lamb, variety meats and by-products, heart, cooked, braised	24.97	7.91	185	1.93
Veal, variety meats and by-products, heart, raw	17.18	3.98	110	0.08
Veal, variety meats and by-products, heart, cooked, braised	29.12	6.75	186	0.13
Lamb, variety meats and by-products, kidneys, raw	15.74	2.95	97	0.82
Lamb, variety meats and by-products, kidneys, cooked, braised	23.65	3.62	137	0.99
Veal, variety meats and by-products, kidneys, raw	15.76	3.12	99	0.85
Veal, variety meats and by-products, kidneys, cooked, braised	26.32	5.66	163	0
Lamb, variety meats and by-products, liver, raw	20.38	5.02	139	1.78
Lamb, variety meats and by-products, liver, cooked, braised	30.57	8.81	220	2.53
Lamb, variety meats and by-products, liver, cooked, pan-fried	25.53	12.65	238	3.78
Veal, variety meats and by-products, liver, raw	19.93	4.85	140	2.91
Veal, variety meats and by-products, liver, cooked, braised	28.42	6.26	192	3.77
Veal, variety meats and by-products, liver, cooked, pan-fried	27.37	6.51	193	4.47
Lamb, variety meats and by-products, lungs, raw	16.7	2.6	95	0
Lamb, variety meats and by-products, lungs, cooked, braised	19.88	3.1	113	0
Veal, variety meats and by-products, lungs, raw	16.3	2.3	90	0
Veal, variety meats and by-products, lungs, cooked, braised	18.74	2.64	104	0
Lamb, variety meats and by-products, mechanically separated, raw	14.97	23.54	276	0
Lamb, variety meats and by-products, pancreas, raw	14.84	9.82	152	0
Lamb, variety meats and by-products, pancreas, cooked, braised	22.83	15.12	234	0
Veal, variety meats and by-products, pancreas, raw	15	13.1	182	0
Veal, variety meats and by-products, pancreas, cooked, braised	29.1	14.6	256	0

Food Name ---> per 100 g	Protein (g)	Fat (g)	Calorie	Net Carb (g)
Lamb, variety meats and by-products, spleen, raw	17.2	3.1	101	0
Lamb, variety meats and by-products, spleen, cooked, braised	26.46	4.77	156	0
Veal, variety meats and by-products, spleen, raw	18.3	2.2	98	0
Veal, variety meats and by-products, spleen, cooked, braised	24.08	2.89	129	0
Veal, variety meats and by-products, thymus, raw	17.21	3.07	101	0
Veal, variety meats and by-products, thymus, cooked, braised	22.67	3.11	125	0
Lamb, variety meats and by-products, tongue, raw	15.7	17.17	222	0
Lamb, variety meats and by-products, tongue, cooked, braised	21.57	20.28	275	0
Veal, variety meats and by-products, tongue, raw	17.18	5.48	131	1.91
Veal, variety meats and by-products, tongue, cooked, braised	25.85	10.1	202	0
Lamb, ground, raw	16.56	23.41	282	0
Lamb, ground, cooked, broiled	24.75	19.65	283	0
Lamb, domestic, composite of trimmed retail cuts, separable lean and fat, trimmed to 1/8" fat, choice, raw	17.54	18.66	243	0
Lamb, domestic, composite of trimmed retail cuts, separable lean and fat, trimmed to 1/8" fat, choice, cooked	25.51	18.01	271	0
Lamb, domestic, foreshank, separable lean and fat, trimmed to 1/8" fat, choice, raw	18.91	13.38	201	0
Lamb, domestic, foreshank, separable lean and fat, trimmed to 1/8" fat, cooked, braised	28.37	13.46	243	0
Lamb, domestic, leg, whole (shank and sirloin), separable lean and fat, trimmed to 1/8" fat, choice, raw	18.47	14.42	209	0
Lamb, domestic, leg, whole (shank and sirloin), separable lean and fat, trimmed to 1/8" fat, choice, cooked, roasted	26.2	14.42	242	0
Lamb, domestic, leg, shank half, separable lean and fat, trimmed to 1/8" fat, choice, raw	18.99	11.5	185	0
Lamb, domestic, leg, shank half, separable lean and fat, trimmed to 1/8" fat, choice, cooked, roasted	26.73	11.4	217	0
Lamb, domestic, leg, sirloin half, separable lean and fat, trimmed to 1/8" fat, choice, raw	17.21	20.8	261	0
Lamb, domestic, leg, sirloin half, separable lean and fat, trimmed to 1/8" fat, choice, cooked, roasted	24.95	19.67	284	0
Lamb, domestic, loin, separable lean and fat, trimmed to 1/8" fat, choice, raw	17.18	22.75	279	0
Lamb, domestic, loin, separable lean and fat, trimmed to 1/8" fat, choice, cooked, broiled	26.06	20.61	297	0

Food Name ---> per 100 g	Protein (g)	Fat (g)	Calorie	Net Carb (g)
Lamb, domestic, loin, separable lean and fat, trimmed to 1/8" fat, choice, cooked, roasted	23.27	21.12	290	0
Lamb, domestic, rib, separable lean and fat, trimmed to 1/8" fat, choice, raw	15.32	30.71	342	0
Lamb, domestic, rib, separable lean and fat, trimmed to 1/8" fat, choice, cooked, broiled	23.06	26.82	340	0
Lamb, domestic, rib, separable lean and fat, trimmed to 1/8" fat, choice, cooked, roasted	21.82	27.53	341	0
Lamb, domestic, shoulder, whole (arm and blade), separable lean and fat, trimmed to 1/8" fat, choice, raw	17.07	18.96	244	0
Lamb, domestic, shoulder, whole (arm and blade), separable lean and fat, trimmed to 1/8" fat, choice, cooked, braised	29.46	23.57	338	0
Lamb, domestic, shoulder, whole (arm and blade), separable lean and fat, trimmed to 1/8" fat, choice, cooked, broiled	23.84	18.39	268	0
Lamb, domestic, shoulder, whole (arm and blade), separable lean and fat, trimmed to 1/8" fat, choice, cooked, roasted	22.7	19.08	269	0
Lamb, domestic, shoulder, arm, separable lean and fat, trimmed to 1/8" fat, choice, raw	17.19	18.94	244	0
Lamb, domestic, shoulder, arm, separable lean and fat, trimmed to 1/8" fat, choice, cooked, braised	31.1	22.65	337	0
Lamb, domestic, shoulder, arm, separable lean and fat, trimmed to 1/8" fat, cooked, broiled	24.91	18.05	269	0
Lamb, domestic, shoulder, arm, separable lean and fat, trimmed to 1/8" fat, choice, roasted	22.93	18.75	267	0
Lamb, domestic, shoulder, blade, separable lean and fat, trimmed to 1/8" fat, choice, raw	17.01	18.97	244	0
Lamb, domestic, shoulder, blade, separable lean and fat, trimmed to 1/8" fat, choice, cooked, braised	28.92	23.88	339	0
Lamb, domestic, shoulder, blade, separable lean and fat, trimmed to 1/8" fat, choice, cooked, broiled	23.48	18.5	267	0
Lamb, domestic, shoulder, blade, separable lean and fat, trimmed to 1/8" fat, choice, cooked, roasted	22.62	19.19	270	0
Lamb, New Zealand, imported, frozen, composite of trimmed retail cuts, separable lean and fat, trimmed to 1/8" fat, raw	17.95	17.2	232	0
Lamb, New Zealand, imported, frozen, composite of trimmed retail cuts, separable lean and fat, trimmed to 1/8" fat, cooked	25.26	17.98	270	0
Lamb, New Zealand, imported, frozen, foreshank, separable lean and fat, trimmed to 1/8" fat, raw	18.04	16.15	223	0

Food Name ---> per 100 g	Protein (g)	Fat (g)	Calorie	Net Carb (g)
Lamb, New Zealand, imported, frozen, foreshank, separable lean and fat, trimmed to 1/8" fat, cooked, braised	26.97	15.83	258	0
Lamb, New Zealand, imported, frozen, leg, whole (shank and sirloin), separable lean and fat, trimmed to 1/8" fat, raw	18.76	13.37	201	0
Lamb, New Zealand, imported, frozen, leg, whole (shank and sirloin), separable lean and fat, trimmed to 1/8" fat, cooked, roasted	25.34	13.95	234	0
Lamb, New Zealand, imported, frozen, loin, separable lean and fat, trimmed to 1/8" fat, raw	17.18	22.1	273	0
Lamb, New Zealand, imported, frozen, loin, separable lean and fat, trimmed to 1/8" fat, cooked, broiled	24.41	21.28	296	0
Lamb, new zealand, imported, frozen, rib, separable lean and fat, trimmed to 1/8" fat, raw	15.87	27	311	0
Lamb, New Zealand, imported, frozen, rib, separable lean and fat, trimmed to 1/8" fat, cooked, roasted	19.86	25.74	317	0
Lamb, New Zealand, imported, frozen, shoulder, whole (arm and blade), separable lean and fat, trimmed to 1/8" fat, raw	17.19	19.74	251	0
Lamb, New Zealand, imported, frozen, shoulder, whole (arm and blade), separable lean and fat, trimmed to 1/8" fat, cooked, braised	29.43	24.03	342	0
Game meat, bison, top sirloin, separable lean only, trimmed to 0" fat, raw	21.4	2.4	113	0
Game meat, bison, ribeye, separable lean only, trimmed to 0" fat, raw	22.1	2.4	116	0
Game meat, bison, shoulder clod, separable lean only, trimmed to 0" fat, raw	21.1	2.1	109	0
Veal, breast, separable fat, cooked	9.4	53.35	521	0
Veal, breast, whole, boneless, separable lean and fat, raw	17.47	14.75	208	0
Veal, breast, whole, boneless, separable lean and fat, cooked, braised	26.97	16.77	266	0
Veal, breast, plate half, boneless, separable lean and fat, cooked, braised	25.93	18.95	282	0
Veal, breast, point half, boneless, separable lean and fat, cooked, braised	28.23	14.16	248	0
Veal, breast, whole, boneless, separable lean only, cooked, braised	30.32	9.8	218	0
Veal, shank (fore and hind), separable lean and fat, raw	19.15	3.48	113	0

Food Name ---> per 100 g	Protein (g)	Fat (g)	Calorie	Net Carb (g)
Veal, shank (fore and hind), separable lean and fat, cooked, braised	31.54	6.2	191	0
Veal, shank (fore and hind), separable lean only, raw	19.28	2.83	108	0
Veal, shank (fore and hind), separable lean only, cooked, braised	32.22	4.33	177	0
Lamb, Australian, imported, fresh, composite of trimmed retail cuts, separable lean and fat, trimmed to 1/8" fat, raw	17.84	16.97	229	0
Lamb, Australian, imported, fresh, composite of trimmed retail cuts, separable lean and fat, trimmed to 1/8" fat, cooked	24.52	16.82	256	0
Lamb, Australian, imported, fresh, composite of trimmed retail cuts, separable lean only, trimmed to 1/8" fat, raw	20.25	6.18	142	0
Lamb, Australian, imported, fresh, composite of trimmed retail cuts, separable lean only, trimmed to 1/8" fat, cooked	26.71	9.63	201	0
Lamb, Australian, imported, fresh, separable fat, raw	6.27	68.87	648	0
Lamb, Australian, imported, fresh, separable fat, cooked	9.42	66.4	639	0
Lamb, Australian, imported, fresh, foreshank, separable lean and fat, trimmed to 1/8" fat, raw	18.85	12.68	195	0
Lamb, Australian, imported, fresh, foreshank, separable lean and fat, trimmed to 1/8" fat, cooked, braised	24.78	14.44	236	0
Lamb, Australian, imported, fresh, foreshank, separable lean only, trimmed to 1/8" fat, raw	20.83	3.81	123	0
Lamb, Australian, imported, fresh, foreshank, separable lean only, trimmed to 1/8" fat, cooked, braised	27.5	5.22	165	0
Lamb, Australian, imported, fresh, leg, whole (shank and sirloin), separable lean and fat, trimmed to 1/8" fat, raw	18.24	15.19	215	0
Lamb, Australian, imported, fresh, leg, whole (shank and sirloin), separable lean and fat, trimmed to 1/8" fat, cooked, roasted	25.16	15.13	244	0
Lamb, Australian, imported, fresh, leg, whole (shank and sirloin), separable lean only, trimmed to 1/8" fat, raw	20.46	5.23	135	0
Lamb, Australian, imported, fresh, leg, whole (shank and sirloin), separable lean only, trimmed to 1/8" fat, cooked, roasted	27.31	8.1	190	0
Lamb, Australian, imported, fresh, leg, shank half, separable lean and fat, trimmed to 1/8" fat, raw	18.59	13.48	201	0
Lamb, Australian, imported, fresh, leg, shank half, separable lean and fat, trimmed to 1/8" fat, cooked, roasted	25.25	13.69	231	0
Lamb, Australian, imported, fresh, leg, shank half, separable lean only, trimmed to 1/8" fat, raw	20.45	5.1	133	0

Food Name ---> per 100 g	Protein (g)	Fat (g)	Calorie	Net Carb (g)
Lamb, Australian, imported, fresh, leg, shank half, separable lean only, trimmed to 1/8" fat, cooked, roasted	27.18	7.27	182	0
Lamb, Australian, imported, fresh, leg, sirloin half, boneless, separable lean and fat, trimmed to 1/8" fat, raw	17.25	20	254	0
Lamb, Australian, imported, fresh, leg, sirloin half, boneless, separable lean and fat, trimmed to 1/8" fat, cooked, roasted	24.88	19.38	281	0
Lamb, Australian, imported, fresh, leg, sirloin half, boneless, separable lean only, trimmed to 1/8" fat, raw	20.48	5.64	138	0
Lamb, Australian, imported, fresh, leg, sirloin half, boneless, separable lean only, trimmed to 1/8" fat, cooked, roasted	27.75	10.65	215	0
Lamb, Australian, imported, fresh, leg, sirloin chops, boneless, separable lean and fat, trimmed to 1/8" fat, raw	18.33	14.38	208	0
Lamb, Australian, imported, fresh, leg, sirloin chops, boneless, separable lean and fat, trimmed to 1/8" fat, cooked, broiled	25.75	13.83	235	0
Lamb, Australian, imported, fresh, leg, sirloin chops, boneless, separable lean only, trimmed to 1/8" fat, raw	20.43	4.91	132	0
Lamb, Australian, imported, fresh, leg, sirloin chops, boneless, separable lean only, trimmed to 1/8" fat, cooked, broiled	27.63	7.8	188	0
Lamb, Australian, imported, fresh, leg, center slice, bone-in, separable lean and fat, trimmed to 1/8" fat, raw	19.17	12.56	195	0
Lamb, Australian, imported, fresh, leg, center slice, bone-in, separable lean and fat, trimmed to 1/8" fat, cooked, broiled	25.54	11.78	215	0
Lamb, Australian, imported, fresh, leg, center slice, bone-in, separable lean only, trimmed to 1/8" fat, raw	20.65	6.08	143	0
Lamb, Australian, imported, fresh, leg, center slice, bone-in, separable lean only, trimmed to 1/8" fat, cooked, broiled	26.75	7.68	183	0
Lamb, Australian, imported, fresh, loin, separable lean and fat, trimmed to 1/8" fat, raw	19.32	13.38	203	0
Lamb, Australian, imported, fresh, loin, separable lean and fat, trimmed to 1/8" fat, cooked, broiled	25.49	12.25	219	0
Lamb, Australian, imported, fresh, loin, separable lean only, trimmed to 1/8" fat, raw	21	6.24	146	0
Lamb, Australian, imported, fresh, loin, separable lean only, trimmed to 1/8" fat, cooked, broiled	26.53	8.75	192	0
Lamb, Australian, imported, fresh, rib chop/rack roast, frenched, bone-in, separable lean and fat, trimmed to 1/8" fat, raw	21.26	16.89	237	0
Lamb, Australian, imported, fresh, rib chop, frenched, bone-in, separable lean and fat, trimmed to 1/8" fat, cooked, grilled	28.48	21.2	305	0

Food Name ---> per 100 g	Protein (g)	Fat (g)	Calorie	Net Carb (g)
Lamb, Australian, imported, fresh, rib chop/rack roast, frenched, bone-in, separable lean only, trimmed to 1/8" fat, raw	24.07	5.59	147	0
Lamb, Australian, imported, fresh, rib chop, frenched, bone-in, separable lean only, trimmed to 1/8" fat, cooked, grilled	32.16	11.68	234	0
Lamb, Australian, imported, fresh, shoulder, whole (arm and blade), separable lean and fat, trimmed to 1/8" fat, raw	16.68	20.47	256	0
Lamb, Australian, imported, fresh, shoulder, whole (arm and blade), separable lean and fat, trimmed to 1/8" fat, cooked	23.58	21.65	296	0
Lamb, Australian, imported, fresh, shoulder, whole (arm and blade), separable lean only, trimmed to 1/8" fat, raw	19.36	8.01	155	0
Lamb, Australian, imported, fresh, shoulder, whole (arm and blade), separable lean only, trimmed to 1/8" fat, cooked	26.18	13.44	233	0
Lamb, Australian, imported, fresh, shoulder, arm, separable lean and fat, trimmed to 1/8" fat, raw	17.06	18.89	243	0
Lamb, Australian, imported, fresh, shoulder, arm, separable lean and fat, trimmed to 1/8" fat, cooked, braised	29.7	20.38	311	0
Lamb, Australian, imported, fresh, shoulder, arm, separable lean only, trimmed to 1/8" fat, raw	19.88	5.81	137	0
Lamb, Australian, imported, fresh, shoulder, arm, separable lean only, trimmed to 1/8" fat, cooked, braised	34.17	10.23	238	0
Lamb, Australian, imported, fresh, shoulder, blade, separable lean and fat, trimmed to 1/8" fat, raw	16.48	21.28	262	0
Lamb, Australian, imported, fresh, shoulder, blade, separable lean and fat, trimmed to 1/8" fat, cooked, broiled	21.71	22.03	291	0
Lamb, Australian, imported, fresh, shoulder, blade, separable lean only, trimmed to 1/8" fat, raw	19.1	9.09	164	0
Lamb, Australian, imported, fresh, shoulder ,blade, separable lean only, trimmed to 1/8" fat, cooked, broiled	23.83	14.38	231	0
Game meat , bison, ground, raw	18.67	15.93	223	0
Game meat, bison, ground, cooked, pan-broiled	23.77	15.13	238	0
Game meat , bison, top sirloin, separable lean only, 1" steak, cooked, broiled	28.05	5.65	171	0
Game meat, bison, chuck, shoulder clod, separable lean only, cooked, braised	33.78	5.43	193	0
Game meat, bison, chuck, shoulder clod, separable lean only, raw	21.12	3.15	119	0
Game meat, bison, ribeye, separable lean only, 1" steak, cooked, broiled	29.45	5.67	177	0

Food Name ---> per 100 g	Protein (g)	Fat (g)	Calorie	Net Carb (g)
Game meat, bison, top round, separable lean only, 1" steak, cooked, broiled	30.18	4.96	174	0
Game meat, bison, top round, separable lean only, 1" steak, raw	23.32	2.43	122	0
Game meat, elk, ground, raw	21.76	8.82	172	0
Game meat, elk, ground, cooked, pan-broiled	26.64	8.74	193	0
Game meat, elk, loin, separable lean only, cooked, broiled	31	3.84	167	0
Game meat, elk, round, separable lean only, cooked, broiled	30.94	2.64	156	0
Game meat, elk, tenderloin, separable lean only, cooked, broiled	30.76	3.41	162	0
Game meat, deer, ground, raw	21.78	7.13	157	0
Game meat, deer, ground, cooked, pan-broiled	26.45	8.22	187	0
Game meat, deer, loin, separable lean only, 1" steak, cooked, broiled	30.2	2.38	150	0
Game meat, deer, shoulder clod, separable lean only, cooked, braised	36.28	3.95	191	0
Game meat, deer, tenderloin, separable lean only, cooked, broiled	29.9	2.35	149	0
Game meat, deer, top round, separable lean only, 1" steak, cooked, broiled	31.47	1.92	152	0
Veal, Australian, shank, fore, bone-in, separable lean only, raw	20.18	4.65	123	0
Veal, Australian, shank, fore, bone-in, separable lean and fat, raw	19.58	7.42	145	0
Veal, Australian, shank, hind, bone-in, separable lean only, raw	20.37	4.47	122	0
Veal, Australian, shank, hind, bone-in, separable lean and fat	19.78	7.2	144	0
Lamb, Australian, ground, 85% lean / 15% fat, raw	17.14	20.71	255	0
Lamb, New Zealand, imported, Intermuscular fat, cooked	8.53	62.44	596	0
Lamb, New Zealand, imported, Intermuscular fat, raw	4.63	68.53	640	1.26
Lamb, New Zealand, imported, subcutaneous fat, raw	3.87	76.16	703	0.55
Lamb, New Zealand, imported, brains, cooked, soaked and fried	14.03	10.92	154	0
Lamb, New Zealand, imported, brains, raw	11.33	8.03	118	0
Lamb, New Zealand, imported, breast, separable lean only, cooked, braised	28.16	17.53	270	0
Lamb, New Zealand, imported, breast, separable lean only, raw	18.31	7.98	149	1.02
Lamb, New Zealand, imported, chump, boneless, separable lean only, cooked, fast roasted	23.69	5.27	142	0
Lamb, New Zealand, imported, subcutaneous fat, cooked	5.24	72.28	674	0.62

Food Name ---> per 100 g	Protein (g)	Fat (g)	Calorie	Net Carb (g)
Lamb, New Zealand, imported, chump, boneless, separable lean only, raw	21.68	3.83	121	0
Lamb, New Zealand, imported, kidney, cooked, soaked and fried	19.78	3.56	112	0.18
Lamb, New Zealand, imported, flap, boneless, separable lean only, cooked, braised	27.88	13.6	234	0
Lamb, New Zealand, imported, flap, boneless, separable lean only, raw	21.72	10.31	180	0
Lamb, New Zealand, imported, kidney, raw	15.21	2.54	84	0.03
Lamb, New Zealand, imported, liver, cooked, soaked and fried	25.8	6.56	168	1.48
Lamb, New Zealand, imported, liver, raw	20.7	4.92	136	2.22
Lamb, New Zealand, imported, ground lamb, cooked, braised	22.6	11.34	192	0
Lamb, New Zealand, imported, ground lamb, raw	20.33	12.41	193	0
Lamb, New Zealand, imported, heart, cooked, soaked and simmered	26.26	6.21	161	0
Lamb, New Zealand, imported, heart, raw	18.09	3.68	105	0
Lamb, New Zealand, imported, sweetbread, cooked, soaked and simmered	21.13	6.61	144	0
Lamb, New Zealand, imported, sweetbread, raw	11	3.16	72	0
Lamb, New Zealand, imported, testes, cooked, soaked and fried	21.01	4.56	125	0
Lamb, New Zealand, imported, testes, raw	11.4	2.38	68	0.14
Lamb, New Zealand, imported, tongue - swiss cut, cooked, soaked and simmered	17.51	22.04	272	0.86
Lamb, New Zealand, imported, tongue - swiss cut, raw	14.27	18.61	225	0
Lamb, New Zealand, imported, tunnel-boned leg, chump off, shank off, separable lean only, cooked, slow roasted	25.29	6.44	159	0
Lamb, New Zealand, imported, tunnel-boned leg, chump off, shank off, separable lean only, raw	20.93	4.09	121	0
Lamb, New Zealand, imported, square-cut shoulder chops, separable lean only, cooked, braised	31.06	14.56	255	0
Lamb, New Zealand, imported, square-cut shoulder chops, separable lean only, raw	20.62	9.08	164	0
Lamb, New Zealand, imported, tenderloin, separable lean only, cooked, fast fried	27.94	4.81	155	0
Lamb, New Zealand, imported, tenderloin, separable lean only, raw	20.53	3.81	116	0

Food Name ---> per 100 g	Protein (g)	Fat (g)	Calorie	Net Carb (g)
Lamb, New Zealand, imported, loin saddle, separable lean only, cooked, fast roasted	25.53	6.7	162	0
Lamb, New Zealand, imported, loin saddle, separable lean only, raw	20.86	5.32	131	0
Lamb, New Zealand, imported, loin, boneless, separable lean only, cooked, fast roasted	28.99	4.49	156	0
Lamb, New Zealand, imported, loin, boneless, separable lean only, raw	21.5	3.77	120	0
Lamb, New Zealand, imported, hind-shank, separable lean only, cooked, braised	32.5	7.37	196	0
Lamb, New Zealand, imported, hind-shank, separable lean only, raw	20.4	3.35	115	0.73
Lamb, New Zealand, imported, neck chops, separable lean only, raw	19.84	7.97	151	0
Lamb, New Zealand, imported, neck chops, separable lean only, cooked, braised	31.4	15.36	264	0
Lamb, New Zealand, imported, netted shoulder, rolled, boneless, separable lean only, cooked, slow roasted	25.14	10.91	199	0
Lamb, New Zealand, imported, netted shoulder, rolled, boneless, separable lean only, raw	20.2	6.88	143	0
Lamb, New Zealand, imported, rack - fully frenched, separable lean only, cooked, fast roasted	24.39	8.38	173	0
Lamb, New Zealand, imported, rack - fully frenched, separable lean only, raw	20.61	7.12	147	0
Lamb, New Zealand, imported, loin chop, separable lean only, cooked, fast fried	27.43	10.7	208	0.41
Lamb, New Zealand, imported, square-cut shoulder, separable lean only, cooked, slow roasted	25.08	10.13	192	0
Lamb, New Zealand, imported, leg chop/steak, bone-in, separable lean only, cooked, fast fried	26.31	6.35	162	0
Lamb, New Zealand, imported, flap, boneless, separable lean and fat, cooked, braised	20.48	32.63	376	0.14
Lamb, New Zealand, imported, flap, boneless, separable lean and fat, raw	16.17	30.14	337	0.27
Lamb, New Zealand, imported, hind-shank, separable lean and fat, cooked, braised	29.59	14.22	247	0.04
Lamb, New Zealand, imported, hind-shank, separable lean and fat, raw	18.39	12.12	186	0.73

Food Name ---> per 100 g	Protein (g)	Fat (g)	Calorie	Net Carb (g)
Lamb, New Zealand, imported, leg chop/steak, bone-in, separable lean and fat, cooked, fast fried	24.26	12.76	212	0.04
Lamb, New Zealand, imported, loin chop, separable lean and fat, cooked, fast fried	21.5	27.11	332	0.41
Lamb, New Zealand, imported, loin saddle, separable lean and fat, cooked, fast roasted	21.13	20.98	274	0.1
Lamb, New Zealand, imported, loin saddle, separable lean and fat, raw	16.56	22.9	273	0.2
Lamb, New Zealand, imported, loin, boneless, separable lean and fat, cooked, fast roasted	28.96	4.57	157	0
Lamb, New Zealand, imported, loin, boneless, separable lean and fat, raw	21.44	3.99	122	0
Lamb, New Zealand, imported, neck chops, separable lean and fat, cooked, braised	28.53	21.43	307	0.03
Lamb, New Zealand, imported, neck chops, separable lean and fat, raw	17.43	17.9	231	0.14
Lamb, New Zealand, imported, netted shoulder, rolled, boneless, separable lean and fat, cooked, slow roasted	21.45	22.33	287	0.05
Lamb, New Zealand, imported, netted shoulder, rolled, boneless, separable lean and fat, raw	16.9	20.36	252	0.2
Lamb, New Zealand, imported, square-cut shoulder chops, separable lean and fat, cooked, braised	26.79	23.86	322	0.05
Lamb, New Zealand, imported, square-cut shoulder chops, separable lean and fat, raw	17.02	22.84	275	0.23
Lamb, New Zealand, imported, square-cut shoulder, separable lean and fat, cooked, slow roasted	20.88	23.39	294	0.03
Lamb, New Zealand, imported, tenderloin, separable lean and fat, cooked, fast fried	27.87	5	157	0
Lamb, New Zealand, imported, rack - fully frenched, separable lean and fat, cooked, fast roasted	23.56	11.2	195	0.01
Lamb, New Zealand, imported, rack - fully frenched, separable lean and fat, raw	19.88	9.96	169	0.05
Lamb, New Zealand, imported, tunnel-boned leg, chump off, shank off, separable lean and fat, cooked, slow roasted	23.41	12.68	208	0.03
Lamb, New Zealand, imported, tunnel-boned leg, chump off, shank off, separable lean and fat, raw	20.93	4.09	121	0
Lamb, New Zealand, imported, tenderloin, separable lean and fat, raw	20.43	4.22	120	0.01

Food Name ---> per 100 g	Protein (g)	Fat (g)	Calorie	Net Carb (g)
Veal, ground, cooked, pan-fried	25.83	11.78	215	1.51
Veal, leg, top round, cap off, cutlet, boneless, cooked, grilled	31.89	2.63	151	0
Veal, leg, top round, cap off, cutlet, boneless, raw	22.07	2.07	107	0
Veal, loin, chop, separable lean only, cooked, grilled	29.75	4.44	159	0.07
Veal, shank, separable lean only, raw	19.77	1.64	94	0
Veal, foreshank, osso buco, separable lean only, cooked, braised	29.12	4.51	157	0
Veal, shoulder, blade chop, separable lean only, cooked, grilled	27.33	5.53	159	0
Veal, external fat only, raw	8.85	51.6	503	0.89
Veal, external fat only, cooked	15.28	53.23	540	0
Veal, seam fat only, raw	12.53	43.75	444	0
Veal, seam fat only, cooked	11.16	50.17	505	2.11
Veal, shank, separable lean and fat, raw	19.28	3.3	107	0
Veal, foreshank, osso buco, separable lean and fat, cooked, braised	27.94	7.77	182	0.11
Veal, loin, chop, separable lean and fat, cooked, grilled	28.04	9.48	198	0.16
Veal, shoulder, blade chop, separable lean and fat, cooked, grilled	25.72	10.57	199	0.15
Lamb, Australian, imported, fresh, leg, bottom, boneless, separable lean only, trimmed to 1/8" fat, cooked, roasted	28.6	8.35	190	0
Lamb, Australian, imported, fresh, leg, hindshank, heel on, bone-in, separable lean only, trimmed to 1/8" fat, cooked, braised	30.73	5.63	174	0
Lamb, Australian, imported, fresh, leg, hindshank, heel on, bone-in, separable lean only, trimmed to 1/8" fat, raw	22.49	3.53	122	0
Lamb, Australian, imported, fresh, tenderloin, boneless, separable lean only, trimmed to 1/8" fat, cooked, roasted	30.97	6.71	184	0
Lamb, Australian, imported, fresh, tenderloin, boneless, separable lean only, trimmed to 1/8" fat, raw	23.42	4.73	136	0
Lamb, Australian, imported, fresh, leg, bottom, boneless, separable lean only, trimmed to 1/8" fat, raw	22.28	5.24	136	0
Lamb, Australian, imported, fresh, leg, trotter off, bone-in, separable lean only, trimmed to 1/8" fat, cooked, roasted	32.08	9.59	215	0
Lamb, Australian, imported, fresh, leg, trotter off, bone-in, separable lean only, trimmed to 1/8" fat, raw	23.11	4.33	131	0
Lamb, Australian, imported, fresh, rack, roast, frenched, denuded, bone-in, separable lean only, trimmed to 0" fat, cooked, roasted	26.52	7.63	175	0

Food Name ---> per 100 g	Protein (g)	Fat (g)	Calorie	Net Carb (g)
Lamb, Australian, imported, fresh, rack, roast, frenched, bone-in, separable lean only, trimmed to 1/8" fat, cooked, roasted	28.01	14.64	244	0
Lamb, Australian, imported, fresh, external fat, cooked	16.9	52.3	538	0
Lamb, Australian, imported, fresh, external fat, raw	12.59	48.5	487	0
Lamb, Australian, imported, fresh, seam fat, cooked	13.81	54.72	554	1.55
Lamb, Australian, imported, fresh, seam fat, raw	15.65	44.01	459	0
Lamb, Australian, imported, fresh, leg, bottom, boneless, separable lean and fat, trimmed to 1/8" fat, cooked, roasted	27.54	12.04	219	0
Lamb, Australian, imported, fresh, leg, bottom, boneless, separable lean and fat, trimmed to 1/8" fat, raw	20.97	11.43	187	0
Lamb, Australian, imported, fresh, leg, hindshank, heel on, bone-in, separable lean and fat, trimmed to 1/8" fat, cooked, braised	29.52	9.5	204	0
Lamb, Australian, imported, fresh, leg, hindshank, heel on, bone-in, separable lean and fat, trimmed to 1/8" fat, raw	20.58	12.68	196	0
Lamb, Australian, imported, fresh, leg, trotter off, bone-in, separable lean and fat, trimmed to 1/8" fat, cooked, roasted	30.15	11.64	226	0.08
Lamb, Australian, imported, fresh, leg, trotter off, bone-in, separable lean and fat, trimmed to 1/8" fat, raw	21.95	9.73	175	0
Lamb, Australian, imported, fresh, tenderloin, boneless, separable lean and fat, trimmed to 1/8" fat, cooked, roasted	30.87	7.02	187	0
Lamb, Australian, imported, fresh, tenderloin, boneless, separable lean and fat, trimmed to 1/8" fat, raw	23.23	5.52	143	0
Lamb, Australian, imported, fresh, rib chop, frenched, denuded, bone-in, separable lean only, trimmed to 0" fat, cooked, grilled	33.17	11.5	236	0
Lamb, Australian, imported, fresh, rack, roast, frenched, denuded, bone-in, separable lean and fat, trimmed to 0" fat, cooked, roasted	25.95	9.91	193	0
Lamb, Australian, imported, fresh, rack, roast, frenched, bone-in, separable lean and fat, trimmed to 1/8" fat, cooked, roasted	25.96	20.77	291	0
Lamb, Australian, imported, fresh, rib chop, frenched, denuded, bone-in, separable lean and fat, trimmed to 0" fat, cooked, grilled	30.9	16.96	276	0

Legumes and Legume Products

Food Name ---> per 100 g	Protein (g)	Fat (g)	Calorie	Net Carb (g)
Beans, adzuki, mature seeds, raw	19.87	0.53	329	50.2
Beans, adzuki, mature seeds, cooked, boiled, without salt	7.52	0.1	128	17.47
Beans, adzuki, mature seeds, canned, sweetened	3.8	0.03	237	55.01
Yokan, prepared from adzuki beans and sugar	3.29	0.12	260	60.72
Beans, baked, home prepared	5.54	5.15	155	16.13
Beans, baked, canned, plain or vegetarian	4.75	0.37	94	17.04
Beans, baked, canned, with beef	6.38	3.45	121	16.91
Beans, baked, canned, with franks	6.75	6.57	142	8.49
Beans, baked, canned, with pork	5.19	1.55	106	14.49
Beans, baked, canned, with pork and sweet sauce	4.52	0.89	105	17.17
Beans, baked, canned, with pork and tomato sauce	5.15	0.93	94	14.69
Beans, black, mature seeds, raw	21.6	1.42	341	46.86
Beans, black, mature seeds, cooked, boiled, without salt	8.86	0.54	132	15.01
Beans, black turtle, mature seeds, raw	21.25	0.9	339	47.75
Beans, black turtle, mature seeds, cooked, boiled, without salt	8.18	0.35	130	16.05
Beans, black turtle, mature seeds, canned	6.03	0.29	91	9.65
Beans, cranberry (roman), mature seeds, raw	23.03	1.23	335	35.35
Beans, cranberry (roman), mature seeds, cooked, boiled, without salt	9.34	0.46	136	15.86
Beans, cranberry (roman), mature seeds, canned	5.54	0.28	83	8.82
Beans, french, mature seeds, raw	18.81	2.02	343	38.91
Beans, french, mature seeds, cooked, boiled, without salt	7.05	0.76	129	14.62
Beans, great northern, mature seeds, raw	21.86	1.14	339	42.17
Beans, great northern, mature seeds, cooked, boiled, without salt	8.33	0.45	118	14.09
Beans, great northern, mature seeds, canned	7.37	0.39	114	16.12
Beans, kidney, all types, mature seeds, raw	23.58	0.83	333	35.11
Beans, kidney, all types, mature seeds, cooked, boiled, without salt	8.67	0.5	127	16.4
Beans, kidney, all types, mature seeds, canned	5.22	0.6	84	10.2

Food Name ---> per 100 g	Protein (g)	Fat (g)	Calorie	Net Carb (g)
Beans, kidney, california red, mature seeds, raw	24.37	0.25	330	34.9
Beans, kidney, california red, mature seeds, cooked, boiled, without salt	9.13	0.09	124	13.11
Beans, kidney, red, mature seeds, raw	22.53	1.06	337	46.09
Beans, kidney, red, mature seeds, cooked, boiled, without salt	8.67	0.5	127	15.4
Beans, kidney, red, mature seeds, canned, solids and liquids	5.22	0.36	81	10.53
Beans, kidney, royal red, mature seeds, raw	25.33	0.45	329	33.43
Beans, kidney, royal red, mature seeds, cooked, boiled, without salt	9.49	0.17	123	12.55
Beans, navy, mature seeds, raw	22.33	1.5	337	45.45
Beans, navy, mature seeds, cooked, boiled, without salt	8.23	0.62	140	15.55
Beans, navy, mature seeds, canned	7.53	0.43	113	15.35
Beans, pink, mature seeds, raw	20.96	1.13	343	51.49
Beans, pink, mature seeds, cooked, boiled, without salt	9.06	0.49	149	22.61
Beans, pinto, mature seeds, raw	21.42	1.23	347	47.05
Beans, pinto, mature seeds, cooked, boiled, without salt	9.01	0.65	143	17.22
Beans, pinto, mature seeds, canned, solids and liquids	4.6	0.56	82	10.58
Beans, small white, mature seeds, raw	21.11	1.18	336	37.35
Beans, small white, mature seeds, cooked, boiled, without salt	8.97	0.64	142	15.41
Beans, yellow, mature seeds, raw	22	2.6	345	35.6
Beans, yellow, mature seeds, cooked, boiled, without salt	9.16	1.08	144	14.88
Beans, white, mature seeds, raw	23.36	0.85	333	45.07
Beans, white, mature seeds, cooked, boiled, without salt	9.73	0.35	139	18.79
Beans, white, mature seeds, canned	7.26	0.29	114	16.4
Broadbeans (fava beans), mature seeds, raw	26.12	1.53	341	33.29
Broadbeans (fava beans), mature seeds, cooked, boiled, without salt	7.6	0.4	110	14.25
Broadbeans (fava beans), mature seeds, canned	5.47	0.22	71	8.71
Carob flour	4.62	0.65	222	49.08
Chickpeas (garbanzo beans, bengal gram), mature seeds, raw	20.47	6.04	378	50.75
Chickpeas (garbanzo beans, bengal gram), mature seeds, cooked, boiled, without salt	8.86	2.59	164	19.82

Food Name ---> per 100 g	Protein (g)	Fat (g)	Calorie	Net Carb (g)
Chickpeas (garbanzo beans, bengal gram), mature seeds, canned, solids and liquids	4.92	1.95	88	9.09
Chili with beans, canned	6.12	3.76	103	9.94
Cowpeas, catjang, mature seeds, raw	23.85	2.07	343	48.94
Cowpeas, catjang, mature seeds, cooked, boiled, without salt	8.13	0.71	117	16.72
Cowpeas, common (blackeyes, crowder, southern), mature seeds, raw	23.52	1.26	336	49.43
Cowpeas, common (blackeyes, crowder, southern), mature seeds, cooked, boiled, without salt	7.73	0.53	116	14.26
Cowpeas, common (blackeyes, crowder, southern), mature seeds, canned, plain	4.74	0.55	77	10.33
Cowpeas, common (blackeyes, crowder, southern), mature seeds, canned with pork	2.74	1.6	83	13.23
Hyacinth beans, mature seeds, raw	23.9	1.69	344	35.14
Hyacinth beans, mature seeds, cooked, boiled, without salt	8.14	0.58	117	20.69
Lentils, raw	24.63	1.06	352	52.65
Lentils, mature seeds, cooked, boiled, without salt	9.02	0.38	116	12.23
Lima beans, large, mature seeds, raw	21.46	0.69	338	44.38
Lima beans, large, mature seeds, cooked, boiled, without salt	7.8	0.38	115	13.88
Lima beans, large, mature seeds, canned	4.93	0.17	79	10.11
Lima beans, thin seeded (baby), mature seeds, raw	20.62	0.93	335	42.23
Lima beans, thin seeded (baby), mature seeds, cooked, boiled, without salt	8.04	0.38	126	15.61
Lupins, mature seeds, raw	36.17	9.74	371	21.47
Lupins, mature seeds, cooked, boiled, without salt	15.57	2.92	119	7.08
Mothbeans, mature seeds, raw	22.94	1.61	343	61.52
Mothbeans, mature seeds, cooked, boiled, without salt	7.81	0.55	117	20.96
Mung beans, mature seeds, raw	23.86	1.15	347	46.32
Mung beans, mature seeds, cooked, boiled, without salt	7.02	0.38	105	11.55
Noodles, chinese, cellophane or long rice (mung beans), dehydrated	0.16	0.06	351	85.59
Mungo beans, mature seeds, raw	25.21	1.64	341	40.69
Mungo beans, mature seeds, cooked, boiled, without salt	7.54	0.55	105	11.94
Peas, green, split, mature seeds, raw	23.82	1.16	352	38.24

Food Name ---> per 100 g	Protein (g)	Fat (g)	Calorie	Net Carb (g)
Peas, split, mature seeds, cooked, boiled, without salt	8.34	0.39	118	12.8
Peanuts, all types, raw	25.8	49.24	567	7.63
Peanuts, all types, cooked, boiled, with salt	13.5	22.01	318	12.46
Peanuts, all types, oil-roasted, with salt	28.03	52.5	599	5.86
Peanuts, all types, dry-roasted, with salt	24.35	49.66	587	12.86
Peanuts, spanish, raw	26.15	49.6	570	6.33
Peanuts, spanish, oil-roasted, with salt	28.01	49.04	579	8.55
Peanuts, valencia, raw	25.09	47.58	570	12.21
Peanuts, valencia, oil-roasted, with salt	27.04	51.24	589	7.4
Peanuts, virginia, raw	25.19	48.75	563	8.04
Peanuts, virginia, oil-roasted, with salt	25.87	48.62	578	10.96
Peanut butter, chunk style, with salt	24.06	49.94	589	13.57
Peanut butter, smooth style, with salt	22.21	51.36	598	17.31
Peanut flour, defatted	52.2	0.55	327	18.9
Peanut flour, low fat	33.8	21.9	428	15.47
Pigeon peas (red gram), mature seeds, raw	21.7	1.49	343	47.78
Pigeon peas (red gram), mature seeds, cooked, boiled, without salt	6.76	0.38	121	16.55
Refried beans, canned, traditional style (includes USDA commodity)	4.98	2.01	90	9.85
Bacon, meatless	11.69	29.52	309	2.71
Meat extender	41.71	2.97	311	17.21
Sausage, meatless	20.28	18.16	255	5.29
Soybeans, mature seeds, raw	36.49	19.94	446	20.86
Soybeans, mature cooked, boiled, without salt	18.21	8.97	172	2.36
Soybeans, mature seeds, roasted, salted	38.55	25.4	469	12.52
Soybeans, mature seeds, dry roasted	43.32	21.62	449	20.88
Miso	12.79	6.01	198	19.97
Natto	19.4	11	211	7.28
Tempeh	20.29	10.8	192	7.64
Soy flour, full-fat, raw	37.81	20.65	434	22.32
Soy flour, full-fat, roasted	38.09	21.86	439	20.68

Food Name ---> per 100 g	Protein (g)	Fat (g)	Calorie	Net Carb (g)
Soy flour, defatted	51.46	1.22	327	16.42
Soy flour, low-fat	49.81	8.9	372	14.63
Soy meal, defatted, raw	49.2	2.39	337	35.89
Soymilk, original and vanilla, unfortified	3.27	1.75	54	5.68
Soy protein concentrate, produced by alcohol extraction	63.63	0.46	328	19.91
Soy protein isolate	88.32	3.39	335	0
Soy sauce made from soy and wheat (shoyu)	8.14	0.57	53	4.13
Soy sauce made from soy (tamari)	10.51	0.1	60	4.77
Soy sauce made from hydrolyzed vegetable protein	7	0.51	60	7.34
Tofu, firm, prepared with calcium sulfate and magnesium chloride (nigari)	9.04	4.17	78	1.95
Tofu, soft, prepared with calcium sulfate and magnesium chloride (nigari)	7.17	3.69	61	0.98
Tofu, dried-frozen (koyadofu)	52.47	30.34	477	2.83
Tofu, fried	18.82	20.18	270	4.96
Okara	3.52	1.73	76	12.23
Tofu, salted and fermented (fuyu)	8.92	8	116	4.38
Yardlong beans, mature seeds, raw	24.33	1.31	347	50.91
Yardlong beans, mature seeds, cooked, boiled, without salt	8.29	0.45	118	17.29
Winged beans, mature seeds, raw	29.65	16.32	409	15.81
Winged beans, mature seeds, cooked, boiled, without salt	10.62	5.84	147	14.94
Hummus, home prepared	4.86	8.59	177	16.12
Falafel, home-prepared	13.31	17.8	333	31.84
Soymilk, original and vanilla, with added calcium, vitamins A and D	2.6	1.47	43	4.72
Lentils, pink or red, raw	23.91	2.17	358	52.3
Beans, kidney, red, mature seeds, canned, drained solids	7.98	1.05	124	15.99
Beans, pinto, canned, drained solids	6.99	0.9	114	14.72
Veggie burgers or soyburgers, unprepared	15.7	6.3	177	9.37
Peanut spread, reduced sugar	24.8	54.89	650	6.43
Peanut butter, smooth, reduced fat	25.9	34	520	30.45
Peanut butter, smooth, vitamin and mineral fortified	25.72	50.81	591	13.15

Food Name ---> per 100 g	Protein (g)	Fat (g)	Calorie	Net Carb (g)
Peanut butter, chunky, vitamin and mineral fortified	26.06	51.47	593	11.99
Chickpea flour (besan)	22.39	6.69	387	47.02
Hummus, commercial	7.9	9.6	166	8.29
Tofu, extra firm, prepared with nigari	9.98	5.26	83	0.18
Tofu, hard, prepared with nigari	12.68	9.99	145	3.79
MORI-NU, Tofu, silken, soft	4.8	2.7	55	2.8
MORI-NU, Tofu, silken, firm	6.9	2.7	62	2.3
MORI-NU, Tofu, silken, extra firm	7.4	1.9	55	1.9
MORI-NU, Tofu, silken, lite firm	6.3	0.8	37	1.1
MORI-NU, Tofu, silken, lite extra firm	7	0.7	38	1
Soymilk, chocolate, unfortified	2.26	1.53	63	9.55
USDA Commodity, Peanut Butter, smooth	21.93	49.54	588	18.28
Soymilk, chocolate, with added calcium, vitamins A and D	2.26	1.53	63	9.55
Refried beans, canned, vegetarian	5.28	0.87	83	8.8
Refried beans, canned, fat-free	5.34	0.45	79	8.8
Frijoles rojos volteados (Refried beans, red, canned)	5	6.93	144	10.77
Tempeh, cooked	19.91	11.38	195	7.62
Campbell's Brown Sugar And Bacon Flavored Baked Beans	3.85	1.92	123	16.88
Campbell's Pork and Beans	4.62	1.15	108	13.83
PACE, Traditional Refried Beans	4.17	0	67	6.63
PACE, Salsa Refried Beans	3.33	0	60	8.37
PACE, Spicy Jalapeno Refried Beans	4.17	0	63	7.47
Vitasoy USA, Nasoya Lite Firm Tofu	8.3	1.7	54	0.7
Vitasoy USA, Organic Nasoya Super Firm Cubed Tofu	12.4	6.3	118	0.8
Vitasoy USA, Organic Nasoya Extra Firm Tofu	10.1	5.2	98	1.3
Vitasoy USA, Organic Nasoya Firm Tofu	8.9	4.4	84	1.5
Vitasoy USA, Organic Nasoya Silken Tofu	4.8	2.5	47	1.1
Vitasoy USA, Vitasoy Organic Creamy Original Soymilk	2.9	1.6	44	4.1
Vitasoy USA, Vitasoy Organic Classic Original Soymilk	3.2	1.8	47	4.1
Vitasoy USA, Vitasoy Light Vanilla Soymilk	1.6	0.82	30	4
Soymilk (all flavors), unsweetened, with added calcium, vitamins A and D	2.86	1.61	33	1.24

Food Name ---> per 100 g	Protein (g)	Fat (g)	Calorie	Net Carb (g)
Soymilk (All flavors), enhanced	2.94	1.99	45	3.05
Soymilk, original and vanilla, light, with added calcium, vitamins A and D	2.38	0.77	30	3.21
Soymilk, chocolate and other flavors, light, with added calcium, vitamins A and D	2.1	0.64	47	7.54
Soymilk, original and vanilla, light, unsweetened, with added calcium, vitamins A and D	2.62	0.85	34	3.25
Soymilk (All flavors), lowfat, with added calcium, vitamins A and D	1.65	0.62	43	6.4
Soymilk (all flavors), nonfat, with added calcium, vitamins A and D	2.47	0.04	28	3.94
Soymilk, chocolate, nonfat, with added calcium, vitamins A and D	2.47	0.04	44	8.31
SILK Plain, soymilk	2.88	1.65	41	2.89
SILK Vanilla, soymilk	2.47	1.44	41	3.72
SILK Chocolate, soymilk	2.06	1.44	58	8.67
SILK Light Plain, soymilk	2.47	0.82	29	2.89
SILK Light Vanilla, soymilk	2.47	0.82	33	3.72
SILK Light Chocolate, soymilk	2.06	0.62	49	8.25
SILK Plus Omega-3 DHA, soymilk	2.88	2.06	45	2.89
SILK Plus for Bone Health, soymilk	2.47	1.44	41	3.73
SILK Plus Fiber, soymilk	2.47	1.44	41	3.66
SILK Unsweetened, soymilk	2.88	1.65	33	1.25
SILK Very Vanilla, soymilk	2.47	1.65	53	7.42
SILK Nog, soymilk	2.46	1.64	74	12.3
SILK Chai, soymilk	2.47	1.44	53	7.82
SILK Mocha, soymilk	2.06	1.44	58	9.05
SILK Coffee, soymilk	2.06	1.44	62	10.29
SILK Vanilla soy yogurt (family size)	2.64	1.76	79	13.26
SILK Vanilla soy yogurt (single serving size)	2.94	1.76	88	14.11
SILK Plain soy yogurt	2.64	1.76	66	9.29
SILK Strawberry soy yogurt	2.35	1.18	94	17.64
SILK Raspberry soy yogurt	2.35	1.18	88	17.05

Food Name ---> per 100 g	Protein (g)	Fat (g)	Calorie	Net Carb (g)
SILK Peach soy yogurt	2.35	1.18	94	18.22
SILK Black Cherry soy yogurt	2.35	1.18	88	16.46
SILK Blueberry soy yogurt	2.35	1.18	88	16.46
SILK Key Lime soy yogurt	2.35	1.18	88	17.05
SILK Banana-Strawberry soy yogurt	2.35	1.18	88	16.46
SILK Original Creamer	0	6.67	100	6.67
SILK French Vanilla Creamer	0	6.67	133	20
SILK Hazelnut Creamer	0	6.67	133	20
Vitasoy USA Organic Nasoya, Soft Tofu	8.76	3.5	70	0.14
Vitasoy USA Nasoya, Lite Silken Tofu	8.21	1.1	43	0
Vitasoy USA Organic Nasoya, Tofu Plus Extra Firm	10.18	4.9	92	0.82
Vitasoy USA Organic Nasoya, Tofu Plus Firm	9.19	3.4	74	0.91
Vitasoy USA Organic Nasoya Sprouted, Tofu Plus Super Firm	13.24	5.9	115	0.96
Vitasoy USA Azumaya, Extra Firm Tofu	10.07	4.6	88	0.63
Vitasoy USA Azumaya, Firm Tofu	9.08	4.2	80	0.92
Vitasoy USA Azumaya, Silken Tofu	4.82	2.4	43	0.38
HOUSE FOODS Premium Soft Tofu	6.38	2.71	59	1.39
HOUSE FOODS Premium Firm Tofu	10.92	4.19	85	0.07
Beans, adzuki, mature seed, cooked, boiled, with salt	7.52	0.1	128	17.47
Beans, black, mature seeds, cooked, boiled, with salt	8.86	0.54	132	15.01
Beans, black, mature seeds, canned, low sodium	6.03	0.29	91	9.65
Beans, black turtle, mature seeds, cooked, boiled, with salt	8.18	0.35	130	16.05
Beans, cranberry (roman), mature seeds, cooked, boiled, with salt	9.34	0.46	136	15.86
Beans, french, mature seeds, cooked, boiled, with salt	7.05	0.76	129	14.62
Beans, great northern, mature seeds, cooked, boiled, with salt	8.33	0.45	118	14.09
Beans, great northern, mature seeds, canned, low sodium	7.37	0.39	114	16.12
Beans, kidney, all types, mature seeds, cooked, boiled, with salt	8.67	0.5	127	16.4
Beans, kidney, california red, mature seeds, cooked, boiled, with salt	9.13	0.09	124	13.11
Beans, kidney, red, mature seeds, cooked, boiled, with salt	8.67	0.5	127	15.4

Food Name ---> per 100 g	Protein (g)	Fat (g)	Calorie	Net Carb (g)
Beans, kidney, red, mature seeds, canned, drained solids, rinsed in tap water	8.12	0.93	121	14.8
Beans, kidney, royal red, mature seeds, cooked, boiled with salt	9.49	0.17	123	12.55
Beans, kidney, red, mature seeds, canned, solids and liquid, low sodium	5.22	0.36	81	9.53
Beans, navy, mature seeds, cooked, boiled, with salt	8.23	0.62	140	15.55
Beans, pink, mature seeds, cooked, boiled, with salt	9.06	0.49	149	22.61
Beans, pinto, mature seeds, cooked, boiled, with salt	9.01	0.65	143	17.22
Beans, pinto, mature seeds, canned, drained solids, rinsed in tap water	7.04	0.97	117	20.77
Beans, small white, mature seeds, cooked, boiled, with salt	8.97	0.64	142	15.41
Beans, pinto, mature seeds, canned, solids and liquids, low sodium	4.6	0.56	82	10.58
Beans, yellow, mature seeds, cooked, boiled, with salt	9.16	1.08	144	14.88
Beans, white, mature seeds, cooked, boiled, with salt	9.73	0.35	139	18.79
Broadbeans (fava beans), mature seeds, cooked, boiled, with salt	7.6	0.4	110	14.25
Chickpeas (garbanzo beans, bengal gram), mature seeds, cooked, boiled, with salt	8.86	2.59	164	19.82
Chickpeas (garbanzo beans, bengal gram), mature seeds, canned, drained solids	7.05	2.77	139	16.13
Chickpeas (garbanzo beans, bengal gram), mature seeds, canned, drained, rinsed in tap water	7.04	2.47	138	16.57
Chickpeas (garbanzo beans, bengal gram), mature seeds, canned, solids and liquids, low sodium	4.92	1.95	88	9.09
Cowpeas, catjang, mature seeds, cooked, boiled, with salt	8.13	0.71	117	16.72
Cowpeas, common (blackeyes, crowder, southern), mature seeds, cooked, boiled, with salt	7.73	0.53	116	14.26
Hyacinth beans, mature seeds, cooked, boiled, with salt	8.14	0.58	117	20.7
Lentils, mature seeds, cooked, boiled, with salt	9.02	0.38	114	11.64
Lima beans, large, mature seeds, cooked, boiled, with salt	7.8	0.38	115	13.88
Lima beans, thin seeded (baby), mature seeds, cooked, boiled, with salt	8.04	0.38	126	15.61
Lupins, mature seeds, cooked, boiled, with salt	15.57	2.92	116	6.49
Mothbeans, mature seeds, cooked, boiled, with salt	7.81	0.55	117	20.96
Mung beans, mature seeds, cooked, boiled, with salt	7.02	0.38	105	11.55

Food Name ---> per 100 g	Protein (g)	Fat (g)	Calorie	Net Carb (g)
Mungo beans, mature seeds, cooked, boiled, with salt	7.54	0.55	105	11.94
Peas, split, mature seeds, cooked, boiled, with salt	8.34	0.39	116	12.21
Peanuts, all types, oil-roasted, without salt	28.03	52.5	599	5.86
Peanuts, all types, dry-roasted, without salt	24.35	49.66	587	12.86
Peanuts, spanish, oil-roasted, without salt	28.01	49.04	579	8.55
Peanuts, valencia, oil-roasted, without salt	27.04	51.24	589	7.4
Peanuts, virginia, oil-roasted, without salt	25.87	48.62	578	10.96
Peanut butter, chunk style, without salt	24.06	49.94	589	13.57
Peanut butter, smooth style, without salt	22.21	51.36	598	17.31
Peanut butter with omega-3, creamy	24.47	54.17	608	10.9
Pigeon peas (red gram), mature seeds, cooked, boiled, with salt	6.76	0.38	121	16.55
Refried beans, canned, traditional, reduced sodium	4.98	2.01	89	9.85
Soybeans, mature seeds, cooked, boiled, with salt	18.21	8.97	172	2.36
Soybeans, mature seeds, roasted, no salt added	38.55	25.4	469	12.52
Soy protein concentrate, produced by acid wash	63.63	0.46	328	19.91
Soy protein isolate, potassium type	88.32	0.53	321	2.59
Soy sauce made from soy and wheat (shoyu), low sodium	9.05	0.3	57	4.89
Soy sauce, reduced sodium, made from hydrolyzed vegetable protein	8.19	0.31	90	14.14
Tofu, raw, firm, prepared with calcium sulfate	17.27	8.72	144	0.48
Tofu, raw, regular, prepared with calcium sulfate	8.08	4.78	76	1.57
Tofu, dried-frozen (koyadofu), prepared with calcium sulfate	52.43	30.34	470	7.1
Tofu, fried, prepared with calcium sulfate	18.82	20.18	270	4.96
Tofu, salted and fermented (fuyu), prepared with calcium sulfate	8.15	8	116	5.15
Yardlong beans, mature seeds, cooked, boiled, with salt	8.29	0.45	118	17.29
Winged beans, mature seeds, cooked, boiled, with salt	10.62	5.84	147	14.94
LOMA LINDA Little Links, canned, unprepared	19.4	13.5	221	1.3
LOMA LINDA Low Fat Big Franks, canned, unprepared	23.1	4.7	154	0.8
LOMA LINDA Tender Rounds with Gravy, canned, unprepared	16.3	5.6	145	3.9
LOMA LINDA Swiss Stake with Gravy, canned, unprepared	10.2	6.2	138	7.2
LOMA LINDA Vege-Burger, canned, unprepared	22.2	1.2	114	1.1
LOMA LINDA Redi-Burger, canned, unprepared	21.9	2.8	146	3.9

Food Name ---> per 100 g	Protein (g)	Fat (g)	Calorie	Net Carb (g)
LOMA LINDA Tender Bits, canned, unprepared	15.1	4.6	135	4
LOMA LINDA Linketts, canned, unprepared	21.3	11.8	209	1.4
WORTHINGTON Chili, canned, unprepared	10.4	4.5	126	7.5
WORTHINGTON Choplets, canned, unprepared	19.4	1	103	1.3
WORTHINGTON Diced Chik, canned, unprepared	14.7	0.7	80	2.3
WORTHINGTON FriChik Original, canned, unprepared	13.4	10.3	160	1.9
WORTHINGTON Low Fat Fri Chik, canned, unprepared	14.3	2.7	102	3.9
WORTHINGTON Low Fat Veja-Links, canned, unprepared	15.8	4.8	123	3.1
WORTHINGTON Multigrain Cutlets, canned, unprepared	23.29	1.5	117	2.8
WORTHINGTON Prime Stakes, canned, unprepared	10.2	7.2	135	6.1
WORTHINGTON Saucettes, canned, unprepared	15	15.2	219	2.8
WORTHINGTON Super Links, canned, unprepared	14.5	15.5	219	3.7
WORTHINGTON Vegetable Skallops, canned, unprepared	19.9	1.2	109	1.2
WORTHINGTON Vegetable Steaks, canned, unprepared	20.7	1.2	113	2.9
WORTHINGTON Vegetarian Burger, canned, unprepared	18.6	2.9	124	3.5
WORTHINGTON Veja-Links, canned, unprepared	14.6	8.9	155	0.8
WORTHINGTON Chic-Ketts, frozen, unprepared	23.6	9.7	200	3.9
WORTHINGTON Meatless Chicken Roll, frozen, unprepared	16.1	8	154	1.9
WORTHINGTON Meatless Corned Beef Roll, frozen, unprepared	18.6	14.5	245	9.9
WORTHINGTON Dinner Roast, frozen, unprepared	16	13.5	213	3.8
WORTHINGTON FriPats, frozen, unprepared	23.7	9.1	209	5.2
WORTHINGTON Prosage Links, frozen, unprepared	20.2	4.7	143	2.2
WORTHINGTON Prosage Roll, frozen, unprepared	19.6	17.6	261	2.5
WORTHINGTON Smoked Turkey Roll, frozen, unprepared	18.5	16.1	251	6.8
WORTHINGTON Stakelets, frozen, unprepared	19.7	10.4	211	6.8
WORTHINGTON Stripples, frozen, unprepared	12.4	26.6	346	9.2
WORTHINGTON Wham (roll), frozen, unprepared	17.8	11.3	196	5.7
MORNINGSTAR FARMS Breakfast Pattie with Organic Soy, frozen, unprepared	23.7	8.3	220	5
MORNINGSTAR FARMS Breakfast Bacon Strips, frozen, unprepared	12.4	26.6	346	9.2

Food Name ---> per 100 g	Protein (g)	Fat (g)	Calorie	Net Carb (g)
MORNINGSTAR FARMS Breakfast Sausage Links, frozen, unprepared	19.2	6.1	159	2.8
MORNINGSTAR FARMS Grillers Original, frozen, unprepared	23.9	9.3	213	4.1
MORNINGSTAR FARMS Grillers Prime, frozen, unprepared	24	13.2	238	3.3
MORNINGSTAR FARMS Asian Veggie Patties, frozen, unprepared	11.4	6.2	158	13.1
MORNINGSTAR FARMS Mushroom Lover's Burger, frozen, unprepared	14.3	8.2	168	4.1
MORNINGSTAR FARMS Tomato & Basil Pizza Burger, frozen, unprepared	15.5	8.6	161	4.9
MORNINGSTAR FARMS Buffalo Wings, frozen, unprepared	14.1	11	232	17.8
MORNINGSTAR FARMS Chik'n Nuggets, frozen, unprepared	14.4	10	221	16.9
MORNINGSTAR FARMS Chik Patties, frozen, unprepared	11.8	7	197	19.9
MORNINGSTAR FARMS Italian Herb Chik'n Pattie, frozen, unprepared	13.6	7	236	27.7
MORNINGSTAR FARMS Corn Dog, frozen, unprepared	11.2	3.5	208	32.2
MORNINGSTAR FARMS Corn Dog Mini, frozen, unprepared	13.2	4.7	219	30
MORNINGSTAR FARMS Sausage Style Recipe Crumbles, frozen, unprepared	20.2	4.6	159	5.3
GARDENBURGER Black Bean Chipotle Burger, frozen, unprepared	6.5	3.9	133	15.9
GARDENBURGER Original, frozen, unprepared	7.2	4.6	155	17.1
GARDENBURGER Flame Grilled Burger, frozen, unprepared	15.2	4.4	122	3.1
GARDENBURGER Savory Portabella Veggie Burger, frozen, unprepared	5.9	3.3	138	15
GARDENBURGER Sun-Dried Tomato Basil Burger, frozen, unprepared	5.5	3.6	137	18.5
GARDENBURGER Veggie Medley Burger, frozen, unprepared	4.1	3.6	121	16.9
MORNINGSTAR FARMS Breakfast Sausage Patties Maple Flavored, frozen, unprepared	26.3	7.2	222	11.6
MORNINGSTAR FARMS Chik'n Grill Veggie Patties, frozen, unprepared	12.8	4.8	118	4.5
MORNINGSTAR FARMS BBQ Riblets, frozen, unprepared	11.4	2.3	150	19.9
WORTHINGTON Leanies, frozen, unprepared	19.5	16.5	251	2.3
MORNINGSTAR FARMS California Turk'y Burger, frozen, unprepared	14.9	7.7	155	5

Food Name ---> per 100 g	Protein (g)	Fat (g)	Calorie	Net Carb (g)
MORNINGSTAR FARMS Hot and Spicy Veggie Sausage Patties, frozen, unprepared	21.8	7.4	185	6.2
MORNINGSTAR FARMS Lasagna with Veggie Sausage, frozen, unprepared	7.1	2.3	96	12.1
MORNINGSTAR FARMS Grillers Quarter Pound Veggie Burger, frozen, unprepared	22.8	10.5	219	6.4
MORNINGSTAR FARMS Sesame Chik'n Entree, frozen, unprepared	5.3	3.5	116	16
MORNINGSTAR FARMS Grillers Chik'n Veggie Patties, frozen, unprepared	12.8	4.8	118	4.5
MORNINGSTAR FARMS Meal Starters Veggie Meatballs, frozen, unprepared	17.7	5.8	158	6.3
MORNINGSTAR FARMS Breakfast Biscuit Sausage, Egg & Cheese, frozen, unprepared	9.3	8.1	257	36
MORNINGSTAR FARMS Mediterranean Chickpea, frozen, unprepared	15.5	6.5	200	9.7
MORNINGSTAR FARMS Buffalo Chik Patties, frozen, unprepared	12.1	12.8	255	20.1
MORNINGSTAR FARMS Chik Patties Original, frozen, unprepared	11.2	9.1	197	16.8
MORNINGSTAR FARMS Breakfast Pattie, frozen, unprepared	23.7	8.3	195	5
MORNINGSTAR FARMS Roasted Garlic & Quinoa Burger, frozen, unprepared	10.7	12.1	192	7.7
MORNINGSTAR FARMS Parmesan Garlic Wings, frozen, unprepared	14.2	8.6	227	21
MORNINGSTAR FARMS Breakfast Sandwich Veggie Sausage Egg & Cheese English Muffin, frozen, unprepared	14.3	9.4	205	14.9
MORNINGSTAR FARMS Breakfast Sandwich Veggie Scramble & Cheese English Muffin, frozen, unprepared	10.4	4.8	149	16
MORNINGSTAR FARMS Chipotle Black Bean Crumbles, frozen, unprepared	14.4	4.1	122	5.9
MORNINGSTAR FARMS Garden Veggie Nuggets, frozen, unprepared	9.6	12.2	197	10
MORNINGSTAR FARMS Spicy Black Bean Enchilada Entree, frozen, unprepared	5.8	5.2	123	13.3
MORNINGSTAR FARMS Spicy Indian Veggie Burger, frozen, unprepared	9.2	11.6	189	9.2

Food Name ---> per 100 g	Protein (g)	Fat (g)	Calorie	Net Carb (g)
MORNINGSTAR FARMS Tuscan Greens & Beans, frozen, unprepared	5.9	6.3	112	7.9
Papad	25.56	3.25	371	41.27
Peanut butter, reduced sodium	24	49.9	590	15.23
Beans, chili, barbecue, ranch style, cooked	5	1	97	12.7
Vermicelli, made from soy	0.1	0.1	331	78.42
Beans, liquid from stewed kidney beans	1.8	3.2	47	2.7
Chicken, meatless	23.64	12.73	224	0.04
Frankfurter, meatless	19.61	13.73	233	3.8
Luncheon slices, meatless	17.78	11.11	189	3.34
Meatballs, meatless	21	9	197	3.4
Vegetarian fillets	23	18	290	2.9
Sandwich spread, meatless	8	9	149	5.7
Vegetarian meatloaf or patties	21	9	197	3.4
Bacon bits, meatless	32	25.9	476	18.4
Soybean, curd cheese	12.5	8.1	151	6.9
Chicken, meatless, breaded, fried	21.28	12.77	234	4.21
Beans, baked, canned, no salt added	4.8	0.4	105	14.99
Tofu yogurt	3.5	1.8	94	15.76

Nuts & Seeds

Food Name ---> per 100 g	Protein (g)	Fat (g)	Calorie	Net Carb (g)
Seeds, breadfruit seeds, raw	7.4	5.59	191	24.04
Seeds, breadfruit seeds, boiled	5.3	2.3	168	27.2
Seeds, breadnut tree seeds, raw	5.97	0.99	217	46.28
Seeds, breadnut tree seeds, dried	8.62	1.68	367	64.49
Seeds, chia seeds, dried	16.54	30.74	486	7.72
Seeds, cottonseed flour, partially defatted (glandless)	40.96	6.2	359	37.54
Seeds, cottonseed flour, low fat (glandless)	49.83	1.41	332	36.1
Seeds, cottonseed meal, partially defatted (glandless)	49.1	4.77	367	38.43
Seeds, hemp seed, hulled	31.56	48.75	553	4.67
Seeds, lotus seeds, dried	15.41	1.97	332	64.47
Seeds, pumpkin and squash seed kernels, dried	30.23	49.05	559	4.71
Seeds, pumpkin and squash seed kernels, roasted, without salt	29.84	49.05	574	8.21
Seeds, safflower seed kernels, dried	16.18	38.45	517	34.29
Seeds, safflower seed meal, partially defatted	35.62	2.39	342	48.73
Seeds, sesame seeds, whole, dried	17.73	49.67	573	11.65
Seeds, sesame seeds, whole, roasted and toasted	16.96	48	565	11.74
Seeds, sesame seed kernels, toasted, without salt added (decorticated)	16.96	48	567	9.14
Seeds, sesame flour, partially defatted	40.32	11.89	382	35.14
Seeds, sesame flour, low-fat	50.14	1.75	333	35.51
Seeds, sesame meal, partially defatted	16.96	48	567	26.04
Seeds, sunflower seed kernels, dried	20.78	51.46	584	11.4
Seeds, sunflower seed kernels, dry roasted, without salt	19.33	49.8	582	12.97
Seeds, sunflower seed kernels, oil roasted, without salt	20.06	51.3	592	12.29
Seeds, sunflower seed kernels, toasted, without salt	17.21	56.8	619	9.09
Seeds, sunflower seed butter, without salt	17.28	55.2	617	17.62
Seeds, sunflower seed flour, partially defatted	48.06	1.61	326	30.63
Nuts, acorns, raw	6.15	23.86	387	40.75
Nuts, acorns, dried	8.1	31.41	509	53.66
Nuts, acorn flour, full fat	7.49	30.17	501	54.65
Nuts, almonds	21.15	49.93	579	9.05
Nuts, almonds, blanched	21.4	52.52	590	8.77

Food Name ---> per 100 g	Protein (g)	Fat (g)	Calorie	Net Carb (g)
Nuts, almonds, dry roasted, without salt added	20.96	52.54	598	10.11
Nuts, almonds, oil roasted, without salt added	21.23	55.17	607	7.18
Nuts, almond paste	9	27.74	458	43.01
Nuts, beechnuts, dried	6.2	50	576	33.5
Nuts, brazilnuts, dried, unblanched	14.32	67.1	659	4.24
Nuts, butternuts, dried	24.9	56.98	612	7.35
Nuts, cashew nuts, dry roasted, without salt added	15.31	46.35	574	29.69
Nuts, cashew nuts, oil roasted, without salt added	16.84	47.77	580	26.57
Nuts, cashew nuts, raw	18.22	43.85	553	26.89
Nuts, cashew butter, plain, without salt added	17.56	49.41	587	25.57
Nuts, chestnuts, chinese, raw	4.2	1.11	224	49.07
Nuts, chestnuts, chinese, dried	6.82	1.81	363	79.76
Nuts, chestnuts, chinese, boiled and steamed	2.88	0.76	153	33.64
Nuts, chestnuts, chinese, roasted	4.48	1.19	239	52.36
Nuts, chestnuts, european, raw, unpeeled	2.42	2.26	213	37.44
Nuts, chestnuts, european, raw, peeled	1.63	1.25	196	44.17
Nuts, chestnuts, european, dried, unpeeled	6.39	4.45	374	65.61
Nuts, chestnuts, european, dried, peeled	5.01	3.91	369	78.43
Nuts, chestnuts, european, boiled and steamed	2	1.38	131	27.76
Nuts, coconut meat, raw	3.33	33.49	354	6.23
Nuts, coconut meat, dried (desiccated), not sweetened	6.88	64.53	660	7.35
Nuts, coconut meat, dried (desiccated), sweetened, flaked, packaged	3.13	27.99	456	41.95
Nuts, coconut meat, dried (desiccated), sweetened, flaked, canned	3.35	31.69	443	36.41
Nuts, coconut meat, dried (desiccated), toasted	5.3	47	592	44.4
Nuts, coconut cream, raw (liquid expressed from grated meat)	3.63	34.68	330	4.45
Nuts, coconut cream, canned, sweetened	1.17	16.31	357	53.01
Nuts, coconut milk, raw (liquid expressed from grated meat and water)	2.29	23.84	230	3.34
Nuts, coconut milk, canned (liquid expressed from grated meat and water)	2.02	21.33	197	2.81
Nuts, coconut water (liquid from coconuts)	0.72	0.2	19	2.61

Food Name ---> per 100 g	Protein (g)	Fat (g)	Calorie	Net Carb (g)
Nuts, hazelnuts or filberts	14.95	60.75	628	7
Nuts, hazelnuts or filberts, blanched	13.7	61.15	629	6
Nuts, hazelnuts or filberts, dry roasted, without salt added	15.03	62.4	646	8.2
Nuts, ginkgo nuts, raw	4.32	1.68	182	37.6
Nuts, ginkgo nuts, dried	10.35	2	348	72.45
Nuts, ginkgo nuts, canned	2.29	1.62	111	12.8
Nuts, hickorynuts, dried	12.72	64.37	657	11.85
Nuts, macadamia nuts, raw	7.91	75.77	718	5.22
Nuts, macadamia nuts, dry roasted, without salt added	7.79	76.08	718	5.38
Nuts, mixed nuts, dry roasted, with peanuts, without salt added	19.5	53.5	607	16.02
Nuts, mixed nuts, dry roasted, with peanuts, salt added, PLANTERS pistachio blend	21.95	49.3	580	14.41
Nuts, mixed nuts, oil roasted, with peanuts, without salt added	20.04	53.95	607	14.05
Nuts, mixed nuts, oil roasted, without peanuts, without salt added	15.52	56.17	615	16.77
Nuts, formulated, wheat-based, unflavored, with salt added	13.82	57.7	622	18.48
Nuts, mixed nuts, dry roasted, with peanuts, salt added, CHOSEN ROASTER	18	58.8	632	11.92
Nuts, pecans	9.17	71.97	691	4.26
Nuts, pecans, dry roasted, without salt added	9.5	74.27	710	4.15
Nuts, pecans, oil roasted, without salt added	9.2	75.23	715	3.51
Nuts, pilinuts, dried	10.8	79.55	719	3.98
Nuts, pine nuts, dried	13.69	68.37	673	9.38
Nuts, pine nuts, pinyon, dried	11.57	60.98	629	8.6
Nuts, pistachio nuts, raw	20.16	45.32	560	16.57
Nuts, pistachio nuts, dry roasted, without salt added	21.05	45.82	572	17.98
Nuts, walnuts, black, dried	24.06	59.33	619	2.78
Nuts, walnuts, english	15.23	65.21	654	7.01
Nuts, walnuts, glazed	8.28	35.71	500	43.99
Nuts, walnuts, dry roasted, with salt added	14.29	60.71	643	10.76
Seeds, breadfruit seeds, roasted	6.2	2.7	207	34.1
Seeds, cottonseed kernels, roasted (glandless)	32.59	36.29	506	16.4

Food Name ---> per 100 g	Protein (g)	Fat (g)	Calorie	Net Carb (g)
Seeds, pumpkin and squash seeds, whole, roasted, without salt	18.55	19.4	446	35.35
Seeds, sesame butter, tahini, from roasted and toasted kernels (most common type)	17	53.76	595	11.89
Nuts, chestnuts, european, roasted	3.17	2.2	245	47.86
Seeds, sesame butter, paste	18.08	50.87	586	18.55
Seeds, sesame flour, high-fat	30.78	37.1	526	26.62
Seeds, sesame butter, tahini, from unroasted kernels (non-chemically removed seed coat)	17.95	56.44	607	8.59
Seeds, watermelon seed kernels, dried	28.33	47.37	557	15.31
Nuts, chestnuts, japanese, dried	5.25	1.24	360	81.43
Nuts, coconut milk, frozen (liquid expressed from grated meat and water)	1.61	20.8	202	5.58
Nuts, coconut meat, dried (desiccated), creamed	5.3	69.08	684	21.52
Nuts, coconut meat, dried (desiccated), sweetened, shredded	2.88	35.49	501	43.17
Seeds, sisymbrium sp. seeds, whole, dried	12.14	4.6	318	58.26
Nuts, almond butter, plain, without salt added	20.96	55.5	614	8.52
Seeds, sesame butter, tahini, from raw and stone ground kernels	17.81	48	570	16.89
Nuts, formulated, wheat-based, all flavors except macadamia, without salt	13.11	62.3	647	15.59
Seeds, sesame seed kernels, dried (decorticated)	20.45	61.21	631	0.13
Nuts, chestnuts, japanese, raw	2.25	0.53	154	34.91
Nuts, chestnuts, japanese, boiled and steamed	0.82	0.19	56	12.64
Nuts, chestnuts, japanese, roasted	2.97	0.8	201	45.13
Seeds, lotus seeds, raw	4.13	0.53	89	17.28
Nuts, almonds, honey roasted, unblanched	18.17	49.9	594	14.2
Seeds, flaxseed	18.29	42.16	534	1.58
Seeds, pumpkin and squash seed kernels, roasted, with salt added	29.84	49.05	574	8.21
Seeds, sesame seed kernels, toasted, with salt added (decorticated)	16.96	48	567	9.14
Seeds, sunflower seed kernels from shell, dry roasted, with salt added	19.33	49.8	546	6.31
Seeds, sunflower seed kernels, dry roasted, with salt added	19.33	49.8	582	15.07
Seeds, sunflower seed kernels, oil roasted, with salt added	20.06	51.3	592	12.29

Food Name ---> per 100 g	Protein (g)	Fat (g)	Calorie	Net Carb (g)
Seeds, sunflower seed kernels, toasted, with salt added	17.21	56.8	619	9.09
Seeds, sunflower seed butter, with salt added	17.28	55.2	617	17.62
Nuts, almonds, dry roasted, with salt added	20.96	52.54	598	10.11
Nuts, almonds, oil roasted, with salt added	21.23	55.17	607	7.18
Nuts, almonds, oil roasted, with salt added, smoke flavor	21.43	55.89	607	7.16
Nuts, cashew nuts, dry roasted, with salt added	15.31	46.35	574	29.69
Nuts, cashew nuts, oil roasted, with salt added	16.84	47.77	581	26.86
Nuts, cashew butter, plain, with salt added	12.12	53.03	609	27.3
Nuts, macadamia nuts, dry roasted, with salt added	7.79	76.08	716	4.83
Nuts, mixed nuts, dry roasted, with peanuts, with salt added	17.3	51.45	594	16.35
Nuts, mixed nuts, oil roasted, with peanuts, with salt added	20.04	53.95	607	14.05
Nuts, mixed nuts, oil roasted, without peanuts, with salt added	15.52	56.17	615	16.77
Nuts, pecans, dry roasted, with salt added	9.5	74.27	710	4.15
Nuts, pecans, oil roasted, with salt added	9.2	75.23	715	3.51
Nuts, pistachio nuts, dry roasted, with salt added	21.05	45.82	569	17.25
Seeds, pumpkin and squash seeds, whole, roasted, with salt added	18.55	19.4	446	35.35
Nuts, almonds, oil roasted, lightly salted	21.23	55.17	607	7.18
Nuts, almond butter, plain, with salt added	20.96	55.5	614	8.52
Seeds, sesame butter, tahini, type of kernels unspecified	17.4	53.01	592	16.8
Nuts, mixed nuts, oil roasted, with peanuts, lightly salted	20.04	53.95	607	14.05
Nuts, mixed nuts, oil roasted, without peanuts, lightly salted	17.86	50	607	17.9

Pork Products

Food Name ---> per 100 g	Protein (g)	Fat (g)	Calories	Net Carb (g)
Pork, fresh, composite of separable fat, with added solution, cooked	10.06	60.42	585	0.32
Pork, fresh, carcass, separable lean and fat, raw	13.91	35.07	376	0
Pork, fresh, composite of trimmed retail cuts (leg, loin, shoulder), separable lean only, raw	21.2	4.86	134	0
Pork, fresh, composite of trimmed leg, loin, shoulder, and spareribs, (includes cuts to be cured), separable lean and fat, raw	18.22	14.79	211	0
Pork, fresh, backfat, raw	2.92	88.69	812	0
Pork, fresh, belly, raw	9.34	53.01	518	0
Pork, fresh, separable fat, raw	9.25	65.7	632	0
Pork, fresh, separable fat, cooked	7.06	66.1	626	0
Pork, fresh, leg (ham), whole, separable lean and fat, raw	17.43	18.87	245	0
Pork, fresh, leg (ham), whole, separable lean and fat, cooked, roasted	26.83	17.61	273	0
Pork, fresh, leg (ham), whole, separable lean only, raw	20.48	5.41	136	0
Pork, fresh, leg (ham), whole, separable lean only, cooked, roasted	29.41	9.44	211	0
Pork, fresh, leg (ham), rump half, separable lean and fat, raw	20.27	10.63	182	0
Pork, fresh, leg (ham), rump half, separable lean and fat, cooked, roasted	27.03	10.32	209	0
Pork, fresh, leg (ham), rump half, separable lean only, raw	21.81	2.93	120	0
Pork, fresh, leg (ham), rump half, separable lean only, cooked, roasted	28.86	4.62	165	0
Pork, fresh, leg (ham), shank half, separable lean and fat, raw	19.87	11.96	193	0
Pork, fresh, leg (ham), shank half, separable lean and fat, cooked, roasted	25.96	13.42	232	0
Pork, fresh, leg (ham), shank half, separable lean only, raw	21.66	2.95	119	0
Pork, fresh, leg (ham), shank half, separable lean only, cooked, roasted	28.69	5.83	175	0
Pork, fresh, loin, whole, separable lean and fat, raw	19.74	12.58	198	0
Pork, fresh, loin, whole, separable lean and fat, cooked, braised	27.23	13.62	239	0

Food Name ---> per 100 g	Protein (g)	Fat (g)	Calories	Net Carb (g)
Pork, fresh, loin, whole, separable lean and fat, cooked, broiled	27.32	13.92	242	0
Pork, fresh, loin, whole, separable lean and fat, cooked, roasted	27.09	14.65	248	0
Pork, fresh, loin, whole, separable lean only, raw	21.43	5.66	143	0
Pork, fresh, loin, whole, separable lean only, cooked, braised	28.57	9.12	204	0
Pork, fresh, loin, whole, separable lean only, cooked, broiled	28.57	9.8	210	0
Pork, fresh, loin, whole, separable lean only, cooked, roasted	28.62	9.63	209	0
Pork, fresh, loin, blade (chops or roasts), bone-in, separable lean and fat, raw	19.56	12.27	194	0
Pork, fresh, loin, blade (chops), bone-in, separable lean and fat, cooked, braised	26.54	15.71	255	0
Pork, fresh, loin, blade (chops), bone-in, separable lean and fat, cooked, broiled	23.72	14.35	231	0
Pork, fresh, loin, blade (roasts), bone-in, separable lean and fat, cooked, roasted	24.29	16.71	254	0
Pork, fresh, loin, blade (chops or roasts), bone-in, separable lean only, raw	21.22	5.84	143	0
Pork, fresh, loin, blade (chops), bone-in, separable lean only, cooked, braised	28.02	11.29	222	0
Pork, fresh, loin, blade (chops), bone-in, separable lean only, cooked, broiled	24.99	9.56	193	0
Pork, fresh, loin, blade (roasts), bone-in, separable lean only, cooked, roasted	25.7	11.89	217	0
Pork, fresh, loin, center loin (chops), bone-in, separable lean and fat, raw	20.71	9.03	170	0
Pork, fresh, loin, center loin (chops), bone-in, separable lean and fat, cooked, braised	28.21	13.51	242	0
Pork, fresh, loin, center loin (chops), bone-in, separable lean and fat, cooked, broiled	25.61	11.06	209	0
Pork, fresh, loin, center loin (roasts), bone-in, separable lean and fat, cooked, roasted	27.01	12.8	231	0
Pork, fresh, loin, center loin (chops), bone-in, separable lean only, raw	21.99	3.71	127	0
Pork, fresh, loin, center loin (chops), bone-in, separable lean only, cooked, braised	30.2	7.86	200	0
Pork, fresh, loin, center loin (chops), bone-in, separable lean only, cooked, broiled	26.76	7.29	180	0

Food Name ---> per 100 g	Protein (g)	Fat (g)	Calories	Net Carb (g)
Pork, fresh, loin, center loin (roasts), bone-in, separable lean only, cooked, roasted	28.58	7.95	194	0
Pork, fresh, loin, center rib (chops or roasts), bone-in, separable lean and fat, raw	20.28	11.04	186	0
Pork, fresh, loin, center rib (chops), bone-in, separable lean and fat, cooked, braised	26.66	16.28	261	0
Pork, fresh, loin, center rib (chops), bone-in, separable lean and fat, cooked, broiled	24.42	13.04	222	0
Pork, fresh, loin, center rib (roasts), bone-in, separable lean and fat, cooked, roasted	26.99	14.68	248	0
Pork, fresh, loin, center rib (chops or roasts), bone-in, separable lean only, raw	21.79	4.8	136	0
Pork, fresh, loin, center rib (chops), bone-in, separable lean only, cooked, braised	29.03	9.32	208	0
Pork, fresh, loin, center rib (chops), bone-in, separable lean only, cooked, broiled	25.79	8.36	186	0
Pork, fresh, loin, center rib (roasts), bone-in, separable lean only, cooked, roasted	28.82	9.21	206	0
Pork, fresh, loin, sirloin (chops or roasts), bone-in, separable lean and fat, raw	20.48	8.96	168	0
Pork, fresh, loin, sirloin (chops), bone-in, separable lean and fat, cooked, braised	28.81	12.31	234	0
Pork, fresh, loin, sirloin (chops), bone-in, separable lean and fat, cooked, broiled	26.96	11.82	222	0
Pork, fresh, loin, sirloin (roasts), bone-in, separable lean and fat, cooked, roasted	26.64	12.87	230	0
Pork, fresh, loin, sirloin (chops or roasts), bone-in, separable lean only, raw	21.65	4.02	129	0
Pork, fresh, loin, sirloin (chops), bone-in, separable lean only, cooked, braised	31	6.9	195	0
Pork, fresh, loin, sirloin (chops), bone-in, separable lean only, cooked, broiled	29.29	5.45	174	0
Pork, fresh, loin, sirloin (roasts), bone-in, separable lean only, cooked, roasted	27.78	9.44	204	0
Pork, fresh, loin, tenderloin, separable lean only, raw	20.95	2.17	109	0
Pork, fresh, loin, tenderloin, separable lean only, cooked, roasted	26.17	3.51	143	0

Food Name ---> per 100 g	Protein (g)	Fat (g)	Calories	Net Carb (g)
Pork, fresh, loin, top loin (chops), boneless, separable lean and fat, raw	21.55	6.94	155	0
Pork, fresh, loin, top loin (chops), boneless, separable lean and fat, cooked, braised	29.2	8.31	200	0
Pork, fresh, loin, top loin (chops), boneless, separable lean and fat, cooked, broiled	26.62	9.14	196	0
Pork, fresh, loin, top loin (roasts), boneless, separable lean and fat, cooked, roasted	26.45	8.82	192	0
Pork, fresh, loin, top loin (chops), boneless, separable lean only, raw	22.41	3.42	127	0
Pork, fresh, loin, top loin (chops), boneless, separable lean only, cooked, braised	30.54	4.34	170	0
Pork, fresh, loin, top loin (chops), boneless, separable lean only, cooked, broiled	27.58	6.08	173	0
Pork, fresh, loin, top loin (roasts), boneless, separable lean only, cooked, roasted	27.23	6.28	173	0
Pork, fresh, spareribs, separable lean and fat, raw	15.47	23.4	277	0
Pork, fresh, spareribs, separable lean and fat, cooked, braised	29.06	30.3	397	0
Pork, fresh, composite of trimmed retail cuts (leg, loin, and shoulder), separable lean only, cooked	27.51	9.21	201	0
Pork, fresh, loin, center loin (chops), boneless, separable lean only, raw	23.75	3.09	123	0
Pork, fresh, variety meats and by-products, brain, raw	10.28	9.21	127	0
Pork, fresh, variety meats and by-products, brain, cooked, braised	12.14	9.51	138	0
Pork, fresh, variety meats and by-products, chitterlings, raw	7.64	16.61	182	0
Pork, fresh, variety meats and by-products, chitterlings, cooked, simmered	12.49	20.32	233	0
Pork, fresh, variety meats and by-products, ears, frozen, raw	22.45	15.1	234	0.6
Pork, fresh, variety meats and by-products, ears, frozen, cooked, simmered	15.95	10.8	166	0.2
Pork, fresh, variety meats and by-products, feet, raw	23.16	12.59	212	0
Pork, fresh, variety meats and by-products, heart, raw	17.27	4.36	118	1.33
Pork, fresh, variety meats and by-products, heart, cooked, braised	23.6	5.05	148	0.4
Pork, fresh, variety meats and by-products, jowl, raw	6.38	69.61	655	0

Food Name ---> per 100 g	Protein (g)	Fat (g)	Calories	Net Carb (g)
Pork, fresh, variety meats and by-products, kidneys, raw	16.46	3.25	100	0
Pork, fresh, variety meats and by-products, kidneys, cooked, braised	25.4	4.7	151	0
Pork, fresh, variety meats and by-products, leaf fat, raw	1.76	94.16	857	0
Pork, fresh, variety meats and by-products, liver, raw	21.39	3.65	134	2.47
Pork, fresh, variety meats and by-products, liver, cooked, braised	26.02	4.4	165	3.76
Pork, fresh, variety meats and by-products, lungs, raw	14.08	2.72	85	0
Pork, fresh, variety meats and by-products, lungs, cooked, braised	16.6	3.1	99	0
Pork, fresh, variety meats and by-products, mechanically separated, raw	15.03	26.54	304	0
Pork, fresh, variety meats and by-products, pancreas, raw	18.56	13.24	199	0
Pork, fresh, variety meats and by-products, pancreas, cooked, braised	28.5	10.8	219	0
Pork, fresh, variety meats and by-products, spleen, raw	17.86	2.59	100	0
Pork, fresh, variety meats and by-products, spleen, cooked, braised	28.2	3.2	149	0
Pork, fresh, variety meats and by-products, stomach, raw	16.85	10.14	159	0
Pork, fresh, loin, blade (chops), bone-in, separable lean only, cooked, pan-fried	26.38	12.14	222	0
Pork, fresh, variety meats and by-products, tongue, raw	16.3	17.2	225	0
Pork, fresh, variety meats and by-products, tongue, cooked, braised	24.1	18.6	271	0
Pork, cured, bacon, unprepared	12.62	39.69	417	1.28
Pork, cured, breakfast strips, raw or unheated	11.74	37.16	388	0.7
Canadian bacon, unprepared	20.31	2.62	110	1.34
Pork, cured, feet, pickled	11.63	10.02	140	0.01
Pork, cured, ham, boneless, extra lean (approximately 5% fat), roasted	20.93	5.53	145	1.5
Pork, cured, ham, boneless, regular (approximately 11% fat), roasted	22.62	9.02	178	0
Pork, cured, ham, extra lean (approximately 4% fat), canned, unheated	18.49	4.56	120	0
Pork, cured, ham, extra lean (approximately 4% fat), canned, roasted	21.16	4.88	136	0.52

Food Name ---> per 100 g	Protein (g)	Fat (g)	Calories	Net Carb (g)
Pork, cured, ham, regular (approximately 13% fat), canned, roasted	20.53	15.2	226	0.42
Pork, cured, ham, center slice, country-style, separable lean only, raw	27.8	8.32	195	0.3
Pork, cured, ham, center slice, separable lean and fat, unheated	20.17	12.9	203	0.05
Pork, cured, ham, patties, unheated	12.78	28.19	315	1.69
Pork, cured, ham, steak, boneless, extra lean, unheated	19.56	4.25	122	0
Pork, cured, ham, whole, separable lean and fat, unheated	18.49	18.52	246	0.06
Pork, cured, ham, whole, separable lean only, unheated	22.32	5.71	147	0.05
Pork, cured, ham, whole, separable lean only, roasted	25.05	5.5	157	0
USDA Commodity, pork, canned	19.4	12.95	196	0.59
Pork, fresh, loin, center loin (chops), boneless, separable lean only, cooked, pan-broiled	30.02	4.65	162	0
Pork, fresh, loin, center loin (chops), boneless, separable lean and fat, raw	21.14	12.96	201	0
Pork, cured, salt pork, raw	5.05	80.5	748	0
Pork, cured, separable fat (from ham and arm picnic), unheated	5.68	61.41	579	0.09
Pork, cured, separable fat (from ham and arm picnic), roasted	7.64	61.86	591	0
Pork, cured, shoulder, arm picnic, separable lean and fat, roasted	20.43	21.35	280	0
Pork, cured, shoulder, arm picnic, separable lean only, roasted	24.94	7.04	170	0
Pork, cured, shoulder, blade roll, separable lean and fat, unheated	16.47	21.98	269	0
Pork, cured, shoulder, blade roll, separable lean and fat, roasted	17.28	23.48	287	0.37
Pork, fresh, variety meats and by-products, feet, cooked, simmered	21.94	16.05	238	0
Pork, fresh, variety meats and by-products, tail, raw	17.75	33.5	378	0
Pork, fresh, variety meats and by-products, tail, cooked, simmered	17	35.8	396	0
Pork, fresh, loin, center loin (chops), bone-in, separable lean only, cooked, pan-fried	29.56	7.66	195	0
Pork, fresh, loin, center rib (chops), bone-in, separable lean only, cooked, pan-fried	28.84	9.73	211	0
Pork, fresh, loin, blade (chops), bone-in, separable lean and fat, cooked, pan-fried	25.02	16.56	256	0

Food Name ---> per 100 g	Protein (g)	Fat (g)	Calories	Net Carb (g)
Pork, fresh, loin, center loin (chops), bone-in, separable lean and fat, cooked, pan-fried	27.63	13.32	238	0
Pork, fresh, loin, center rib (chops), bone-in, separable lean and fat, cooked, pan-fried	26.81	15.71	256	0
Pork, fresh, loin, top loin (chops), boneless, separable lean only, cooked, pan-fried	30.46	4.62	172	0
Pork, cured, ham, boneless, extra lean and regular, unheated	18.26	8.39	162	2.28
Pork, cured, ham, boneless, extra lean and regular, roasted	21.97	7.66	165	0.5
Pork, cured, ham, extra lean and regular, canned, unheated	17.97	7.46	144	0
Pork, cured, ham, extra lean and regular, canned, roasted	20.94	8.43	167	0.49
Pork, fresh, loin, top loin (chops), boneless, separable lean and fat, cooked, pan-fried	29.36	7.86	196	0
Pork, fresh, composite of trimmed retail cuts (leg, loin, shoulder, and spareribs), separable lean and fat, raw	18.95	14.95	216	0
Pork, fresh, composite of trimmed retail cuts (leg, loin, shoulder, and spareribs), separable lean and fat, cooked	26.36	13.89	238	0
Pork, fresh, loin, center loin (chops), boneless, separable lean and fat, cooked, pan-broiled	26.68	13.6	229	0
Pork, fresh, backribs, separable lean and fat, raw	19.07	16.33	224	0
Pork, fresh, backribs, separable lean and fat, cooked, roasted	23.01	21.51	292	0
Pork, fresh, loin, center rib (chops or roasts), boneless, separable lean and fat, raw	19.9	14.01	211	0
Pork, fresh, loin, center rib (chops), boneless, separable lean and fat, cooked, braised	26.29	15.79	255	0
Pork, fresh, loin, center rib (chops), boneless, separable lean and fat, cooked, broiled	27.63	15.76	260	0
Pork, fresh, loin, center rib (chops), boneless, separable lean and fat, cooked, pan-fried	25.82	18.05	273	0
Pork, fresh, loin, center rib (roasts), boneless, separable lean and fat, cooked, roasted	26.99	15.15	252	0
Pork, fresh, loin, center rib (chops or roasts), boneless, separable lean only, raw	21.8	6.48	152	0
Pork, fresh, loin, center rib (chops), boneless, separable lean only, cooked, braised	27.95	10.14	211	0
Pork, fresh, loin, center rib (chops), boneless, separable lean only, cooked, broiled	29.46	10.05	216	0

Food Name ---> per 100 g	Protein (g)	Fat (g)	Calories	Net Carb (g)
Pork, fresh, loin, center rib (chops), boneless, separable lean only, cooked, pan-fried	27.68	11.8	224	0
Pork, fresh, loin, center rib (roasts), boneless, separable lean only, cooked, roasted	28.81	10.13	214	0
Pork, fresh, loin, country-style ribs, separable lean and fat, raw	19.34	11.82	189	0
Pork, fresh, loin, country-style ribs, separable lean and fat, cooked, braised	26.49	17.71	273	0
Pork, fresh, loin, country-style ribs, separable lean and fat, bone-in, cooked, roasted	21.75	29.46	359	0
Pork, fresh, loin, country-style ribs, separable lean only, raw	20.76	5.64	140	0
Pork, fresh, loin, country-style ribs, separable lean only, cooked, braised	27.74	14.26	247	0
Pork, fresh, loin, country-style ribs, separable lean only, bone-in, cooked, roasted	29.2	11.38	227	0
Pork, fresh, loin, sirloin (chops or roasts), boneless, separable lean and fat, raw	22.49	4.05	133	0
Pork, fresh, loin, sirloin (chops), boneless, separable lean and fat, cooked, braised	28.41	5.47	171	0
Pork, fresh, loin, sirloin (chops), boneless, separable lean and fat, cooked, broiled	28.19	5.53	170	0
Pork, fresh, loin, sirloin (roasts), boneless, separable lean and fat, cooked, roasted	29.62	7.32	192	0
Pork, fresh, loin, sirloin (chops or roasts), boneless, separable lean only, raw	22.81	2.59	121	0
Pork, fresh, loin, sirloin (chops), boneless, separable lean only, cooked, braised	28.75	4.5	163	0
Pork, fresh, loin, sirloin (chops), boneless, separable lean only, cooked, broiled	28.6	4.36	161	0
Pork, fresh, loin, sirloin (roasts), boneless, separable lean only, cooked, roasted	30.39	5.31	178	0
Pork, fresh, loin, tenderloin, separable lean and fat, raw	20.65	3.53	120	0
Pork, fresh, ground, raw	16.88	21.19	263	0
Pork, fresh, ground, cooked	25.69	20.77	297	0
Pork, fresh, loin, tenderloin, separable lean and fat, cooked, broiled	29.86	8.11	201	0
Pork, fresh, loin, tenderloin, separable lean and fat, cooked, roasted	26.04	3.96	147	0

Food Name ---> per 100 g	Protein (g)	Fat (g)	Calories	Net Carb (g)
Pork, fresh, loin, tenderloin, separable lean only, cooked, broiled	30.42	6.33	187	0
Pork, fresh, loin, top loin (roasts), boneless, separable lean and fat, raw	21.34	8.33	166	0
Pork, fresh, loin, top loin (roasts), boneless, separable lean only, raw	22.39	4.06	132	0
Pork, fresh, composite of trimmed retail cuts (loin and shoulder blade), separable lean and fat, raw	20.08	10.14	177	0
Pork, fresh, composite of trimmed retail cuts (loin and shoulder blade), separable lean and fat, cooked	26.07	13.66	235	0
Pork, fresh, composite of trimmed retail cuts (loin and shoulder blade), separable lean only, raw	21.23	5.88	144	0
Pork, fresh, composite of trimmed retail cuts (loin and shoulder blade), separable lean only, cooked	29.47	9.44	211	0
USDA Commodity, pork, cured, ham, boneless, cooked, heated	18.84	7.62	149	0
USDA Commodity, pork, ground, fine/coarse, frozen, cooked	23.55	18.19	265	0
USDA Commodity, pork, cured, ham, boneless, cooked, unheated	17.44	6.16	133	0.69
USDA Commodity, pork, ground, fine/coarse, frozen, raw	15.41	17.18	221	0
HORMEL, Cure 81 Ham	18.43	3.59	106	0.21
HORMEL ALWAYS TENDER, Pork Tenderloin, Teriyaki-Flavored	18.2	3.07	119	4.63
HORMEL ALWAYS TENDER, Pork Tenderloin, Peppercorn-Flavored	17.21	3.8	110	1.82
HORMEL ALWAYS TENDER, Pork Loin Filets, Lemon Garlic-Flavored	17.83	4.16	118	1.79
HORMEL ALWAYS TENDER, Center Cut Chops, Fresh Pork	18.74	9.62	167	0.84
HORMEL ALWAYS TENDER, Boneless Pork Loin, Fresh Pork	19.02	7.18	145	0.76
HORMEL Canadian Style Bacon	16.88	4.94	122	1.87
Pork, fresh, loin, top loin (chops), boneless, separable lean only, with added solution, cooked, pan-broiled	28.95	5	169	0
Pork, fresh, loin, top loin (chops), boneless, separable lean and fat, with added solution, cooked, pan-broiled	28.35	7.66	190	0
Pork, cured, bacon, cooked, baked	35.73	43.27	548	1.35
Pork, cured, bacon, cooked, microwaved	39.01	34.12	476	0.48
Pork, cured, bacon, pre-sliced, cooked, pan-fried	33.92	35.09	468	1.7

Food Name ---> per 100 g	Protein (g)	Fat (g)	Calories	Net Carb (g)
Pork, fresh, variety meats and by-products, stomach, cooked, simmered	21.4	7.26	157	0.09
Pork, bacon, rendered fat, cooked	0.07	99.5	898	0
Pork, cured, ham -- water added, rump, bone-in, separable lean only, heated, roasted	21.41	3.56	121	0.87
Pork, cured, ham -- water added, rump, bone-in, separable lean only, unheated	15.43	3.48	95	0.67
Pork, cured, ham -- water added, shank, bone-in, separable lean only, heated, roasted	20.92	4.43	128	1.2
Pork, cured, ham -- water added, slice, bone-in, separable lean only, heated, pan-broil	22.04	4.3	131	1.48
Pork, cured, ham and water product, slice, bone-in, separable lean only, heated, pan-broil	20.9	3.63	122	1.35
Pork, cured, ham and water product, slice, boneless, separable lean only, heated, pan-broil	15.09	5.06	123	4.69
Pork, cured, ham and water product, whole, boneless, separable lean only, heated, roasted	13.88	5.46	123	4.61
Pork, cured, ham and water product, whole, boneless, separable lean only, unheated	14.07	4.86	116	4.22
Pork, cured, ham with natural juices, rump, bone-in, separable lean only, heated, roasted	24.14	4.25	137	0.48
Pork, cured, ham with natural juices, shank, bone-in, separable lean only, heated, roasted	24.95	4.97	145	0.34
Pork, cured, ham with natural juices, slice, bone-in, separable lean only, heated, pan-broil	27.75	4.38	150	0
Pork, cured, ham with natural juices, spiral slice, meat only, boneless, separable lean only, heated, roasted	22.56	3.78	126	1.08
Pork, cured, ham and water product, rump, bone-in, separable lean only, heated, roasted	21.28	4.7	131	1.15
Pork, cured, ham -- water added, slice, boneless, separable lean only, heated, pan-broil	18.82	4.09	119	1.75
Pork, cured, ham -- water added, whole, boneless, separable lean only, heated, roasted	17.99	4.39	117	1.57
Pork, cured, ham -- water added, whole, boneless, separable lean only, unheated	17.34	3.97	110	1.45
Pork, cured, ham and water product, shank, bone-in, separable lean only, heated, roasted	21.69	4.45	132	1.26

Food Name ---> per 100 g	Protein (g)	Fat (g)	Calories	Net Carb (g)
Pork, cured, ham with natural juices, slice, boneless, separable lean only, heated, pan-broil	20.95	3.16	116	1.05
Pork, cured, ham with natural juices, whole, boneless, separable lean only, heated, roasted	20.57	3.01	113	0.84
Pork, cured, ham with natural juices, whole, boneless, separable lean only, unheated	19.44	3.21	111	1.03
Pork, cured, ham -- water added, shank, bone-in, separable lean only, unheated	18.65	1.87	91	0.71
Pork, cured, ham -- water added, slice, bone-in, separable lean only, unheated	17.38	2.29	95	1.23
Pork, cured, ham and water product, rump, bone-in, separable lean only, unheated	17.93	3.38	107	1.24
Pork, cured, ham and water product, slice, bone-in, separable lean only, unheated	14.47	3.78	103	2.82
Pork, cured, ham and water product, shank, bone-in, unheated, separable lean only	17.53	4.18	113	1.2
Pork, cured, ham with natural juices, rump, bone-in, separable lean only, unheated	22.71	3.47	122	0.43
Pork, cured, ham with natural juices, shank, bone-in, separable lean only, unheated	25.11	3.33	130	0.3
Pork, cured, ham with natural juices, slice, bone-in, separable lean only, unheated	24.34	2.87	123	0
Pork, cured, ham with natural juices, spiral slice, boneless, separable lean only, unheated	19.25	3.26	109	1.22
Pork, cured, ham, separable fat, boneless, heated	8.77	51.57	507	2
Pork, cured, ham, separable fat, boneless, unheated	7.5	53	515	1.87
Pork, pickled pork hocks	19.11	10.54	171	0
Pork, cured, ham, slice, bone-in, separable lean only, heated, pan-broil	27.18	4.09	148	0.74
Pork, cured, ham with natural juices, whole, boneless, separable lean and fat, unheated	19.38	3.43	112	1.02
Pork, cured, ham with natural juices, spiral slice, boneless, separable lean and fat, unheated	18.66	5.75	129	1.18
Pork, cured, ham with natural juices, slice, bone-in, separable lean and fat, unheated	22.82	7.4	159	0.17
Pork, cured, ham with natural juices, shank, bone-in, separable lean and fat, unheated	22.35	11.11	191	0.32

Food Name ---> per 100 g	Protein (g)	Fat (g)	Calories	Net Carb (g)
Pork, cured, ham with natural juices, rump, bone-in, separable lean and fat, unheated	19.7	13.26	200	0.43
Pork, cured, ham and water product, whole, boneless, separable lean and fat, unheated	14.05	4.99	117	4.21
Pork, cured, ham and water product, slice, bone-in, separable lean and fat, unheated	13.69	9.29	149	2.72
Pork, cured, ham and water product, shank, bone-in, separable lean and fat, unheated	14.28	20	243	1.42
Pork, cured, ham and water product, rump, bone-in, separable lean and fat, unheated	16.09	12.13	179	1.35
Pork, cured, ham -- water added, whole, boneless, separable lean and fat, unheated	17.06	5.38	121	1.42
Pork, cured, ham -- water added, slice, bone-in, separable lean and fat, unheated	15.73	10.77	164	1.1
Pork, cured, ham -- water added, shank, bone-in, separable lean and fat, unheated	16.65	11.02	167	0.66
Pork, cured, ham -- water added, rump, bone-in, separable lean and fat, unheated	13.99	12.5	172	0.8
Pork, cured, ham -- water added, rump, bone-in, separable lean and fat, heated, roasted	20.1	8.56	161	0.99
Pork, cured, ham -- water added, shank, bone-in, separable lean and fat, heated, roasted	18.62	13.37	200	1.35
Pork, cured, ham -- water added, slice, bone-in, separable lean and fat, heated, pan-broil	20.8	8.73	166	1.54
Pork, cured, ham -- water added, slice, boneless, separable lean and fat, heated, pan-broil	18.62	5.05	125	1.72
Pork, cured, ham -- water added, whole, boneless, separable lean and fat, heated, roasted	17.77	5.48	126	1.54
Pork, cured, ham and water product, rump, bone-in, separable lean and fat, heated, roasted	19.46	11.48	186	1.15
Pork, cured, ham and water product, shank, bone-in, separable lean and fat, heated, roasted	18.17	17.29	234	1.42
Pork, cured, ham and water product, slice, bone-in, separable lean and fat, heated, pan-broil	19.85	7.78	155	1.41
Pork, cured, ham and water product, slice, boneless, separable lean and fat, heated, pan-broil	15.08	5.13	124	4.69
Pork, cured, ham and water product, whole, boneless, separable lean and fat, heated, roasted	13.88	5.46	123	4.61

Food Name ---> per 100 g	Protein (g)	Fat (g)	Calories	Net Carb (g)
Pork, cured, ham with natural juices, rump, bone-in, separable lean and fat, heated, roasted	22.47	9.39	177	0.6
Pork, cured, ham with natural juices, shank, bone-in, separable lean and fat, heated, roasted	22.88	10.93	191	0.33
Pork, cured, ham with natural juices, slice, bone-in, separable lean and fat, heated, pan-broil	26.18	8.28	180	0.17
Pork, cured, ham with natural juices, slice, boneless, separable lean and fat, heated, pan-broil	20.89	3.4	118	1.04
Pork, cured, ham with natural juices, spiral slice, boneless, separable lean and fat, heated, roasted	22.18	5.1	139	1.06
Pork, cured, ham with natural juices, whole, boneless, separable lean and fat, heated, roasted	20.54	3.13	114	0.84
Pork, cured, ham, rump, bone-in, separable lean and fat, heated, roasted	23.95	8.88	177	0.64
Pork, cured, ham, rump, bone-in, separable lean only, heated, roasted	26.02	3.07	132	0.68
Pork, cured, ham, rump, bone-in, separable lean only, unheated	24.46	2.92	125	0.32
Pork, cured, ham, shank, bone-in, separable lean only, heated, roasted	26.49	3.68	139	0.68
Pork, cured, ham, shank, bone-in, separable lean only, unheated	23.79	3.19	125	0.18
Pork, cured, ham, shank, bone-in, separable lean and fat, heated, roasted	24.39	9.35	191	0.64
Pork, cured, ham, shank, bone-in, separable lean and fat, unheated	21.61	9.85	177	0.41
Pork, cured, ham, slice, bone-in, separable lean and fat, heated, pan-broil	25.48	8.48	181	0.7
Pork, cured, ham, slice, bone-in, separable lean only, unheated	24.36	3.59	130	0
Pork, cured, ham, slice, bone-in, separable lean and fat, unheated	22.45	9.17	173	0.21
Pork, fresh, spareribs, separable lean and fat, cooked, roasted	20.89	30.86	361	0
Pork, fresh, composite of separable fat, with added solution, raw	9.27	52.33	508	0
Pork, fresh, loin, tenderloin, separable lean only, with added solution, cooked, roasted	21.61	3.15	116	0.31
Pork, fresh, enhanced, loin, tenderloin, separable lean only, raw	20.39	2.09	106	0
Pork, fresh, shoulder, (Boston butt), blade (steaks), separable lean only, with added solution cooked, braised	27.58	12.14	227	0

Food Name ---> per 100 g	Protein (g)	Fat (g)	Calories	Net Carb (g)
Pork, fresh, shoulder, (Boston butt), blade (steaks), separable lean only, with added solution, raw	18.29	5.36	122	0.18
Pork, fresh, loin, top loin (chops), boneless, separable lean only, with added solution, cooked, broiled	29.65	5.73	170	0
Pork, fresh, loin, top loin (chops), boneless, separable lean only, with added solution, raw	21.09	3.48	117	0.22
Pork, fresh, loin, top loin (chops), boneless, separable lean and fat, with added solution, raw	19.45	10.26	171	0
Pork, fresh, loin, top loin (chops), boneless, separable lean and fat, with added solution, cooked, broiled	28.33	9.42	198	0.02
Pork, fresh, loin, tenderloin, separable lean and fat, with added solution, raw	20.16	3.14	114	0
Pork, fresh, loin, tenderloin, separable lean and fat, with added solution, cooked, roasted	21.5	3.7	121	0.31
Pork, fresh, shoulder, (Boston butt), blade (steaks), separable lean and fat, with added solution, raw	17.19	11.12	169	0.16
Pork, fresh, shoulder, (Boston butt), blade (steaks), separable lean and fat, with added solution, cooked, braised	25.84	16.94	263	0.03
Pork, cured, ham, rump, bone-in, separable lean and fat, unheated	22.27	9.38	176	0.52
Pork, loin, leg cap steak, boneless, separable lean and fat, cooked, broiled	27.57	4.41	158	0
Pork, Leg Cap Steak, boneless, separable lean and fat, raw	21.64	3.39	123	0
Pork, Shoulder breast, boneless, separable lean and fat, raw	22.54	3.4	127	0
Pork, Shoulder breast, boneless, separable lean and fat, cooked, broiled	28.47	4.49	162	0
Pork, shoulder, petite tender, boneless, separable lean and fat, cooked, broiled	27.47	4.23	155	0
Pork, Shoulder petite tender, boneless, separable lean and fat, raw	21.65	3.91	128	0
Pork, Leg sirloin tip roast, boneless, separable lean and fat, cooked, braised	31.11	2.56	156	0
Pork, Leg sirloin tip roast, boneless, separable lean and fat, raw	22.88	1.71	113	0
Pork, ground, 84% lean / 16% fat, raw	17.99	16	218	0.44
Pork, ground, 96% lean / 4% fat, raw	21.1	4	121	0.21
Pork, ground, 72% lean / 28% fat, cooked, crumbles	22.83	32.93	393	1.39
Pork, ground, 84% lean / 16% fat, cooked, crumbles	26.69	20.04	289	0.58

Food Name ---> per 100 g	Protein (g)	Fat (g)	Calories	Net Carb (g)
Pork, ground, 96% lean / 4% fat, cooked, crumbles	30.55	7.15	187	0
Pork, ground, 72% lean / 28% fat, cooked, pan-broiled	22.59	31.42	377	1.08
Pork, ground, 84% lean / 16% fat, cooked, pan-broiled	27.14	21.39	301	0
Pork, ground, 96% lean / 4% fat, cooked, pan-broiled	31.69	6.2	185	0.57
Pork loin, fresh, backribs, bone-in, raw, lean only	20.85	9.84	172	0
Pork loin, fresh, backribs, bone-in, cooked-roasted, lean only	24.15	17.65	255	0
Pork, fresh, loin, blade (chops or roasts), boneless, separable lean only, raw	21.35	3.78	123	0.82
Pork, fresh, loin, blade (roasts), boneless, separable lean only, cooked, roasted	27.58	7.14	175	0
Pork, fresh, loin, blade (chops), boneless, separable lean only, boneless, cooked, broiled	26.14	6.74	169	0.89
Pork, fresh, loin, country-style ribs, separable lean only, boneless, cooked, broiled	27.83	11.65	216	0
Pork, fresh, loin, country-style ribs, separable lean only, bone-in, cooked, broiled	27.83	11.65	216	0
Pork, fresh, loin, country-style ribs, separable lean only, boneless, cooked, roasted	29.2	11.38	219	0
Pork, fresh, blade, (chops), boneless, separable lean and fat, cooked, broiled	24.73	11.13	202	0.83
Pork, fresh, loin, blade (chops or roasts), boneless, separable lean and fat only, raw	20.54	7.94	157	0.76
Pork, fresh, loin, blade (roasts), boneless, separable lean and fat, cooked, roasted	26.48	10.32	199	0
Pork, fresh, loin, country-style ribs, separable lean and fat, boneless, cooked, broiled	26.28	15.73	247	0
Pork, fresh, loin, country-style ribs, separable lean and fat, bone-in, cooked, broiled	25.58	17.56	260	0
Pork, fresh, loin, country-style ribs, separable lean and fat, boneless, cooked, roasted	26.4	18.31	270	0
Bacon, pre-sliced, reduced/low sodium, unprepared	12.53	39.27	407	0.83
Canadian bacon, cooked, pan-fried	28.31	2.78	146	1.8
Pork, oriental style, dehydrated	11.8	62.4	615	1.4
Pork, cured, ham, boneless, low sodium, extra lean and regular, roasted	22	7.7	165	0.5
Pork, cured, ham, low sodium, lean and fat, cooked	22.3	8.3	172	0.3

Food Name ---> per 100 g	Protein (g)	Fat (g)	Calories	Net Carb (g)
Pork, cured, ham, boneless, low sodium, extra lean (approximately 5% fat), roasted	20.9	5.5	145	1.5
Pork, cured, bacon, cooked, broiled, pan-fried or roasted, reduced sodium	37.04	41.78	541	1.43

Poultry Products

Food Name ---> per 100 g	Protein (g)	Fat (g)	Calorie	Net Carb (g)
Chicken, broiler, rotisserie, BBQ, breast meat only	28.04	3.57	144	0
Chicken, broilers or fryers, meat and skin and giblets and neck, raw	18.33	14.83	213	0.13
Chicken, broilers or fryers, meat and skin and giblets and neck, cooked, fried, batter	22.84	17.53	291	9.03
Chicken, broilers or fryers, meat and skin and giblets and neck, cooked, fried, flour	28.57	15.27	272	3.27
Chicken, broilers or fryers, meat and skin and giblets and neck, roasted	26.78	13.27	234	0.06
Chicken, broilers or fryers, meat and skin and giblets and neck, stewed	24.49	12.37	216	0.06
Chicken, broilers or fryers, meat and skin, raw	18.6	15.06	215	0
Chicken, broilers or fryers, meat and skin, cooked, fried, batter	22.54	17.35	289	9.12
Chicken, broilers or fryers, meat and skin, cooked, fried, flour	28.56	14.92	269	3.05
Chicken, broilers or fryers, meat and skin, cooked, roasted	27.3	13.6	239	0
Chicken, broilers or fryers, meat and skin, cooked, stewed	24.68	12.56	219	0
Chicken, broilers or fryers, meat only, raw	21.39	3.08	119	0
Chicken, broilers or fryers, meat only, cooked, fried	30.57	9.12	219	1.59
Chicken, broilers or fryers, meat only, roasted	28.93	7.41	190	0
Chicken, broilers or fryers, meat only, stewed	27.29	6.71	177	0
Chicken, broilers or fryers, skin only, raw	13.33	32.35	349	0
Chicken, broilers or fryers, skin only, cooked, fried, batter	10.32	28.83	394	23.15
Chicken, broilers or fryers, skin only, cooked, fried, flour	19.09	42.58	502	9.34
Chicken, broilers or fryers, skin only, cooked, roasted	20.36	40.68	454	0
Chicken, broilers or fryers, skin only, cooked, stewed	15.22	33.04	363	0
Chicken, broilers or fryers, giblets, raw	17.88	4.47	124	1.8
Chicken, broilers or fryers, giblets, cooked, fried	32.54	13.46	277	4.35
Chicken, broilers or fryers, giblets, cooked, simmered	27.15	4.5	157	0
Chicken, gizzard, all classes, raw	17.66	2.06	94	0
Chicken, gizzard, all classes, cooked, simmered	30.39	2.68	154	0
Chicken, heart, all classes, raw	15.55	9.33	153	0.71

Food Name ---> per 100 g	Protein (g)	Fat (g)	Calorie	Net Carb (g)
Chicken, heart, all classes, cooked, simmered	26.41	7.92	185	0.1
Chicken, liver, all classes, raw	16.92	4.83	119	0.73
Chicken, liver, all classes, cooked, simmered	24.46	6.51	167	0.87
Chicken, broilers or fryers, light meat, meat and skin, raw	20.27	11.07	186	0
Chicken, broilers or fryers, light meat, meat and skin, cooked, fried, batter	23.55	15.44	277	9.5
Chicken, broilers or fryers, light meat, meat and skin, cooked, fried, flour	30.45	12.09	246	1.72
Chicken, broilers or fryers, light meat, meat and skin, cooked, roasted	29.02	10.85	222	0
Chicken, broilers or fryers, light meat, meat and skin, cooked, stewed	26.14	9.97	201	0
Chicken, broilers or fryers, dark meat, meat and skin, raw	16.69	18.34	237	0
Chicken, broilers or fryers, dark meat, meat and skin, cooked, fried, batter	21.85	18.64	298	9.38
Chicken, broilers or fryers, dark meat, meat and skin, cooked, fried, flour	27.22	16.91	285	4.08
Chicken, broilers or fryers, dark meat, meat and skin, cooked, roasted	25.97	15.78	253	0
Chicken, broilers or fryers, dark meat, meat and skin, cooked, stewed	23.5	14.66	233	0
Chicken, broilers or fryers, light meat, meat only, raw	23.2	1.65	114	0
Chicken, broilers or fryers, light meat, meat only, cooked, fried	32.82	5.54	192	0.42
Chicken, broilers or fryers, light meat, meat only, cooked, roasted	30.91	4.51	173	0
Chicken, broilers or fryers, light meat, meat only, cooked, stewed	28.88	3.99	159	0
Chicken, broilers or fryers, dark meat, meat only, raw	20.08	4.31	125	0
Chicken, broilers or fryers, dark meat, meat only, cooked, fried	28.99	11.62	239	2.59
Chicken, broilers or fryers, dark meat, meat only, cooked, roasted	27.37	9.73	205	0
Chicken, broilers or fryers, dark meat, meat only, cooked, stewed	25.97	8.98	192	0
Chicken, broilers or fryers, separable fat, raw	3.73	67.95	629	0
Chicken, broilers or fryers, back, meat and skin, raw	14.05	28.74	319	0
Chicken, broilers or fryers, back, meat and skin, cooked, fried, batter	21.97	21.91	331	10.25
Chicken, broilers or fryers, back, meat and skin, cooked, fried, flour	27.79	20.74	331	6.5
Chicken, broilers or fryers, back, meat and skin, cooked, roasted	25.95	20.97	300	0
Chicken, broilers or fryers, back, meat and skin, cooked, stewed	22.18	18.14	258	0

Food Name ---> per 100 g	Protein (g)	Fat (g)	Calorie	Net Carb (g)
Chicken, broilers or fryers, back, meat only, raw	19.56	5.92	137	0
Chicken, broilers or fryers, back, meat only, cooked, fried	29.99	15.32	288	5.68
Chicken, broilers or fryers, back, meat only, cooked, roasted	28.19	13.16	239	0
Chicken, broilers or fryers, back, meat only, cooked, stewed	25.31	11.19	209	0
Chicken, broilers or fryers, breast, meat and skin, raw	20.85	9.25	172	0
Chicken, broilers or fryers, breast, meat and skin, cooked, fried, batter	24.84	13.2	260	8.69
Chicken, broilers or fryers, breast, meat and skin, cooked, fried, flour	31.84	8.87	222	1.54
Chicken, broilers or fryers, breast, meat and skin, cooked, roasted	29.8	7.78	197	0
Chicken, broilers or fryers, breast, meat and skin, cooked, stewed	27.39	7.42	184	0
Chicken, broiler or fryers, breast, skinless, boneless, meat only, raw	22.5	2.62	120	0
Chicken, broilers or fryers, breast, meat only, cooked, fried	33.44	4.71	187	0.51
Chicken, broilers or fryers, breast, meat only, cooked, roasted	31.02	3.57	165	0
Chicken, broilers or fryers, breast, meat only, cooked, stewed	28.98	3.03	151	0
Chicken, broilers or fryers, drumstick, meat and skin, raw	18.08	9.2	161	0.11
Chicken, broilers or fryers, drumstick, meat and skin, cooked, fried, batter	21.95	15.75	268	7.98
Chicken, broilers or fryers, drumstick, meat and skin, cooked, fried, flour	26.96	13.72	245	1.53
Chicken, broilers or fryers, drumstick, meat and skin, cooked, roasted	23.35	10.15	191	0
Chicken, broilers or fryers, drumstick, meat and skin, cooked, stewed	25.32	10.64	204	0
Chicken, broilers or fryers, dark meat, drumstick, meat only, raw	19.41	3.71	116	0
Chicken, broilers or fryers, drumstick, meat only, cooked, fried	28.62	8.08	195	0
Chicken, broilers or fryers, dark meat, drumstick, meat only, cooked, roasted	24.24	5.7	155	0
Chicken, broilers or fryers, drumstick, meat only, cooked, stewed	27.5	5.71	169	0
Chicken, broilers or fryers, leg, meat and skin, raw	16.37	15.95	214	0.17
Chicken, broilers or fryers, leg, meat and skin, cooked, fried, batter	21.77	16.17	273	8.42
Chicken, broilers or fryers, leg, meat and skin, cooked, fried, flour	26.84	14.43	254	2.4
Chicken, broilers or fryers, leg, meat and skin, cooked, roasted	24.03	8.99	184	0
Chicken, broilers or fryers, leg, meat and skin, cooked, stewed	24.17	12.92	220	0
Chicken, broilers or fryers, leg, meat only, raw	19.16	4.22	120	0

Food Name ---> per 100 g	Protein (g)	Fat (g)	Calorie	Net Carb (g)
Chicken, broilers or fryers, leg, meat only, cooked, fried	28.38	9.32	208	0.65
Chicken, broilers or fryers, leg, meat only, cooked, roasted	24.22	7.8	174	0
Chicken, broilers or fryers, leg, meat only, cooked, stewed	26.26	8.06	185	0
Chicken, broilers or fryers, neck, meat and skin, raw	14.07	26.24	297	0
Chicken, broilers or fryers, neck, meat and skin, cooked, fried, batter	19.82	23.52	330	8.7
Chicken, broilers or fryers, neck, meat and skin, cooked, fried, flour	24.01	23.61	332	4.24
Chicken, broilers or fryers, neck, meat and skin, cooked simmered	19.61	18.1	247	0
Chicken, broilers or fryers, neck, meat only, raw	17.55	8.78	154	0
Chicken, broilers or fryers, neck, meat only, cooked, fried	26.87	11.88	229	1.77
Chicken, broilers or fryers, neck, meat only, cooked, simmered	24.56	8.18	179	0
Chicken, broilers or fryers, thigh, meat and skin, raw	16.52	16.61	221	0.25
Chicken, broilers or fryers, thigh, meat and skin, cooked, fried, batter	21.61	16.53	277	8.78
Chicken, broilers or fryers, thigh, meat and skin, cooked, fried, flour	26.75	14.98	262	3.08
Chicken, broilers or fryers, thigh, meat and skin, cooked, roasted	23.26	14.71	232	0
Chicken, broilers or fryers, thigh, meat and skin, cooked, stewed	23.26	14.74	232	0
Chicken, broilers or fryers, dark meat, thigh, meat only, raw	19.66	4.12	121	0
Chicken, broilers or fryers, thigh, meat only, cooked, fried	28.18	10.3	218	1.18
Chicken, broilers or fryers, thigh, meat only, cooked, roasted	24.76	8.15	179	0
Chicken, broilers or fryers, thigh, meat only, cooked, stewed	25	9.79	195	0
Chicken, broilers or fryers, wing, meat and skin, raw	17.52	12.85	191	0
Chicken, broilers or fryers, wing, meat and skin, cooked, fried, batter	19.87	21.81	324	10.64
Chicken, broilers or fryers, wing, meat and skin, cooked, fried, flour	26.11	22.16	321	2.29
Chicken, broilers or fryers, wing, meat and skin, cooked, roasted	23.79	16.87	254	0
Chicken, broilers or fryers, wing, meat and skin, cooked, stewed	22.78	16.82	249	0
Chicken, broilers or fryers, wing, meat only, raw	21.97	3.54	126	0
Chicken, broilers or fryers, wing, meat only, cooked, fried	30.15	9.15	211	0
Chicken, broilers or fryers, wing, meat only, cooked, roasted	30.46	8.13	203	0
Chicken, broilers or fryers, wing, meat only, cooked, stewed	27.18	7.18	181	0
Chicken, roasting, meat and skin and giblets and neck, raw	17.09	15.46	213	0.09

Food Name ---> per 100 g	Protein (g)	Fat (g)	Calorie	Net Carb (g)
Chicken, roasting, meat and skin and giblets and neck, cooked, roasted	23.96	13.07	220	0.05
Canada Goose, breast meat, skinless, raw	24.31	4.02	133	0
Chicken, roasting, meat and skin, cooked, roasted	23.97	13.39	223	0
Chicken, roasting, meat only, raw	20.33	2.7	111	0
Chicken, roasting, meat only, cooked, roasted	25.01	6.63	167	0
Chicken, roasting, giblets, raw	18.14	5.04	127	1.14
Chicken, roasting, giblets, cooked, simmered	26.77	5.22	165	0.86
Chicken, roasting, light meat, meat only, raw	22.2	1.63	109	0
Chicken, roasting, light meat, meat only, cooked, roasted	27.13	4.07	153	0
Chicken, roasting, dark meat, meat only, raw	18.74	3.61	113	0
Chicken, roasting, dark meat, meat only, cooked, roasted	23.25	8.75	178	0
Chicken, stewing, meat and skin, and giblets and neck, raw	17.48	19.52	251	0.19
Chicken, stewing, meat and skin, and giblets and neck, cooked, stewed	24.88	11.91	214	0
Chicken, stewing, meat and skin, raw	17.55	20.33	258	0
Chicken, stewing, meat and skin, cooked, stewed	26.88	18.87	285	0
Chicken, stewing, meat only, raw	21.26	6.32	148	0
Chicken, stewing, meat only, cooked, stewed	30.42	11.89	237	0
Chicken, stewing, giblets, raw	17.89	9.21	168	2.13
Chicken, stewing, giblets, cooked, simmered	25.73	9.3	194	0.11
Chicken, stewing, light meat, meat only, raw	23.1	4.21	137	0
Chicken, stewing, light meat, meat only, cooked, stewed	33.04	7.98	213	0
Chicken, stewing, dark meat, meat only, raw	19.7	8.12	157	0
Chicken, stewing, dark meat, meat only, cooked, stewed	28.14	15.28	258	0
Chicken, capons, meat and skin and giblets and neck, raw	18.51	16.9	232	0.08
Chicken, capons, meat and skin and giblets and neck, cooked, roasted	28.35	11.67	226	0.04
Chicken, capons, meat and skin, raw	18.77	17.07	234	0
Chicken, capons, meat and skin, cooked, roasted	28.96	11.65	229	0
Chicken, capons, giblets, raw	18.28	5.18	130	1.42
Chicken, capons, giblets, cooked, simmered	26.39	5.4	164	0.76
Duck, domesticated, meat and skin, raw	11.49	39.34	404	0
Duck, domesticated, meat and skin, cooked, roasted	18.99	28.35	337	0

Food Name ---> per 100 g	Protein (g)	Fat (g)	Calorie	Net Carb (g)
Duck, domesticated, meat only, raw	18.28	5.95	135	0.94
Duck, domesticated, meat only, cooked, roasted	23.48	11.2	201	0
Duck, domesticated, liver, raw	18.74	4.64	136	3.53
Duck, wild, meat and skin, raw	17.42	15.2	211	0
Duck, wild, breast, meat only, raw	19.85	4.25	123	0
Goose, domesticated, meat and skin, raw	15.86	33.62	371	0
Goose, domesticated, meat and skin, cooked, roasted	25.16	21.92	305	0
Goose, domesticated, meat only, raw	22.75	7.13	161	0
Goose, domesticated, meat only, cooked, roasted	28.97	12.67	238	0
Goose, liver, raw	16.37	4.28	133	6.32
Turkey, whole, giblets, raw	18.18	5.09	124	0.07
Turkey, whole, giblets, cooked, simmered	26.44	6.61	173	0
Turkey, gizzard, all classes, raw	18.8	3.37	111	0
Turkey, gizzard, all classes, cooked, simmered	26.45	4.64	155	0
Turkey, heart, all classes, raw	16.7	7.44	140	0.4
Turkey, heart, all classes, cooked, simmered	24.88	7.52	174	0
Turkey, liver, all classes, raw	18.26	5.5	128	0
Turkey, liver, all classes, cooked, simmered	27	8.18	189	0
Turkey from whole, neck, meat only, raw	16.51	6.04	125	0
Turkey from whole, neck, meat only, cooked, simmered	22.48	7.36	162	0
Turkey from whole, light meat, meat and skin, raw	21.96	7.43	161	0.15
Turkey from whole, light meat, meat and skin, cooked, roasted	29.55	5.57	177	0.05
Turkey, dark meat, meat and skin, raw	19.81	8.97	161	0.15
Turkey, dark meat from whole, meat and skin, cooked, roasted	27.27	9.95	206	0.07
Turkey from whole, light meat, raw	23.66	1.48	114	0.14
Turkey, all classes, light meat, cooked, roasted	30.13	2.08	147	0
Turkey from whole, dark meat, meat only, raw	21.28	2.5	108	0.15
Turkey, from whole, dark meat, cooked, roasted	27.71	6.04	173	0
Turkey, all classes, back, meat and skin, cooked, roasted	26.59	14.38	244	0.16
Turkey, all classes, breast, meat and skin, raw	21.89	7.02	157	0
Turkey, all classes, breast, meat and skin, cooked, roasted	28.71	7.41	189	0
Turkey, all classes, leg, meat and skin, raw	19.54	6.72	144	0
Turkey, all classes, leg, meat and skin, cooked, roasted	27.87	9.82	208	0

Food Name ---> per 100 g	Protein (g)	Fat (g)	Calorie	Net Carb (g)
Turkey, all classes, wing, meat and skin, raw	20.22	12.32	197	0
Turkey, all classes, wing, meat and skin, cooked, roasted	27.38	12.43	229	0
Turkey, fryer-roasters, meat and skin, cooked, roasted	28.26	5.72	172	0
Turkey, back from whole bird, meat only, raw	21.28	2.5	113	0.15
Turkey, back, from whole bird, meat only, roasted	27.71	6.04	173	0
Turkey, breast, from whole bird, meat only, raw	23.66	1.48	114	0.14
Turkey, breast, from whole bird, meat only, roasted	30.13	2.08	147	0
Turkey, wing, from whole bird, meat only, raw	23.66	1.48	114	0.14
Turkey, wing, from whole bird, meat only, roasted	30.13	2.08	147	0
Turkey, young hen, skin only, cooked, roasted	19.03	44.45	482	0
Chicken, canned, meat only, with broth	21.77	7.95	165	0
Pate de foie gras, canned (goose liver pate), smoked	11.4	43.84	462	4.67
Turkey, canned, meat only, with broth	23.68	6.86	169	1.47
Turkey, diced, light and dark meat, seasoned	18.7	6	138	1
Turkey and gravy, frozen	5.88	2.63	67	4.61
Turkey breast, pre-basted, meat and skin, cooked, roasted	22.16	3.46	126	0
Turkey thigh, pre-basted, meat and skin, cooked, roasted	18.8	8.54	157	0
Turkey roast, boneless, frozen, seasoned, light and dark meat, raw	17.6	2.2	120	6.4
Turkey sticks, breaded, battered, fried	14.2	16.9	279	17
Poultry, mechanically deboned, from backs and necks with skin, raw	11.39	24.73	272	0
Poultry, mechanically deboned, from backs and necks without skin, raw	13.79	15.48	199	0
Poultry, mechanically deboned, from mature hens, raw	14.72	19.98	243	0
Turkey, mechanically deboned, from turkey frames, raw	13.29	15.96	201	0
Ground turkey, raw	19.66	7.66	148	0
Ground turkey, cooked	27.37	10.4	203	0
Duck, young duckling, domesticated, White Pekin, breast, meat and skin, boneless, cooked, roasted	24.5	10.85	202	0
Duck, young duckling, domesticated, White Pekin, breast, meat only, boneless, cooked without skin, broiled	27.6	2.5	140	0
Duck, young duckling, domesticated, White Pekin, leg, meat and skin, bone in, cooked, roasted	26.75	11.4	217	0
Duck, young duckling, domesticated, White Pekin, leg, meat only, bone in, cooked without skin, braised	29.1	5.96	178	0

Food Name ---> per 100 g	Protein (g)	Fat (g)	Calorie	Net Carb (g)
Chicken, broiler, rotisserie, BBQ, drumstick, meat only	27.71	6.76	172	0
Chicken, wing, frozen, glazed, barbecue flavored, heated (conventional oven)	22.24	14.87	242	2.86
Chicken patty, frozen, uncooked	14.33	20.04	292	12.41
Chicken patty, frozen, cooked	14.85	19.58	287	12.54
Chicken breast tenders, breaded, cooked, microwaved	16.35	12.89	252	17.56
Chicken breast tenders, breaded, uncooked	14.73	15.75	263	13.91
Chicken, ground, raw	17.44	8.1	143	0.04
Chicken, ground, crumbles, cooked, pan-browned	23.28	10.92	189	0
Chicken, broiler, rotisserie, BBQ, thigh, meat only	24.09	10.74	193	0
Chicken, feet, boiled	19.4	14.6	215	0.2
USDA Commodity Chicken, canned, meat only, drained	27.52	5.72	162	0
USDA Commodity, Chicken, canned, meat only, with water	22.02	4.58	129	0
USDA Commodity, Chicken, canned, meat only, with broth	22.41	4.69	133	0.23
Chicken, broiler, rotisserie, BBQ, wing, meat only	28.34	7.79	184	0.54
Chicken, broilers or fryers, back, meat only, cooked, rotisserie, original seasoning	25.34	11.54	205	0
Chicken, broilers or fryers, breast, meat only, cooked, rotisserie, original seasoning	28	2.79	137	0
Chicken, broilers or fryers, drumstick, meat only, cooked, rotisserie, original seasoning	28.74	6.81	176	0
Chicken, broilers or fryers, skin only, cooked, rotisserie, original seasoning	17.66	37.24	406	0.11
Chicken, broilers or fryers, thigh, meat only, cooked, rotisserie, original seasoning	24.06	11.09	196	0
Chicken, broilers or fryers, wing, meat only, cooked, rotisserie, original seasoning	27.69	9.53	197	0
Chicken, broilers or fryers, back, meat and skin, cooked, rotisserie, original seasoning	23.23	18.59	260	0.03
Chicken, broilers or fryers, breast, meat and skin, cooked, rotisserie, original seasoning	27.48	8.18	184	0.02
Chicken, broilers or fryers, drumstick, meat and skin, cooked, rotisserie, original seasoning	26.86	11.98	215	0.02
Chicken, broilers or fryers, thigh, meat and skin, cooked, rotisserie, original seasoning	22.93	15.7	233	0.02
Chicken, broilers or fryers, wing, meat and skin, cooked, rotisserie, original seasoning	24.34	18.77	266	0.04

Food Name ---> per 100 g	Protein (g)	Fat (g)	Calorie	Net Carb (g)
USDA Commodity, chicken fajita strips, frozen	18.56	5.73	135	2.23
USDA Commodity, turkey taco meat, frozen, cooked	16.8	7.58	148	3.03
Chicken, broiler, rotisserie, BBQ, skin	15.19	35.15	378	0.7
Chicken, broiler, rotisserie, BBQ, back meat and skin	20.29	18.86	251	0.4
Chicken, broiler, rotisserie, BBQ, breast meat and skin	26.37	7.67	175	0.09
Chicken, broiler, rotisserie, BBQ, drumstick meat and skin	25.65	11.46	206	0.12
Chicken, broiler, rotisserie, BBQ, thigh meat and skin	22.51	15.08	226	0.12
Chicken, broiler, rotisserie, BBQ, wing meat and skin	23.42	18.04	257	0.6
Ruffed Grouse, breast meat, skinless, raw	25.94	0.88	112	0
USDA Commodity, turkey ham, dark meat, smoked, frozen	16.3	4	118	3.1
Chicken, liver, all classes, cooked, pan-fried	25.78	6.43	172	1.11
Ground turkey, fat free, raw	23.57	1.95	112	0
Ground turkey, fat free, pan-broiled crumbles	31.69	2.71	151	0
Ground turkey, fat free, patties, broiled	28.99	2.48	138	0
Ground turkey, 93% lean, 7% fat, raw	18.73	8.34	150	0
Ground turkey, 93% lean, 7% fat, pan-broiled crumbles	27.1	11.6	213	0
Ground turkey, 93% lean, 7% fat, patties, broiled	25.86	11.45	207	0
Ground turkey, 85% lean, 15% fat, raw	16.9	12.54	180	0
Ground turkey, 85% lean, 15% fat, pan-broiled crumbles	25.11	17.45	258	0
Ground turkey, 85% lean, 15% fat, patties, broiled	25.88	16.2	249	0
Chicken, broilers or fryers, dark meat, drumstick, meat only, cooked, braised	23.93	5.95	149	0
Chicken, broilers or fryers, dark meat, thigh, meat only, cooked, braised	24.55	8.63	176	0
Chicken, skin (drumsticks and thighs), cooked, braised	14.61	42.76	443	0
Chicken, skin (drumsticks and thighs), raw	9.58	44.23	440	0.79
Chicken, skin (drumsticks and thighs), cooked, roasted	16.57	43.99	462	0
Chicken, broilers or fryers, dark meat, drumstick, meat and skin, cooked, braised	22.72	10.73	187	0
Chicken, broilers or fryers, dark meat, thigh, meat and skin, cooked, braised	22.57	15.43	229	0
Chicken, dark meat, drumstick, meat only, with added solution, raw	19.19	3.26	106	0
Chicken, dark meat, drumstick, meat only, with added solution, cooked, roasted	25.34	5	146	0

Food Name ---> per 100 g	Protein (g)	Fat (g)	Calorie	Net Carb (g)
Chicken, dark meat, drumstick, meat only, with added solution, cooked, braised	22.99	6.33	149	0
Chicken, dark meat, thigh, meat only, with added solution, cooked, braised	23	7.96	164	0
Chicken, dark meat, thigh, meat only, with added solution, raw	19.11	3.69	110	0
Chicken, dark meat, thigh, meat only, with added solution, cooked, roasted	24.23	7.73	164	0
Chicken, skin (drumsticks and thighs), with added solution, cooked, braised	12.26	38.94	403	1
Chicken, skin (drumsticks and thighs), with added solution, raw	11.11	37.9	386	0.01
Chicken, skin (drumsticks and thighs), with added solution, cooked, roasted	20.31	37.6	421	0.44
Chicken, dark meat, drumstick, meat and skin, with added solution, cooked, braised	21.55	10.71	183	0.13
Chicken, dark meat, drumstick, meat and skin, with added solution, raw	18.03	8.24	146	0
Chicken, dark meat, drumstick, meat and skin, with added solution, cooked, roasted	24.72	9	180	0.05
Chicken, dark meat, thigh, meat and skin, with added solution, cooked, braised	20.7	14.62	215	0.21
Chicken, dark meat, thigh, meat and skin, with added solution, raw	16.56	14.58	197	0
Chicken, dark meat, thigh, meat and skin, with added solution, cooked, roasted	23.47	13.81	214	0.09
Chicken, broiler, rotisserie, BBQ, back meat only	21.85	13.87	212	0.31
Turkey, dark meat from whole, meat only, with added solution, raw	19.27	4.12	115	0.1
Turkey, dark meat, meat only, with added solution, cooked, roasted	26.1	6	158	0
Turkey from whole, light meat, meat only, with added solution, raw	21.54	1.66	101	0
Turkey from whole, light meat, meat only, with added solution, cooked, roasted	26.97	2.08	127	0
Turkey, skin from whole (light and dark), with added solution, raw	12.29	36.8	381	0.21
Turkey, skin from whole, (light and dark), with added solution, roasted	22.15	40.31	451	0
Turkey, dark meat from whole, meat and skin, with added solution, raw	17.84	10.83	169	0.15
Turkey, dark meat from whole, meat and skin, with added solution, cooked, roasted	25.55	10.81	199	0
Turkey from whole, light meat, meat and skin, with added solution, raw	20.02	7.42	147	0.14

Food Name ---> per 100 g	Protein (g)	Fat (g)	Calorie	Net Carb (g)
Turkey from whole, light meat, meat and skin, with added solution, cooked, roasted	26.52	5.64	157	0
Turkey, whole, meat only, with added solution, raw	20.87	2.39	105	0.14
Turkey, whole, meat only, with added solution, roasted	26.61	3.7	140	0
Turkey, whole, meat and skin, with added solution, raw	19.03	9.1	158	0.15
Turkey, whole, meat and skin, with added solution, roasted	26.09	8.01	176	0
Turkey, retail parts, breast, meat only, with added solution, raw	21.99	2.53	111	0
Turkey, retail parts, breast, meat only, with added solution, cooked, roasted	27.94	2.08	130	0
Turkey, retail parts, breast, meat only, raw	23.34	2.33	114	0
Turkey, retail parts, breast, meat only, cooked, roasted	29.51	1.97	136	0
Turkey, retail parts, wing, meat only, raw	22.48	2.49	112	0
Turkey, retail parts, wing, meat only, cooked, roasted	30.17	5.51	170	0
Turkey, skin, from retail parts, from dark meat, raw	14.35	35.83	380	0
Turkey, skin, from retail parts, from dark meat, cooked, roasted	24.58	35.03	414	0
Turkey, retail parts, drumstick, meat only, raw	20.52	3.97	118	0
Turkey, retail parts, thigh, meat only, raw	20.6	3.69	116	0
Turkey, breast, from whole bird, meat only, with added solution, roasted	26.97	2.08	127	0
Turkey, back, from whole bird, meat only, with added solution, raw	19.27	4.12	115	0.15
Turkey, back, from whole bird, meat only, with added solution, roasted	26.97	2.08	127	0
Turkey, breast, from whole bird, meat only, with added solution, raw	21.54	1.66	102	0.14
Turkey, retail parts, thigh, meat only, cooked, roasted	25.14	6.25	159	0.46
Turkey, retail parts, drumstick, meat only, cooked, roasted	28.61	6.52	173	0
Turkey, drumstick, from whole bird, meat only, with added solution, raw	19.27	4.12	115	0.15
Turkey, drumstick, from whole bird, meat only, with added solution, roasted	26.1	6	158	0
Turkey, thigh, from whole bird, meat only, with added solution, raw	19.27	4.12	115	0.15
Turkey, retail parts, breast, meat and skin, with added solution, raw	20.79	6.75	144	0.03
Turkey, thigh, from whole bird, meat only, with added solution, roasted	26.1	6	158	0
Turkey, wing, from whole bird, meat only, with added solution, raw	21.54	1.66	102	0.14

Food Name ---> per 100 g	Protein (g)	Fat (g)	Calorie	Net Carb (g)
Turkey, wing, from whole bird, meat only, with added solution, roasted	26.97	2.08	127	0
Turkey, retail parts, breast, meat and skin, raw	21.88	7.45	155	0
Turkey, retail parts, breast, meat and skin, cooked, roasted	29.01	5.33	164	0.05
Turkey, retail parts, wing, meat and skin, raw	19.53	13.79	202	0.05
Turkey, retail parts, wing, meat and skin, cooked, roasted	28.74	13.29	235	0.13
Turkey, retail parts, drumstick, meat and skin, raw	19.96	6.84	141	0
Turkey, retail parts, drumstick, meat and skin, cooked, roasted	28.21	9.37	197	0
Turkey, drumstick, from whole bird, meat only, raw	23.66	1.48	109	0.14
Turkey, drumstick, from whole bird, meat only, roasted	30.13	2.08	139	0
Turkey, thigh, from whole bird, meat only, raw	21.28	2.5	108	0.15
Turkey, thigh, from whole bird, meat only, roasted	27.71	6.04	165	0
Turkey, retail parts, thigh, meat and skin, raw	19.54	9.16	161	0
Turkey, retail parts, thigh, meat and skin, cooked, roasted	23.95	9.5	183	0.41
Turkey, back, from whole bird, meat and skin, with added solution, raw	16.86	15.41	206	0.15
Turkey, back, from whole bird, meat and skin, with added solution, roasted	25.8	11.36	205	0
Chicken, broiler or fryers, breast, skinless, boneless, meat only, cooked, braised	32.06	3.24	157	0
Chicken, broiler or fryers, breast, skinless, boneless, meat only, cooked, grilled	30.54	3.17	151	0
Chicken, broiler or fryers, breast, skinless, boneless, meat only, with added solution, cooked, braised	28.24	3.61	145	0
Chicken, broiler or fryers, breast, skinless, boneless, meat only, with added solution, cooked, grilled	29.5	3.39	148	0
Quail, cooked, total edible	25.1	14.1	227	0
Pheasant, cooked, total edible	32.4	12.1	239	0
Dove, cooked (includes squab)	23.9	13	213	0
Turkey, wing, smoked, cooked, with skin, bone removed	27.4	12.41	221	0
Turkey, drumstick, smoked, cooked, with skin, bone removed	27.9	9.8	208	0
Turkey, light or dark meat, smoked, cooked, with skin, bone removed	28.1	9.7	208	0
Turkey, light or dark meat, smoked, cooked, skin and bone removed	29.3	5	170	0

Sausages and Luncheon Meats

Food Name ---> per 100 g	Protein (g)	Fat (g)	Calorie	Net Carbs
Sausage, Berliner, pork, beef	15.27	17.2	230	2.59
Blood sausage	14.6	34.5	379	1.29
Bockwurst, pork, veal, raw	14.03	25.87	301	1.95
Bologna, beef	10.91	26.13	299	4.29
Bologna, beef and pork	15.2	24.59	308	5.49
Bologna, pork	15.3	19.87	247	0.73
Bologna, turkey	11.42	16.05	209	4.18
Bratwurst, pork, cooked	13.72	29.18	333	2.85
Braunschweiger (a liver sausage), pork	14.5	28.5	327	3.1
Brotwurst, pork, beef, link	14.3	27.8	323	2.98
Cheesefurter, cheese smokie, pork, beef	14.1	29	328	1.51
Chicken spread	18.01	17.56	158	3.75
Chorizo, pork and beef	24.1	38.27	455	1.86
Corned beef loaf, jellied	22.9	6.1	153	0
Dutch brand loaf, chicken, pork and beef	12	22.91	273	3.63
Frankfurter, beef, unheated	11.16	28.3	316	3.36
Frankfurter, chicken	15.51	16.19	223	2.74
Frankfurter, turkey	12.23	17.29	223	3.81
Ham, chopped, canned	16.06	18.83	239	0.26
Ham, chopped, not canned	16.5	10.3	180	4.2
Ham, sliced, packaged (96% fat free, water added)	16.9	3.4	100	0.55
Ham, sliced, regular (approximately 11% fat)	16.6	8.6	163	2.53
Ham, minced	16.28	20.68	263	1.84
Ham salad spread	8.68	15.53	216	10.64
Ham and cheese loaf or roll	13.6	18.7	241	4
Ham and cheese spread	16.18	18.53	245	2.28
Headcheese, pork	13.83	10.9	157	0
Sausage, Italian, pork, raw	14.25	31.33	346	0.65

Food Name ---> per 100 g	Protein (g)	Fat (g)	Calorie	Net Carbs
Knackwurst, knockwurst, pork, beef	11.1	27.7	307	3.2
Lebanon bologna, beef	19.03	10.44	172	0.44
Liver cheese, pork	15.2	25.6	304	2.1
Liver sausage, liverwurst, pork	14.1	28.5	326	2.2
Roast beef, deli style, prepackaged, sliced	18.62	3.69	115	0.64
USDA Commodity, luncheon meat, canned	17.5	12.77	189	1.04
Luncheon meat, pork, canned	12.5	30.3	334	2.1
Turkey breast, low salt, prepackaged or deli, luncheon meat	21.81	0.83	109	3.01
Mortadella, beef, pork	16.37	25.39	311	3.05
Olive loaf, pork	11.8	16.5	235	9.2
Pastrami, turkey	16.3	6.21	139	3.24
Pate, chicken liver, canned	13.45	13.1	201	6.55
Pate, goose liver, smoked, canned	11.4	43.84	462	4.67
Pate, liver, not specified, canned	14.2	28	319	1.5
Peppered loaf, pork, beef	17.3	6.37	149	4.53
Pepperoni, beef and pork, sliced	19.25	46.28	504	1.18
Pickle and pimiento loaf, pork	11.23	15.95	225	6.96
Polish sausage, pork	14.1	28.72	326	1.63
Luxury loaf, pork	18.4	4.8	141	4.9
Mother's loaf, pork	12.07	22.3	282	7.53
Picnic loaf, pork, beef	14.92	16.64	232	4.76
Pork sausage, link/patty, unprepared	15.39	24.8	288	0.93
Pork sausage, link/patty, cooked, pan-fried	18.53	27.25	325	1.42
Pork and beef sausage, fresh, cooked	13.8	36.25	396	2.7
Turkey sausage, reduced fat, brown and serve, cooked (include BUTTERBALL breakfast links turkey sausage)	17	10.3	204	10.62
Poultry salad sandwich spread	11.64	13.52	200	7.41
Salami, cooked, beef	12.6	22.2	261	1.9
Salami, cooked, beef and pork	21.85	25.9	336	2.4
Salami, cooked, turkey	19.2	9.21	172	1.45
Salami, dry or hard, pork	22.58	33.72	407	1.6
Salami, dry or hard, pork, beef	21.07	31.65	378	0.72

Food Name ---> per 100 g	Protein (g)	Fat (g)	Calorie	Net Carbs
Sandwich spread, pork, beef	7.66	17.34	235	11.74
Smoked link sausage, pork	11.98	28.23	309	0.94
Sausage, smoked link sausage, pork and beef	12	28.73	320	2.42
Smoked link sausage, pork and beef, nonfat dry milk added	13.28	27.61	313	1.92
Thuringer, cervelat, summer sausage, beef, pork	17.45	30.43	362	3.33
Turkey breast, sliced, prepackaged	16.33	2.37	100	2.34
Sausage, Vienna, canned, chicken, beef, pork	10.5	19.4	230	2.6
Honey roll sausage, beef	18.58	10.5	182	2.18
Sausage, Italian, pork, cooked	19.12	27.31	344	4.17
Luncheon sausage, pork and beef	15.38	20.9	260	1.58
New england brand sausage, pork, beef	17.27	7.58	161	4.83
Turkey bacon, unprepared	15.94	16.93	226	1.89
HORMEL Pillow Pak Sliced Turkey Pepperoni	30.99	11.52	243	3.78
Turkey, pork, and beef sausage, low fat, smoked	8	2.5	101	10.94
USDA Commodity, pork, sausage, bulk/links/patties, frozen, cooked	19.76	20.26	267	0
Frankfurter, beef, pork, and turkey, fat free	12.5	1.59	109	11.21
Luncheon meat, pork, ham, and chicken, minced, canned, reduced sodium, added ascorbic acid, includes SPAM, 25% less sodium	12.5	25.1	293	3.4
USDA Commodity, pork sausage, bulk/links/patties, frozen, raw	14.95	18.56	231	0
Luncheon meat, pork with ham, minced, canned, includes SPAM (Hormel)	13.4	26.6	315	4.6
Luncheon meat, pork and chicken, minced, canned, includes SPAM Lite	15.23	13.9	196	1.35
Bratwurst, veal, cooked	13.99	31.7	341	0
Liverwurst spread	12.38	25.45	305	3.39
Roast beef spread	15.27	16.28	223	3.53
Salami, pork, beef, less sodium	15.01	30.5	396	15.18
Sausage, Italian, sweet, links	16.13	8.42	149	2.1
Sausage, Polish, beef with chicken, hot	17.6	19.4	259	3.6
Sausage, Polish, pork and beef, smoked	12.07	26.56	301	1.98

Food Name ---> per 100 g	Protein (g)	Fat (g)	Calorie	Net Carbs
Sausage, pork and beef, with cheddar cheese, smoked	12.89	25.84	296	2.13
Sausage, summer, pork and beef, sticks, with cheddar cheese	19.43	37.91	426	1.62
Sausage, turkey, breakfast links, mild	15.42	18.09	235	1.56
Swisswurst, pork and beef, with swiss cheese, smoked	12.69	27.37	307	1.6
Bacon and beef sticks	29.1	44.2	517	0.8
Bratwurst, beef and pork, smoked	12.2	26.34	297	2
Bratwurst, chicken, cooked	19.44	10.35	176	0
Bratwurst, pork, beef and turkey, lite, smoked	14.45	13.53	186	1.62
Pastrami, beef, 98% fat-free	19.6	1.16	95	1.54
Salami, Italian, pork	21.7	37	425	1.2
Sausage, Italian, turkey, smoked	15.05	8.75	158	3.75
Sausage, chicken, beef, pork, skinless, smoked	13.6	14.3	216	8.1
Sausage, turkey, hot, smoked	15.05	8.75	158	4.35
Yachtwurst, with pistachio nuts, cooked	14.8	22.6	268	1.4
Beerwurst, pork and beef	14	22.53	276	3.37
Chicken breast, fat-free, mesquite flavor, sliced	16.8	0.39	80	2.25
Chicken breast, oven-roasted, fat-free, sliced	16.79	0.39	79	2.17
Kielbasa, Polish, turkey and beef, smoked	13.1	17.6	226	3.9
Oven-roasted chicken breast roll	14.59	7.65	134	1.79
Bologna, pork and turkey, lite	13.06	16.06	211	3.45
Bologna, pork, turkey and beef	11.56	29.25	336	6.66
Ham, honey, smoked, cooked	17.93	2.37	122	7.27
Frankfurter, pork	12.81	23.68	269	0.18
Macaroni and cheese loaf, chicken, pork and beef	11.76	14.96	228	11.63
Salami, Italian, pork and beef, dry, sliced, 50% less sodium	21.8	26.4	350	6.4
Pate, truffle flavor	11.2	28.5	327	6.3
Turkey, breast, smoked, lemon pepper flavor, 97% fat-free	20.9	0.69	95	1.31
Turkey, white, rotisserie, deli cut	13.5	3	112	7.3
Frankfurter, beef, heated	11.69	29.36	322	2.66
Frankfurter, meat, heated	9.77	24.31	278	4.9
Frankfurter, meat	10.26	25.76	290	4.17

Food Name ---> per 100 g	Protein (g)	Fat (g)	Calorie	Net Carbs
Scrapple, pork	8.06	13.87	213	13.76
Bologna, chicken, turkey, pork	9.88	26.18	298	5.65
Pork sausage, link/patty, fully cooked, microwaved	15.12	41.66	438	0.62
Beef sausage, pre-cooked	15.5	37.57	405	0.03
Turkey sausage, fresh, raw	18.79	8.08	155	0.47
Beef sausage, fresh, cooked	18.21	27.98	332	0.35
Pork and turkey sausage, pre-cooked	12.05	30.64	342	3.63
Turkey sausage, fresh, cooked	23.89	10.44	196	0
Bologna, chicken, pork, beef	11.33	22.73	272	5.61
Bologna, chicken, pork	10.31	30.61	336	4.19
Chicken breast, deli, rotisserie seasoned, sliced, prepackaged	17.4	1.86	98	2.92
Frankfurter, meat and poultry, unheated	9.72	24.18	277	5.02
Frankfurter, meat and poultry, cooked, boiled	10.31	26.28	298	4.96
Frankfurter, meat and poultry, cooked, grilled	10.67	26.43	302	5.24
Pork sausage, link/patty, reduced fat, unprepared	16.75	16.55	217	0.2
Pork sausage, link/patty, reduced fat, cooked, pan-fried	20.94	20.32	267	0.15
Pork sausage, link/patty, fully cooked, unheated	13.46	37.25	392	0.69
Kielbasa, fully cooked, grilled	12.45	29.68	337	5.03
Kielbasa, fully cooked, pan-fried	12.36	29.43	333	4.78
Kielbasa, fully cooked, unheated	10.84	29.63	325	3.72
Bologna, meat and poultry	10.34	23.77	281	6.31
Meatballs, frozen, Italian style	14.4	22.21	286	5.76
Turkey bacon, microwaved	29.5	25.87	368	4.24
Bacon, turkey, low sodium	13.33	20	253	4.8
Sausage, chicken or turkey, Italian style, lower sodium	21.43	4.46	183	14.25
Ham, smoked, extra lean, low sodium	18.52	2.71	141	10.7
Pork sausage, reduced sodium, cooked	9.41	22.35	271	8.13
Sausage, pork, turkey, and beef, reduced sodium	10.71	26.79	284	0.01
Beef, cured, corned beef, canned	27.1	14.93	250	0
Beef, cured, dried	31.1	1.94	153	2.76
Beef, cured, luncheon meat, jellied	19	3.3	111	0

Food Name ---> per 100 g	Protein (g)	Fat (g)	Calorie	Net Carbs
Beef, cured, pastrami	21.8	5.82	147	0.36
Beef, cured, sausage, cooked, smoked	14.11	26.91	312	2.42
Beef, cured, smoked, chopped beef	20.19	4.42	133	1.86
Turkey ham, sliced, extra lean, prepackaged or deli-sliced	19.6	3.8	124	2.93
Bologna, beef and pork, low fat	11.5	19.3	230	2.6
Bologna, beef, low fat	11.8	14.8	204	5.2
Turkey and pork sausage, fresh, bulk, patty or link, cooked	22.7	23	307	0.7
Frankfurter, beef, low fat	12	9.5	233	1.6
Pork sausage rice links, brown and serve, cooked	13.7	37.63	407	2.36
Frankfurter, meat and poultry, low fat	15.5	2.8	121	8.3
Beef, bologna, reduced sodium	11.7	28.4	310	2
Frankfurter, low sodium	12	28.51	312	1.8

Snacks

Food Name ---> per 100 g	Protein (g)	Fat (g)	Calorie	Net Carb (g)
Snacks, beef jerky, chopped and formed	33.2	25.6	410	9.2
Snacks, corn-based, extruded, chips, plain	6.17	33.36	538	52.9
Snacks, corn-based, extruded, chips, barbecue-flavor	7	32.7	523	51
Snacks, corn-based, extruded, cones, plain	5.8	26.9	510	61.8
Snacks, corn-based, extruded, onion-flavor	7.7	22.6	499	61.2
Snacks, corn-based, extruded, puffs or twists, cheese-flavor	5.85	36.01	560	52.13
Snacks, KRAFT, CORNNUTS, plain	8.5	15.64	446	64.96
Snacks, crisped rice bar, chocolate chip	5.1	13.5	404	70.8
Snacks, granola bars, hard, plain	10.1	19.8	471	59.1
Snacks, granola bars, hard, almond	7.7	25.5	495	57.2
Snacks, granola bars, hard, chocolate chip	7.3	16.3	438	67.7
Snacks, granola bars, soft, uncoated, plain	7.4	17.2	443	62.7
Snacks, granola bars, soft, uncoated, peanut butter	10.5	15.8	426	60.1
Snacks, granola bars, soft, uncoated, raisin	7.6	17.8	448	62.2
Snacks, granola bars, soft, coated, milk chocolate coating, chocolate chip	5.8	24.9	466	60.4
Snacks, granola bars, soft, coated, milk chocolate coating, peanut butter	10.2	31.1	508	50.6
Snacks, granola bars, soft, uncoated, peanut butter and chocolate chip	9.8	20	432	58
Snacks, oriental mix, rice-based	17.31	25.58	506	38.42
Snacks, GENERAL MILLS, CHEX MIX, traditional flavor	8.83	10	428	69.89
Snacks, popcorn, air-popped	12.94	4.54	387	63.28
Snacks, popcorn, oil-popped, microwave, regular flavor, no trans fat	7.29	43.55	583	36.96
Snacks, popcorn, cakes	9.7	3.1	384	77.2
Snacks, popcorn, caramel-coated, with peanuts	6.4	7.8	400	76.9
Snacks, popcorn, caramel-coated, without peanuts	3.8	12.8	431	73.9
Snacks, popcorn, cheese-flavor	9.3	33.2	526	41.7
Snacks, pork skins, plain	61.3	31.3	544	0

Food Name ---> per 100 g	Protein (g)	Fat (g)	Calorie	Net Carb (g)
Snacks, potato chips, barbecue-flavor	6.51	31.06	487	52.12
Snacks, potato chips, sour-cream-and-onion-flavor	8.1	33.9	531	46.3
Snacks, potato chips, made from dried potatoes, reduced fat	4.56	26.14	502	61.56
Snacks, potato chips, made from dried potatoes, sour-cream and onion-flavor	6.6	37	547	50.1
Snacks, pretzels, hard, plain, salted	10.04	2.93	384	76.99
Snacks, pretzels, hard, confectioner's coating, chocolate-flavor	7.5	16.7	457	68.5
Snacks, M&M MARS, COMBOS Snacks Cheddar Cheese Pretzel	9.85	16.92	463	62.9
Snacks, pretzels, hard, whole-wheat including both salted and unsalted	11.1	2.6	362	73.6
Snacks, rice cracker brown rice, plain	8.2	2.8	387	77.3
Snacks, rice cakes, brown rice, buckwheat	9	3.5	380	76.3
Snacks, rice cakes, brown rice, sesame seed	7.6	3.8	392	76.1
Snacks, tortilla chips, plain, white corn, salted	7.1	20.68	472	62.38
Snacks, tortilla chips, nacho cheese	7.36	27.42	519	55.71
Snacks, tortilla chips, ranch-flavor	7.19	24.63	501	58.74
Snacks, trail mix, regular	13.8	29.4	462	44.9
Snacks, trail mix, tropical	6.3	17.1	442	65.6
Snacks, trail mix, regular, with chocolate chips, salted nuts and seeds	14.2	31.9	484	39.9
Snacks, tortilla chips, taco-flavor	7.9	24.2	480	57.8
Snacks, GENERAL MILLS, BETTY CROCKER Fruit Roll Ups, berry flavored, with vitamin C	0.1	3.5	373	85.2
Snacks, FARLEY CANDY, FARLEY Fruit Snacks, with vitamins A, C, and E	4.4	0	341	80.9
Snacks, SUNKIST, SUNKIST Fruit Roll, strawberry, with vitamins A, C, and E	0.6	1	342	75
Snacks, fruit leather, pieces, with vitamin C	0.1	3.5	373	81.7
Snacks, banana chips	2.3	33.6	519	50.7
Snacks, cornnuts, barbecue-flavor	9	14.3	436	63.3
Snacks, crisped rice bar, almond	7	20.4	458	61
Snacks, granola bars, soft, uncoated, chocolate chip	5.65	16.57	418	66.4
Snacks, granola bars, soft, uncoated, chocolate chip, graham and marshmallow	6.1	15.5	427	66.8

Food Name ---> per 100 g	Protein (g)	Fat (g)	Calorie	Net Carb (g)
Snacks, granola bars, soft, uncoated, nut and raisin	8	20.4	454	58
Snacks, beef sticks, smoked	21.5	49.6	550	5.4
Snacks, pork skins, barbecue-flavor	57.9	31.8	538	1.6
Snack, potato chips, made from dried potatoes, plain	4.62	35.28	545	52.48
Snacks, potato chips, plain, salted	6.39	33.98	532	50.73
Snacks, potato chips, made from dried potatoes, cheese-flavor	7	37	551	47.2
Snacks, rice cakes, brown rice, corn	8.4	3.2	385	78.3
Snacks, rice cakes, brown rice, multigrain	8.5	3.5	387	77.1
Snacks, potato sticks	6.7	34.4	522	49.9
Snacks, rice cakes, brown rice, rye	8.1	3.8	386	75.9
Snacks, sesame sticks, wheat-based, salted	10.9	36.7	541	43.7
Snacks, corn cakes	8.1	2.4	387	81.5
Snacks, granola bars, hard, peanut butter	9.8	23.8	483	59.4
Snacks, potato chips, cheese-flavor	8.5	27.2	496	52.5
Snacks, potato chips, reduced fat	7.1	20.8	471	61
Snacks, potato chips, fat-free, made with olestra	7.74	0.7	274	58.2
Snacks, tortilla chips, nacho-flavor, reduced fat	8.7	15.2	445	66.8
Tortilla chips, low fat, baked without fat	11	5.7	415	74.7
Cheese puffs and twists, corn based, baked, low fat	8.5	12.1	432	68.75
Snacks, granola bar, fruit-filled, nonfat	5.9	0.9	342	70.2
Popcorn, sugar syrup/caramel, fat-free	2	1.4	381	87.56
Snacks, potato chips, fat free, salted	9.64	0.6	379	76.26
Snacks, KELLOGG, KELLOGG'S RICE KRISPIES TREATS Squares	3.4	9	414	80.5
Snacks, KELLOGG, KELLOGG'S Low Fat Granola Bar, Crunchy Almond/Brown Sugar	8	7.4	390	71.8
Snacks, M&M MARS, KUDOS Whole Grain Bar, chocolate chip	4.47	13.02	420	69.71
Snacks, KELLOGG'S, NUTRI-GRAIN Cereal Bars, fruit	4.22	8.67	365	64.61
Snacks, tortilla chips, low fat, made with olestra, nacho cheese	8.44	3.53	318	58.82
Snacks, potato chips, made from dried potatoes, fat-free, made with olestra	5.06	0.93	253	48.7
Snacks, taro chips	2.3	24.9	498	60.9

Food Name ---> per 100 g	Protein (g)	Fat (g)	Calorie	Net Carb (g)
Snacks, corn cakes, very low sodium	8.1	2.4	387	83.4
Snacks, corn-based, extruded, puffs or twists, cheese-flavor, unenriched	5.76	35.76	558	51.9
Snacks, corn-based, extruded, chips, barbecue-flavor, made with enriched masa flour	7	32.7	523	56.2
Snacks, popcorn, air-popped (Unsalted)	12	4.2	382	62.8
Snacks, popcorn, oil-popped, white popcorn, salt added	9	28.1	500	47.2
Snacks, potato chips, plain, made with partially hydrogenated soybean oil, salted	7	34.6	536	48.1
Snacks, potato chips, plain, made with partially hydrogenated soybean oil, unsalted	7	34.6	536	48.1
Snacks, potato chips, plain, unsalted	7	34.6	536	48.1
Snacks, pretzels, hard, plain, made with unenriched flour, salted	9.1	3.5	381	76.4
Snacks, pretzels, hard, plain, made with unenriched flour, unsalted	9.1	3.5	381	76.4
Snacks, pretzels, hard, plain, made with enriched flour, unsalted	9.1	3.5	381	76.4
Snacks, rice cakes, brown rice, plain, unsalted	8.2	2.8	387	77.3
Snacks, rice cakes, brown rice, buckwheat, unsalted	9	3.5	380	80.1
Snacks, rice cakes, brown rice, multigrain, unsalted	8.5	3.5	387	80.1
Snacks, rice cakes, brown rice, sesame seed, unsalted	7.6	3.8	392	81.5
Snacks, sesame sticks, wheat-based, unsalted	10.9	36.7	541	46.5
Snacks, trail mix, regular, unsalted	13.8	29.4	462	44.9
Snacks, trail mix, regular, with chocolate chips, unsalted nuts and seeds	14.2	31.9	484	44.9
Potato chips, without salt, reduced fat	7.1	20.8	487	61.7
Snacks, tortilla chips, low fat, unsalted	11	5.7	416	74.8
Snacks, tortilla chips, nacho-flavor, made with enriched masa flour	7.8	25.6	498	57.1
Snacks, popcorn, microwave, 94% fat free	10.72	6.1	402	62.44
Snacks, popcorn, microwave, low fat	12.6	9.5	424	57.8
Snacks, candy rolls, yogurt-covered, fruit flavored with high vitamin C	0.46	6.53	359	71.34
Formulated bar, MARS SNACKFOOD US, SNICKERS MARATHON Chewy Chocolate Peanut Bar	24.29	13.12	396	44.74

Food Name ---> per 100 g	Protein (g)	Fat (g)	Calorie	Net Carb (g)
Formulated bar, MARS SNACKFOOD US, SNICKERS MARATHON MULTIGRAIN CRUNCH BAR	18.49	13.18	422	54.47
Formulated bar, MARS SNACKFOOD US, SNICKERS MARATHON Double Chocolate Nut Bar	22.35	8.99	343	41.97
Snacks, M&M MARS, KUDOS Whole Grain Bars, peanut butter	5.88	20.78	463	62.09
Formulated bar, MARS SNACKFOOD US, SNICKERS MARATHON Honey Nut Oat Bar	22.5	7.87	378	43.3
Snacks, M&M MARS, KUDOS Whole Grain Bar, M&M's milk chocolate	3.78	11.95	415	70.61
Formulated bar, MARS SNACKFOOD US, COCOAVIA, Chocolate Almond Snack Bar	7.72	14.19	347	46.48
Snacks, sweet potato chips, unsalted	2.94	32.35	532	48.02
Snacks, FRITOLAY, SUNCHIPS, Multigrain Snack, original flavor	7.95	21.11	491	58.46
Snacks, popcorn, microwave, regular (butter) flavor, made with partially hydrogenated oil	7.5	34.02	557	45.16
Formulated bar, MARS SNACKFOOD US, SNICKERS MARATHON Protein Performance Bar, Caramel Nut Rush	25	12.5	415	38
Formulated bar, MARS SNACKFOOD US, SNICKERS MARATHON Energy Bar, all flavors	21.91	10.79	386	43.6
Formulated bar, POWER BAR, chocolate	14.15	3.11	363	63.93
Formulated bar, MARS SNACKFOOD US, COCOAVIA, Chocolate Blueberry Snack Bar	6.21	9.27	325	53.27
Formulated bar, SLIM-FAST OPTIMA meal bar, milk chocolate peanut	16.19	8.92	386	55.11
Formulated bar, LUNA BAR, NUTZ OVER CHOCOLATE	20.75	12.19	403	48.19
Snacks, FRITOLAY, SUNCHIPS, multigrain, French onion flavor	8.68	22.15	496	57.69
Snacks, FRITOLAY, SUNCHIPS, Multigrain Snack, Harvest Cheddar flavor	8.08	22.22	491	56.6
Pretzels, soft, unsalted	8.2	3.1	345	69.34
Snacks, soy chips or crisps, salted	26.5	7.35	385	49.65
Popcorn, microwave, regular (butter) flavor, made with palm oil	8.38	30.22	535	47.26
Snacks, plantain chips, salted	2.28	29.59	531	60.34
Tortilla chips, yellow, plain, salted	6.62	22.33	497	62.68

Food Name ---> per 100 g	Protein (g)	Fat (g)	Calorie	Net Carb (g)
Snacks, vegetable chips, HAIN CELESTIAL GROUP, TERRA CHIPS	4.13	29.81	517	47.07
Formulated bar, ZONE PERFECT CLASSIC CRUNCH BAR, mixed flavors	30	14	422	43
Snacks, granola bar, KASHI GOLEAN, chewy, mixed flavors	16.67	7.69	390	55.72
Snacks, granola bar, KASHI TLC Bar, chewy, mixed flavors	18.57	15.71	429	41.86
Snacks, granola bar, KASHI GOLEAN, crunchy, mixed flavors	17.88	9.23	393	53.68
Snacks, granola bar, chewy, reduced sugar, all flavors	5.55	12.5	412	66.3
Snacks, granola bites, mixed flavors	7.17	17.5	451	60.57
Snacks, pita chips, salted	11.79	15.2	457	64.46
Snacks, granola bars, soft, almond, confectioners coating	8.6	20	455	55.83
Snacks, granola bars, QUAKER OATMEAL TO GO, all flavors	6.67	6.67	389	70.87
Snacks, vegetable chips, made from garden vegetables	5.32	23.3	473	55.73
Snacks, granola bar, KASHI TLC Bar, crunchy, mixed flavors	15	15	446	52.78
Snacks, candy bits, yogurt covered with vitamin C	0	7.5	415	86.7
Formulated bar, high fiber, chewy, oats and chocolate	5	10	350	47.28
Snacks, bagel chips, plain	12.34	15.14	451	62.26
Snacks, NUTRI-GRAIN FRUIT AND NUT BAR	9.38	10.93	403	59.22
Snacks, yucca (cassava) chips, salted	1.34	25.91	515	65.53
Snacks, CLIF BAR, mixed flavors	14.71	5.88	346	58.04
Snacks, granola bar, QUAKER, chewy, 90 Calorie Bar	4.17	8.33	408	74.97
Snacks, granola bar, GENERAL MILLS NATURE VALLEY, SWEET&SALTY NUT, peanut	9.14	22.86	487	58.24
Snacks, granola bar, GENERAL MILLS, NATURE VALLEY, with yogurt coating	5.71	11.43	423	69.89
Snacks, granola bar, GENERAL MILLS, NATURE VALLEY, CHEWY TRAIL MIX	5.71	11.43	415	68.47
Snacks, granola bar, QUAKER, DIPPS, all flavors	7.52	20.42	480	61.76
Snacks, brown rice chips	8.2	2.8	384	77.3
Snack, Pretzel, hard chocolate coated	7.05	17.64	467	66.57
Snack, Mixed Berry Bar	13.16	10.53	383	50.94
Snacks, potato chips, made from dried potatoes (preformed), multigrain	5.3	24.74	505	62.64

Food Name ---> per 100 g	Protein (g)	Fat (g)	Calorie	Net Carb (g)
Snacks, potato chips, lightly salted	6.72	35.39	560	49.34
Snacks, Pretzels, gluten- free made with cornstarch and potato flour	3.52	6.67	389	75.32
Snacks, peas, roasted, wasabi-flavored	14.11	14.11	432	58.4
Formulated Bar, SOUTH BEACH protein bar	30.34	15.17	412	31.1
Snack, BALANCE, original bar	28	12	415	45.63
Snacks, shrimp cracker	7.14	17.86	426	53.49
Rice crackers	10	5	416	82.64
Granola bar, soft, milk chocolate coated, peanut butter	9.6	31.2	536	50.3
Rice cake, cracker (include hain mini rice cakes)	7.1	4.3	392	76.9
Snacks, popcorn, home-prepared, oil-popped, unsalted	9	28.1	500	48.1
Snacks, granola bar, with coconut, chocolate coated	5.2	32.2	531	49
Snacks, potato chips, white, restructured, baked	5	18.2	469	66.6
Breakfast bars, oats, sugar, raisins, coconut (include granola bar)	9.8	17.6	464	63.6
Pretzels, soft	8.2	3.1	338	67.69
Snacks, tortilla chips, unsalted, white corn	7.79	23.36	503	60.02
Snacks, corn-based, extruded, chips, unsalted	6.6	33.4	557	53
Snacks, tortilla chips, light (baked with less oil)	8.7	15.2	465	67.7
Popcorn, microwave, low fat and sodium	12.6	9.5	429	59.19
Breakfast bar, corn flake crust with fruit	4.4	7.5	377	70.8

Soups, Sauces, and Gravies

Food Name ---> per 100 g	Protein (g)	Fat (g)	Calorie	Net Carb (g)
Soup, egg drop, Chinese restaurant	1.16	0.61	27	3.89
Soup, hot and sour, Chinese restaurant	2.58	1.21	39	3.85
Soup, wonton, Chinese restaurant	2.08	0.26	32	5.05
CAMPBELL'S CHUNKY Soups, HEALTHY REQUEST Microwavable Bowls, Chicken Noodle Soup	2.86	1.02	49	6.54
CAMPBELL'S CHUNKY Soups, HEALTHY REQUEST Microwavable Bowls, Grilled Chicken & Sausage Gumbo Soup	2.86	1.22	53	6.55
CAMPBELL'S CHUNKY Soups, HEALTHY REQUEST New England Clam Chowder	2.04	1.22	53	7.36
CAMPBELL'S Red and White, Chicken Barley with Mushrooms Soup, condensed	3.17	1.19	71	10.3
CAMPBELL'S Red and White, Italian Style Wedding Soup, condensed	3.17	1.98	71	7.12
CAMPBELL'S Red and White, PHINEAS and FERB Soup, condensed	2.38	1.59	56	7.93
CAMPBELL'S Homestyle Microwaveable Bowls, HEALTHY REQUEST Italian Wedding Soup	2.45	1.02	41	4.51
CAMPBELL'S Homestyle Microwaveable Bowls, HEALTHY REQUEST Mexican Style Tortilla	2.86	1.02	53	6.56
CAMPBELL'S Homestyle Harvest Tomato with Basil Soup	0.82	0.41	45	8.59
CAMPBELL'S Homestyle HEALTHY REQUEST Chicken with Whole Grain Pasta Soup	3.8	0.82	40	3.58
CAMPBELL'S Soup on the GO, HEALTHY REQUEST Chicken with Mini Noodles Soup	0.98	0.66	20	1.92
CAMPBELL'S Soup on the Go, HEALTHY REQUEST Classic Tomato Soup	0.98	0	39	8.48
PACE, Pico De Gallo	0	0	31	9.38
PACE, Salsa Verde	0	1.56	47	6.25
PACE, Tequila Lime Salsa	0	0	47	9.38
PACE, Triple Pepper Salsa	3.13	0	47	6.28

Food Name ---> per 100 g	Protein (g)	Fat (g)	Calorie	Net Carb (g)
CAMPBELL'S Red and White, Lentil Soup, condensed	6.35	0.79	111	15.05
PREGO Pasta, Heart Smart- Traditional Sauce, ready-to-serve	1.54	1.15	54	7.7
CAMPBELL'S, 98% Fat Free Cream of Mushroom Soup, condensed	1.1	1.98	53	6.43
Soup, ramen noodle, dry, any flavor, reduced fat, reduced sodium	10.89	2.5	350	68.25
Soup, clam chowder, new england, canned, ready-to-serve	2.61	3.94	79	7.28
Soup, clam chowder, new england, reduced sodium, canned, ready-to-serve	2.33	4.23	70	4.88
Soup, chicken noodle, reduced sodium, canned, ready-to-serve	3.29	1.34	41	3.04
Soup, beef and vegetables, reduced sodium, canned, ready-to-serve	3.26	0.95	42	4.19
Sauce, duck, ready-to-serve	0.36	0.13	245	60.01
Sauce, salsa, verde, ready-to-serve	1.13	0.89	38	4.46
Sauce, steak, tomato based	1.25	0.23	95	20.54
Sauce, tartar, ready-to-serve	1	16.7	211	12.8
Sauce, sweet and sour, ready-to-serve	0.27	0.02	150	38.12
Sauce, cocktail, ready-to-serve	1.36	1.05	124	26.42
Dip, salsa con queso, cheese and salsa- medium	3.14	9.51	143	10.44
Dip, OLD EL PASO, Cheese 'n Salsa, medium	2.7	8.43	129	10.05
Dip, TOSTITOS, salsa con queso, medium	2.92	8.26	133	11.12
Sauce, barbecue, SWEET BABY RAY'S, original	0.95	0.43	192	44.78
Sauce, barbecue, BULL'S-EYE, original	0.91	0.67	170	38.95
Sauce, barbecue, KC MASTERPIECE, original	1	0.52	160	36.52
Sauce, barbecue, OPEN PIT, original	0.44	1.41	132	28.95
Sauce, peanut, made from peanut butter, water, soy sauce	6.31	16.02	257	20.22
Soup, chunky vegetable, reduced sodium, canned, ready-to-serve	1.16	0.51	50	9.18
Gravy, HEINZ Home Style, classic chicken	0.67	2.57	46	5.01
Soup, beef barley, ready to serve	2.81	0.96	52	7.04
Sauce, enchilada, red, mild, ready to serve	0.62	0.91	30	4.37
Wasabi	2.23	10.9	292	40.03
Dip, bean, original flavor	5.44	3.7	119	10.99

Food Name ---> per 100 g	Protein (g)	Fat (g)	Calorie	Net Carb (g)
Sauce, horseradish	1.09	50.89	503	9.05
Sauce, OLD EL PASO, enchilada, red, mild, ready to serve	0.59	0.67	29	4.44
Dip, FRITO'S, bean, original flavor	5.44	3.7	119	10.99

Spices and Herbs

Food Name ---> per 100 g	Protein (g)	Fat (g)	Calories	Net Carbs
Spices, allspice, ground	6.09	8.69	263	50.52
Spices, anise seed	17.6	15.9	337	35.42
Spices, basil, dried	22.98	4.07	233	10.05
Spices, bay leaf	7.61	8.36	313	48.67
Spices, caraway seed	19.77	14.59	333	11.9
Spices, cardamom	10.76	6.7	311	40.47
Spices, celery seed	18.07	25.27	392	29.55
Spices, chervil, dried	23.2	3.9	237	37.8
Spices, chili powder	13.46	14.28	282	14.9
Spices, cinnamon, ground	3.99	1.24	247	27.49
Spices, cloves, ground	5.97	13	274	31.63
Spices, coriander leaf, dried	21.93	4.78	279	41.7
Spices, coriander seed	12.37	17.77	298	13.09
Spices, cumin seed	17.81	22.27	375	33.74
Spices, curry powder	14.29	14.01	325	2.63
Spices, dill seed	15.98	14.54	305	34.07
Spices, dill weed, dried	19.96	4.36	253	42.22
Spices, fennel seed	15.8	14.87	345	12.49
Spices, fenugreek seed	23	6.41	323	33.75
Spices, garlic powder	16.55	0.73	331	63.73
Spices, ginger, ground	8.98	4.24	335	57.52
Spices, mace, ground	6.71	32.38	475	30.3
Spices, marjoram, dried	12.66	7.04	271	20.26
Spices, mustard seed, ground	26.08	36.24	508	15.89
Spices, nutmeg, ground	5.84	36.31	525	28.49
Spices, onion powder	10.41	1.04	341	63.92
Spices, oregano, dried	9	4.28	265	26.42
Spices, paprika	14.14	12.89	282	19.09
Spices, parsley, dried	26.63	5.48	292	23.94

Food Name ---> per 100 g	Protein (g)	Fat (g)	Calories	Net Carbs
Spices, pepper, black	10.39	3.26	251	38.65
Spices, pepper, red or cayenne	12.01	17.27	318	29.43
Spices, pepper, white	10.4	2.12	296	42.41
Spices, poppy seed	17.99	41.56	525	8.63
Spices, poultry seasoning	9.59	7.53	307	54.29
Spices, pumpkin pie spice	5.76	12.6	342	54.48
Spices, rosemary, dried	4.88	15.22	331	21.46
Spices, saffron	11.43	5.85	310	61.47
Spices, sage, ground	10.63	12.75	315	20.43
Spices, savory, ground	6.73	5.91	272	23.03
Spices, tarragon, dried	22.77	7.24	295	42.82
Spices, thyme, dried	9.11	7.43	276	26.94
Spices, turmeric, ground	9.68	3.25	312	44.44
Basil, fresh	3.15	0.64	23	1.05
Dill weed, fresh	3.46	1.12	43	4.92
Mustard, prepared, yellow	3.74	3.34	60	1.83
Salt, table	0	0	0	0
Vinegar, cider	0	0	21	0.93
Thyme, fresh	5.56	1.68	101	10.45
Vanilla extract	0.06	0.06	288	12.65
Vanilla extract, imitation, alcohol	0.05	0	237	2.41
Vanilla extract, imitation, no alcohol	0.03	0	56	14.4
Vinegar, distilled	0	0	18	0.04
Capers, canned	2.36	0.86	23	1.69
Horseradish, prepared	1.18	0.69	48	7.99
Rosemary, fresh	3.31	5.86	131	6.6
Peppermint, fresh	3.75	0.94	70	6.89
Spearmint, fresh	3.29	0.73	44	1.61
Spearmint, dried	19.93	6.03	285	22.24
Vinegar, red wine	0.04	0	19	0.27
Vinegar, balsamic	0.49	0	88	17.03

Food Name ---> per 100 g	Protein (g)	Fat (g)	Calories	Net Carbs
PACE, Dry Taco Seasoning Mix	0	0	188	37.49
Seasoning mix, dry, sazon, coriander & annatto	0	0	0	0
Seasoning mix, dry, taco, original	4.5	0	322	44.7
Seasoning mix, dry, chili, original	10.82	7.3	335	45.76

Sweets

Food Name ---> per 100 g	Protein (g)	Fat (g)	Calories	Net Carb (g)
SCHIFF, TIGER'S MILK BAR	16.8	14.29	422	54.16
Candies, TOBLERONE, milk chocolate with honey and almond nougat	5.71	28.57	525	58.71
Snacks, fruit leather, pieces	1	2.68	359	82.82
Snacks, fruit leather, rolls	0.1	3	371	85.8
Fruit syrup	0	0	341	85.03
Candies, honey-combed, with peanut butter	8.72	20.18	486	65.51
Topping, SMUCKER'S MAGIC SHELL	2.94	44.1	609	47.17
Syrup, fruit flavored	0	0.02	261	65.1
Candies, TOOTSIE ROLL, chocolate-flavor roll	1.59	3.31	387	87.63
Candies, ALMOND JOY Candy Bar	4.13	26.93	479	54.51
Candies, TWIZZLERS CHERRY BITES	2.97	1.7	338	79.28
Candies, NESTLE, BIT-O'-HONEY Candy Chews	2	7.5	375	80.69
Candies, NESTLE, BUTTERFINGER Bar	5.4	18.9	459	70.9
Candies, butterscotch	0.03	3.3	391	90.4
Candies, carob, unsweetened	8.15	31.36	540	52.49
Candies, caramels	4.6	8.1	382	77
Candies, CARAMELLO Candy Bar	6.19	21.19	462	62.61
Candies, caramels, chocolate-flavor roll	1.59	3.31	387	87.63
Baking chocolate, unsweetened, liquid	12.1	47.7	472	18.1
Baking chocolate, unsweetened, squares	14.32	52.31	642	11.82
Candies, confectioner's coating, yogurt	5.87	27	522	63.94
Candies, semisweet chocolate	4.2	30	480	58
Candies, sweet chocolate	3.9	34.2	507	54.9
Candies, sweet chocolate coated fondant	2.2	9.3	366	78.3
Candies, HERSHEY'S GOLDEN ALMOND SOLITAIRES	11.97	37.13	569	42.45
Candies, confectioner's coating, butterscotch	2.2	29.05	539	67.1
Candies, confectioner's coating, peanut butter	18.3	29.8	529	41.88
Candies, white chocolate	5.87	32.09	539	59.04

Food Name ---> per 100 g	Protein (g)	Fat (g)	Calories	Net Carb (g)
Ice creams, vanilla, light	4.78	4.83	180	29.16
Ice creams, vanilla, rich	3.5	16.2	249	22.29
Ice creams, french vanilla, soft-serve	4.1	13	222	21.5
Candies, YORK Peppermint Pattie	2.19	7.17	384	78.99
Candies, TWIZZLERS NIBS CHERRY BITS	2.3	2.64	347	78.77
Candies, SYMPHONY Milk Chocolate Bar	8.51	30.57	531	56.31
Desserts, flan, caramel custard, prepared-from-recipe	4.53	4.03	145	22.78
Ice creams, vanilla	3.5	11	207	22.9
Ice creams, vanilla, light, soft-serve	4.9	2.6	126	21.8
Sherbet, orange	1.1	2	144	29.1
Candies, 5TH AVENUE Candy Bar	8.78	23.98	482	59.58
Candies, fondant, prepared-from-recipe	0	0.02	373	93.18
Candies, fudge, chocolate, prepared-from-recipe	2.39	10.41	411	74.74
Candies, fudge, chocolate, with nuts, prepared-from-recipe	4.38	18.93	461	65.43
Candies, fudge, peanut butter, prepared-from-recipe	3.78	6.59	387	77.05
Candies, fudge, vanilla, prepared-from-recipe	1.05	5.45	383	82.15
Candies, fudge, vanilla with nuts	3	13.69	435	73.71
Candies, NESTLE, GOOBERS Chocolate Covered Peanuts	9.7	34	512	43.3
Candies, gumdrops, starch jelly pieces	0	0	396	98.8
Candies, hard	0	0.2	394	98
Candies, jellybeans	0	0.05	375	93.35
Candies, KIT KAT Wafer Bar	6.51	25.99	518	63.59
Candies, KRACKEL Chocolate Bar	6.62	26.58	512	61.76
Candies, NESTLE, BABY RUTH Bar	5.4	21.6	459	62.8
Candies, TWIZZLERS Strawberry Twists Candy	2.56	2.32	348	79.16
Syrups, table blends, pancake, with butter	0	0.09	291	72.43
Ice creams, chocolate, light	5	7.19	187	24.9
Candies, MARS SNACKFOOD US, MARS Almond Bar	8.1	23	467	60.7
Candies, marshmallows	1.8	0.2	318	81.2
Candies, halavah, plain	12.49	21.52	469	55.99
Candies, NESTLE, OH HENRY! Bar	7.7	23	462	63.6

Food Name ---> per 100 g	Protein (g)	Fat (g)	Calories	Net Carb (g)
Candies, NESTLE, CHUNKY Bar	7.5	27.5	475	57.5
Candies, milk chocolate	7.65	29.66	535	56
Puddings, banana, dry mix, instant, prepared with 2% milk	2.76	1.7	105	19.74
Puddings, banana, dry mix, regular, prepared with 2% milk	2.9	1.73	101	18.43
Puddings, chocolate, dry mix, instant, prepared with 2% milk	3.15	1.92	105	18.49
Baking chocolate, mexican, squares	3.64	15.59	426	73.41
Chocolate-flavored hazelnut spread	5.41	29.73	541	56.76
Candies, milk chocolate coated peanuts	13.1	33.5	519	45
Candies, milk chocolate coated raisins	4.1	14.8	390	65.3
Syrups, table blends, pancake, reduced-calorie	0	0	165	44.55
Syrups, table blends, pancake	0	0	234	61.47
Candies, HERSHEY'S POT OF GOLD Almond Bar	12.82	38.46	577	41.09
Candies, milk chocolate, with almonds	9	34.4	526	47.2
Candies, milk chocolate, with rice cereal	7.64	29.37	511	56.37
Candies, MARS SNACKFOOD US, MILKY WAY Bar	4.01	17.23	456	70.17
Candies, HERSHEY'S SKOR Toffee Bar	3.13	30.37	541	62.43
Toppings, strawberry	0.2	0.1	254	65.6
Candies, truffles, prepared-from-recipe	6.21	33.76	510	42.38
Baking chocolate, MARS SNACKFOOD US, M&M's Semisweet Chocolate Mini Baking Bits	4.44	26.15	517	59.26
Candies, MARS SNACKFOOD US, M&M's Peanut Chocolate Candies	9.57	26.13	515	56.78
Candies, MARS SNACKFOOD US, M&M's Milk Chocolate Candies	4.33	21.13	492	68.39
Candies, MOUNDS Candy Bar	4.6	26.6	486	54.89
Candies, MR. GOODBAR Chocolate Bar	10.22	33.21	538	50.54
Candies, NESTLE, 100 GRAND Bar	2.5	19.33	468	69.97
Candies, NESTLE, CRUNCH Bar and Dessert Topping	5	26	500	65.1
Baking chocolate, MARS SNACKFOOD US, M&M's Milk Chocolate Mini Baking Bits	4.78	23.36	502	65.7
Candies, peanut bar	15.5	33.7	522	43.3
Candies, peanut brittle, prepared-from-recipe	7.57	18.98	486	68.74
Candies, NESTLE, RAISINETS Chocolate Covered Raisins	4.4	17	422	68.8

Food Name ---> per 100 g	Protein (g)	Fat (g)	Calories	Net Carb (g)
Candies, REESE'S Peanut Butter Cups	10.24	30.53	515	51.76
Candies, REESE'S PIECES Candy	12.46	24.77	497	56.86
Candies, ROLO Caramels in Milk Chocolate	5.08	20.93	474	67.05
Candies, NESTLE, AFTER EIGHT Mints	1.67	11.9	432	77.13
Candies, sesame crunch	11.6	33.3	516	42.6
Candies, MARS SNACKFOOD US, SNICKERS Bar	7.53	23.85	491	59.21
Candies, MARS SNACKFOOD US, STARBURST Fruit Chews, Original fruits	0.41	8.21	408	82.57
Candies, MARS SNACKFOOD US, M&M's MINIs Milk Chocolate Candies	4.78	23.36	502	65.7
Candies, MARS SNACKFOOD US, 3 MUSKETEERS Bar	2.6	12.75	436	76.27
Candies, MARS SNACKFOOD US, TWIX Caramel Cookie Bars	4.91	24.85	502	63.7
Candies, MARS SNACKFOOD US, TWIX Peanut Butter Cookie Bars	9.18	32.67	536	51.05
Candies, WHATCHAMACALLIT Candy Bar	8.04	23.68	494	61.33
Chewing gum	0	0.3	360	94.3
Candies, SPECIAL DARK Chocolate Bar	5.54	32.4	556	53.99
Cocoa, dry powder, unsweetened	19.6	13.7	228	20.9
Cocoa, dry powder, unsweetened, processed with alkali	18.1	13.1	220	28.5
Desserts, egg custard, baked, prepared-from-recipe	5.02	4.58	104	11
Egg custards, dry mix	6.9	6.4	410	82.8
Egg custards, dry mix, prepared with whole milk	3.99	4	122	17.6
Cocoa, dry powder, unsweetened, HERSHEY'S European Style Cocoa	20	10	410	40
Gelatin desserts, dry mix	7.8	0	381	90.5
Gelatin desserts, dry mix, prepared with water	1.22	0	62	14.19
Gelatin desserts, dry mix, reduced calorie, with aspartame	15.67	0	198	80.11
Gelatin desserts, dry mix, reduced calorie, with aspartame, prepared with water	0.83	0	20	4.22
Gelatins, dry powder, unsweetened	85.6	0.1	335	0
Candies, YORK BITES	1.78	7.32	394	79.64
Desserts, mousse, chocolate, prepared-from-recipe	4.14	16	225	15.47

Food Name ---> per 100 g	Protein (g)	Fat (g)	Calories	Net Carb (g)
Puddings, chocolate, ready-to-eat	2.09	4.6	142	23.01
Puddings, chocolate, dry mix, instant	2.3	1.9	378	84.3
Puddings, chocolate, dry mix, instant, prepared with whole milk	3.1	3.1	111	17.8
Desserts, apple crisp, prepared-from-recipe	1.75	3.43	161	29.44
Flan, caramel custard, dry mix	0	0	348	91.6
Puddings, chocolate, dry mix, regular	2.6	2.1	362	84.8
Puddings, chocolate, dry mix, regular, prepared with whole milk	3.16	3.15	120	18.84
Puddings, chocolate, dry mix, regular, prepared with 2% milk	3.28	2.06	111	18.96
Puddings, coconut cream, dry mix, instant, prepared with 2% milk	2.9	2.3	107	19.1
Puddings, rice, ready-to-eat	3.23	2.15	108	18.09
Puddings, rice, dry mix	2.7	0.1	376	90.5
Puddings, rice, dry mix, prepared with whole milk	3.25	2.82	121	20.58
Puddings, tapioca, dry mix	0.1	0.1	369	94.1
Puddings, tapioca, dry mix, prepared with whole milk	2.84	2.89	115	19.43
Puddings, vanilla, ready-to-eat	1.45	3.78	130	22.6
Puddings, vanilla, dry mix, instant	0	0.6	377	92.9
Puddings, vanilla, dry mix, instant, prepared with whole milk	2.7	2.9	114	19.7
Puddings, lemon, dry mix, instant, prepared with 2% milk	2.76	1.71	107	20.2
Egg custards, dry mix, prepared with 2% milk	4.13	2.83	112	17.61
Puddings, vanilla, dry mix, regular	0.3	0.4	379	92.9
Puddings, vanilla, dry mix, regular, prepared with whole milk	2.8	2.9	113	18.82
Puddings, rice, dry mix, prepared with 2% milk	3.29	1.63	111	20.71
Puddings, tapioca, dry mix, prepared with 2% milk	2.88	1.67	105	19.56
Puddings, vanilla, dry mix, regular, prepared with 2% milk	2.94	1.73	101	18.53
Rennin, chocolate, dry mix, prepared with 2% milk	3.24	2.06	85	12.97
Rennin, vanilla, dry mix, prepared with 2% milk	3.06	1.77	77	12.34
Candies, praline, prepared-from-recipe	3.3	25.9	485	56.09
Frozen novelties, ice type, fruit, no sugar added	0.5	0.1	24	6.2

Food Name ---> per 100 g	Protein (g)	Fat (g)	Calories	Net Carb (g)
Puddings, tapioca, ready-to-eat	1.95	3.88	130	21.69
Puddings, coconut cream, dry mix, regular, prepared with 2% milk	3.1	2.5	104	17.6
Desserts, rennin, chocolate, dry mix	2.4	3.3	363	86.4
Rennin, chocolate, dry mix, prepared with whole milk	3.2	3.34	96	12.84
Desserts, rennin, vanilla, dry mix	0	0	383	99
Rennin, vanilla, dry mix, prepared with whole milk	3.03	3.07	89	12.21
Desserts, rennin, tablets, unsweetened	1	0.1	84	19.8
Frostings, chocolate, creamy, ready-to-eat	1.1	17.6	397	62.3
Frostings, coconut-nut, ready-to-eat	1.5	24	433	50.2
Frostings, cream cheese-flavor, ready-to-eat	0.1	17.3	415	67.32
Frostings, vanilla, creamy, ready-to-eat	0	16.23	418	67.89
Flan, caramel custard, dry mix, prepared with 2% milk	2.99	1.72	103	18.82
Flan, caramel custard, dry mix, prepared with whole milk	2.95	3	113	18.68
Puddings, vanilla, ready-to-eat, fat free	2.02	0	89	20.16
Puddings, tapioca, ready-to-eat, fat free	1.44	0.35	94	21.31
Puddings, chocolate, ready-to-eat, fat free	1.93	0.3	93	20.57
Candies, HERSHEY'S MILK CHOCOLATE WITH ALMOND BITES	9.76	35.73	568	48.12
Candies, REESE'S BITES	11.34	29.85	521	52.08
Candies, REESE'S NUTRAGEOUS Candy Bar	11.28	32.09	517	48.9
Frostings, chocolate, creamy, dry mix	1.3	5.2	389	89.6
Frostings, chocolate, creamy, dry mix, prepared with butter	1.11	13.06	408	69.9
Candies, HEATH BITES	3.94	30.38	530	61.39
Frostings, vanilla, creamy, dry mix	0.3	4.9	410	93.7
Frostings, white, fluffy, dry mix	2.3	0	371	94.9
Frostings, white, fluffy, dry mix, prepared with water	1.5	0	244	62.6
Candies, HERSHEY'S, ALMOND JOY BITES	5.58	34.5	563	53.24
Candies, HERSHEY, REESESTICKS crispy wafers, peanut butter, milk chocolate	9.53	31.34	521	52.08
Candies, HERSHEY, KIT KAT BIG KAT Bar	6.24	27.84	520	61.74
Candies, REESE'S, FAST BREAK, milk chocolate peanut butter and soft nougats	8.66	23.42	474	58.7

Food Name ---> per 100 g	Protein (g)	Fat (g)	Calories	Net Carb (g)
Candies, MARS SNACKFOOD US, DOVE Milk Chocolate	5.94	31.72	546	57.38
Candies, MARS SNACKFOOD US, DOVE Dark Chocolate	5.19	32.45	520	51.8
Candies, MARS SNACKFOOD US, MILKY WAY Caramels, milk chocolate covered	4.28	19.17	463	67.79
Candies, MARS SNACKFOOD US, MILKY WAY Caramels, dark chocolate covered	3.82	20.42	458	64.76
Ice creams, vanilla, light, no sugar added	3.97	7.45	169	21.42
Frozen novelties, fruit and juice bars	1.2	0.1	87	19.2
Ice creams, chocolate, light, no sugar added	3.54	5.74	173	25.89
Candies, dark chocolate coated coffee beans	7.5	30	540	52.45
Ice creams, chocolate	3.8	11	216	27
Ice creams, strawberry	3.2	8.4	192	26.7
Candies, milk chocolate coated coffee beans	7.41	33.18	549	49.55
Frozen novelties, ice type, lime	0.4	0	128	32.6
Frozen novelties, ice type, italian, restaurant-prepared	0.03	0.02	53	13.5
Frozen novelties, ice type, pop	0	0.24	79	19.23
Candies, MARS SNACKFOOD US, M&M's Crispy Chocolate Candies	4.28	19.32	475	70.4
Frozen yogurts, vanilla, soft-serve	4	5.6	159	24.2
Fruit butters, apple	0.39	0.3	173	40.97
Candies, MARS SNACKFOOD US, SNICKERS MUNCH bar	15.25	36.22	536	38.94
Honey	0.3	0	304	82.2
Jams and preserves	0.37	0.07	278	67.76
Jellies	0.15	0.02	266	68.95
Candies, fudge, chocolate marshmallow, with nuts, prepared-by-recipe	3.24	21.11	474	65.59
Candies, MARS SNACKFOOD US, SNICKERS Almond bar	5.4	22.4	472	62.07
Marmalade, orange	0.3	0	246	65.6
Molasses	0	0.1	290	74.73
Candies, MARS SNACKFOOD US, POP'ABLES SNICKERS Brand Bite Size Candies	7.15	24.32	480	58.77
Candies, MARS SNACKFOOD US, POP'ABLES MILKY WAY Brand Bite Size Candies	3.3	18	463	70.85

Food Name ---> per 100 g	Protein (g)	Fat (g)	Calories	Net Carb (g)
Candies, MARS SNACKFOOD US, POP'ABLES 3 MUSKETEERS Brand Bite Size Candies	2.59	15.17	443	74.64
Candies, MARS SNACKFOOD US, STARBURST Fruit Chews, Fruit and Creme	0.41	8.36	408	82.43
Pectin, unsweetened, dry mix	0.3	0.3	325	81.8
Pie fillings, apple, canned	0.1	0.1	100	25.1
Candies, MARS SNACKFOOD US, STARBURST Fruit Chews, Tropical fruits	0.41	8.31	409	82.76
Pie fillings, canned, cherry	0.37	0.07	115	27.4
Candies, MARS SNACKFOOD US, STARBURST Sour Fruit Chews	0.39	7.78	400	79.73
Puddings, banana, dry mix, instant	0	0.6	367	92.7
Puddings, banana, dry mix, instant, prepared with whole milk	2.62	2.8	115	19.76
Puddings, banana, dry mix, regular	0	0.4	366	92.7
Puddings, banana, dry mix, regular, prepared with whole milk	2.74	2.89	111	18.44
Puddings, coconut cream, dry mix, instant	0.9	10	415	79.5
Puddings, coconut cream, dry mix, instant, prepared with whole milk	2.9	3.5	117	19
Puddings, coconut cream, dry mix, regular	1	11.36	434	80.24
Puddings, coconut cream, dry mix, regular, prepared with whole milk	3	3.8	114	17.5
Candies, MARS SNACKFOOD US, COCOAVIA Chocolate Bar	5.81	29.3	539	54.29
Candies, MARS SNACKFOOD US, COCOAVIA Blueberry and Almond Chocolate Bar	6.35	28.68	525	51.27
Candies, MARS SNACKFOOD US, COCOAVIA Crispy Chocolate Bar	8.21	26.23	517	54.26
Puddings, lemon, dry mix, instant	0	0.7	378	95.4
Puddings, lemon, dry mix, instant, prepared with whole milk	2.7	2.9	115	20.1
Puddings, lemon, dry mix, regular	0.1	0.5	363	91.7
Pudding, lemon, dry mix, regular, prepared with sugar, egg yolk and water	0.65	1.12	109	24.2
Sugars, brown	0.12	0	380	98.09
Sugars, granulated	0	0	387	99.98

Food Name ---> per 100 g	Protein (g)	Fat (g)	Calories	Net Carb (g)
Sugars, powdered	0	0	389	99.77
Sweeteners, tabletop, aspartame, EQUAL, packets	2.17	0	365	89.08
Sugars, maple	0.1	0.2	354	90.9
Syrups, chocolate, HERSHEY'S Genuine Chocolate Flavored Lite Syrup	1.4	0.97	153	34.56
Syrups, chocolate, fudge-type	4.6	8.9	350	60.1
Syrups, corn, dark	0	0	286	77.59
Syrups, corn, light	0	0.2	283	76.79
Syrups, corn, high-fructose	0	0	281	76
Syrups, malt	6.2	0	318	71.3
Syrups, maple	0.04	0.06	260	67.04
Syrups, sorghum	0	0	290	74.9
Candies, MARS SNACKFOOD US, SNICKERS CRUNCHER	6.86	24.38	488	60.95
Syrups, table blends, pancake, with 2% maple	0	0.1	265	69.6
Syrups, table blends, cane and 15% maple	0	0.1	278	69.42
Syrups, table blends, corn, refiner, and sugar	0	0	319	83.9
Candies, MARS SNACKFOOD US, SKITTLES Wild Berry Bite Size Candies	0.19	4.25	402	90.76
Toppings, butterscotch or caramel	1.21	0	216	57.01
Toppings, marshmallow cream	0.8	0.3	322	78.9
Toppings, pineapple	0.1	0.1	253	66
Toppings, nuts in syrup	4.5	22	448	55.78
Candies, MARS SNACKFOOD US, SKITTLES Tropical Bite Size Candies	0.19	4.34	405	90.77
Candies, MARS SNACKFOOD US, SKITTLES Sours Original	0.18	4	401	91.02
Candies, MARS SNACKFOOD US, SKITTLES Original Bite Size Candies	0.19	4.37	405	90.78
Frostings, vanilla, creamy, dry mix, prepared with margarine	0.34	12.74	413	74.18
Frostings, chocolate, creamy, dry mix, prepared with margarine	1.1	12.87	404	69.12
Frostings, glaze, prepared-from-recipe	0.44	0.53	341	83.65
Candies, fudge, chocolate marshmallow, prepared-from-recipe	2.26	17.48	453	69.64

Food Name ---> per 100 g	Protein (g)	Fat (g)	Calories	Net Carb (g)
Candies, taffy, prepared-from-recipe	0.03	3.33	397	91.56
Candies, toffee, prepared-from-recipe	1.07	32.75	560	64.72
Candies, divinity, prepared-from-recipe	1.32	0.06	364	89.05
Frozen novelties, ice type, pineapple-coconut	0	2.6	113	23.2
Frozen yogurts, chocolate, soft-serve	4	6	160	22.7
Frostings, glaze, chocolate, prepared-from-recipe, with butter, NFSMI Recipe No. C-32	1.42	7.17	359	71.08
Candies, semisweet chocolate, made with butter	4.2	29.7	477	57.5
Gelatin desserts, dry mix, with added ascorbic acid, sodium-citrate and salt	7.8	0	381	90.5
Gelatin desserts, dry mix, reduced calorie, with aspartame, added phosphorus, potassium, sodium, vitamin C	55.3	0	345	33.3
Gelatin desserts, dry mix, reduced calorie, with aspartame, no added sodium	55.3	0	345	33.3
Puddings, banana, dry mix, instant, with added oil	0	4.4	386	89
Puddings, banana, dry mix, regular, with added oil	0	5	387	88.1
Puddings, lemon, dry mix, regular, with added oil, potassium, sodium	0.1	1.5	366	90.2
Puddings, tapioca, dry mix, with no added salt	0.1	0.1	369	94.1
Puddings, vanilla, dry mix, regular, with added oil	0.3	1.1	369	92.4
Jams and preserves, apricot	0.7	0.2	242	64.1
Syrups, table blends, pancake, with 2% maple, with added potassium	0	0.1	265	69.6
Frozen novelties, juice type, POPSICLE SCRIBBLERS	0	0.24	81	19.68
Candies, sugar-coated almonds	10	17.93	474	65.76
Cocoa, dry powder, hi-fat or breakfast, plain	16.8	23.71	486	21.59
Cocoa, dry powder, hi-fat or breakfast, processed with alkali	16.8	23.71	479	15.81
Candies, soft fruit and nut squares	2.31	9.52	390	71.41
Ice creams, vanilla, fat free	4.48	0	138	29.06
Sweeteners, tabletop, sucralose, SPLENDA packets	0	0	336	91.17
Frozen novelties, No Sugar Added, FUDGSICLE pops	3.67	1.87	124	21.61
Frozen novelties, ice type, sugar free, orange, cherry, and grape POPSICLE pops	0	0	21	5.14

Food Name ---> per 100 g	Protein (g)	Fat (g)	Calories	Net Carb (g)
Frozen novelties, KLONDIKE, SLIM-A-BEAR Fudge Bar, 98% fat free, no sugar added	4.31	1.88	124	24.07
Ice creams, BREYERS, All Natural Light Vanilla	4.84	4.59	162	25.1
Ice creams, BREYERS, All Natural Light French Vanilla	4.82	5.56	173	25.83
Ice creams, BREYERS, 98% Fat Free Vanilla	3.3	2.2	137	25.11
Ice creams, BREYERS, All Natural Light Vanilla Chocolate Strawberry	4.69	4.35	161	25.66
Ice creams, BREYERS, All Natural Light Mint Chocolate Chip	4.69	7.09	196	27.79
Ice creams, BREYERS, No Sugar Added, Butter Pecan	3.99	10.3	180	20.4
Ice creams, BREYERS, No Sugar Added, French Vanilla	4.5	7.05	154	20.25
Ice creams, BREYERS, No Sugar Added, Vanilla	3.68	6.2	143	21.42
Ice creams, BREYERS, No Sugar Added, Vanilla Fudge Twirl	3.53	5.68	153	24.83
Ice creams, BREYERS, No Sugar Added, Vanilla Chocolate Strawberry	3.71	6.26	143	21
Frozen novelties, KLONDIKE, SLIM-A-BEAR Chocolate Cone	4.09	4.1	224	41.02
Frozen novelties, KLONDIKE, SLIM-A-BEAR Vanilla Sandwich	3.9	5.85	239	38.45
Frozen novelties, KLONDIKE, SLIM-A-BEAR, No Sugar Added, Stickless Bar	5.2	13	242	22.08
Frozen novelties, No Sugar Added CREAMSICLE Pops	3.69	0.61	72	9.28
Frozen novelties, Sugar Free, CREAMSICLE Pops	1.37	2.33	49	4.45
Ice creams, BREYERS, All Natural Light French Chocolate	5.3	7.28	201	28.68
Ice creams, BREYERS, 98% Fat Free Chocolate	3.89	2.17	136	24.38
Ice creams, BREYERS, No Sugar Added, Chocolate Caramel	3.54	5.8	151	24.17
Candies, REESE's Fast Break, milk chocolate, peanut butter, soft nougats, candy bar	8.93	23.21	495	60.3
Candies, MARS SNACKFOOD US, COCOAVIA Chocolate Covered Almonds	9.51	37.07	573	39.82
Ice creams, regular, low carbohydrate, vanilla	3.17	12.7	216	17.43
Ice creams, regular, low carbohydrate, chocolate	3.8	12.7	237	22
Chocolate, dark, 45- 59% cacao solids	4.88	31.28	546	54.17
Chocolate, dark, 60-69% cacao solids	6.12	38.31	579	44.42
Chocolate, dark, 70-85% cacao solids	7.79	42.63	598	35

Food Name ---> per 100 g	Protein (g)	Fat (g)	Calories	Net Carb (g)
Candies, chocolate, dark, NFS (45-59% cacao solids 90%; 60-69% cacao solids 5%; 70-85% cacao solids 5%)	5.09	32.2	550	52.77
Sweeteners, for baking, brown, contains sugar and sucralose	0	0	388	97.11
Sweeteners, for baking, contains sugar and sucralose	0	0	398	99.53
Sugar, turbinado	0	0	399	99.8
Sweeteners, sugar substitute, granulated, brown	2.06	0	347	84.17
Candies, crispy bar with peanut butter filling	9.53	31.34	542	52.23
Syrup, maple, Canadian	0	0	270	67.38
Sweetener, syrup, agave	0.09	0.45	310	76.17
Candies, NESTLE, BUTTERFINGER Crisp	6.67	18.33	465	66.75
Candies, M&M MARS 3 MUSKETEERS Truffle Crisp	6.41	28.85	538	63.15
Syrups, chocolate, HERSHEY'S Sugar free, Genuine Chocolate Flavored, Lite Syrup	2.87	2.03	43	11.3
Candies, M&M MARS Pretzel Chocolate Candies	5	15	447	70.44
Sweetener, herbal extract powder from Stevia leaf	0	0	0	100
Candies, fruit snacks, with high vitamin C	0.08	0	352	87.97
Jams, preserves, marmalades, sweetened with fruit juice	0	0	212	52.03
Candies, Tamarind	0	0	368	89.46
Candies, coconut bar, not chocolate covered	2.13	27.65	481	49.47
Candies, HERSHEYS, PAYDAY Bar	13.44	25	490	49.08
Syrup, NESTLE, chocolate	0	0	269	67.21
Syrups, grenadine	0	0	268	66.91
Pectin, liquid	0	0	11	0
Frozen novelties, ice cream type, vanilla ice cream, light, no sugar added, chocolate coated	6.4	10.1	221	25.31
Milk dessert, frozen, milk-fat free, chocolate	4.3	1	167	37.7
Candies, MARS SNACKFOOD US, M&M's Peanut Butter Chocolate Candies	10.16	29.32	529	52.89
Candies, MARS SNACKFOOD US, TWIX chocolate fudge cookie bars	7.3	33.3	550	53
Frozen yogurts, chocolate, nonfat milk, sweetened without sugar	4.4	0.8	107	17.7
Frozen yogurts, chocolate	3	3.6	127	19.3

Food Name ---> per 100 g	Protein (g)	Fat (g)	Calories	Net Carb (g)
Frozen yogurts, flavors other than chocolate	3	3.6	127	21.6
Candies, MARS SNACKFOOD US, MILKY WAY Midnight Bar	3.2	17.5	443	68.32
Candies, MARS SNACKFOOD US, M&M's Almond Chocolate Candies	7.53	27.76	522	54.9
Gums, seed gums (includes locust bean, guar)	4.6	0.5	332	0
Syrups, sugar free	0.8	0	52	11.43
Jellies, no sugar (with sodium saccharin), any flavors	0.55	0	121	27.4
Jams and preserves, no sugar (with sodium saccharin), any flavor	0.3	0.3	132	50.92
Candies, chocolate covered, caramel with nuts	9.5	21	470	56.37
Candies, nougat, with almonds	3.33	1.67	398	89.09
Candies, gum drops, no sugar or low calorie (sorbitol)	0	0.2	354	88.1
Candies, hard, dietetic or low calorie (sorbitol)	0	0	394	98.6
Candies, chocolate covered, low sugar or low calorie	12.39	43.27	590	34.18
Chewing gum, sugarless	0	0.4	268	92.4
Pie fillings, cherry, low calorie	0.82	0.16	53	10.78
Sweeteners, tabletop, saccharin (sodium saccharin)	0.94	0	360	89.11
Sweeteners, tabletop, fructose, dry, powder	0	0	368	100
Frozen novelties, ice cream type, sundae, prepackaged	4.3	6	185	29.1
Jams, preserves, marmalade, reduced sugar	0	0.1	151	36.1
Frozen novelties, juice type, orange	0.5	0	95	23.07
Frozen novelties, juice type, juice with cream	1.41	1.41	115	24.01
Frozen novelties, ice cream type, chocolate or caramel covered, with nuts	4.4	20.2	323	30.3
Frozen novelties, ice type, pop, with low calorie sweetener	0	0	24	5.92
Ice creams, chocolate, rich	4.72	16.98	251	18.88
Sweeteners, tabletop, fructose, liquid	0	0	279	76
Puddings, chocolate flavor, low calorie, instant, dry mix	5.3	2.4	356	72.1
Jellies, reduced sugar, home preserved	0.3	0.03	179	45.3
Pie fillings, blueberry, canned	0.41	0.2	181	41.78
Puddings, chocolate flavor, low calorie, regular, dry mix	10.08	3	365	64.32

Food Name ---> per 100 g	Protein (g)	Fat (g)	Calories	Net Carb (g)
Puddings, all flavors except chocolate, low calorie, regular, dry mix	1.6	0.1	351	85.14
Puddings, all flavors except chocolate, low calorie, instant, dry mix	0.81	0.9	350	83.86
Syrup, Cane	0	0	269	73.14

Vegetables and Vegetable Products

Food Name ---> per 100 g	Protein (g)	Fat (g)	Calories	Net Carb (g)
Alfalfa seeds, sprouted, raw	3.99	0.69	23	0.2
Amaranth leaves, raw	2.46	0.33	23	4.02
Amaranth leaves, cooked, boiled, drained, without salt	2.11	0.18	21	4.11
Arrowhead, raw	5.33	0.29	99	20.23
Arrowhead, cooked, boiled, drained, without salt	4.49	0.1	78	16.14
Artichokes, (globe or french), raw	3.27	0.15	47	5.11
Artichokes, (globe or french), cooked, boiled, drained, without salt	2.89	0.34	53	6.25
Artichokes, (globe or french), frozen, unprepared	2.63	0.43	38	3.85
Artichokes, (globe or french), frozen, cooked, boiled, drained, without salt	3.11	0.5	45	4.58
Asparagus, raw	2.2	0.12	20	1.78
Asparagus, cooked, boiled, drained	2.4	0.22	22	2.11
Asparagus, canned, regular pack, solids and liquids	1.8	0.18	15	1.48
Asparagus, canned, drained solids	2.14	0.65	19	0.86
Asparagus, frozen, unprepared	3.23	0.23	24	2.2
Asparagus, frozen, cooked, boiled, drained, without salt	2.95	0.42	18	0.32
Balsam-pear (bitter gourd), leafy tips, raw	5.3	0.69	30	3.29
Balsam-pear (bitter gourd), leafy tips, cooked, boiled, drained, without salt	3.6	0.2	34	4.78
Balsam-pear (bitter gourd), pods, raw	1	0.17	17	0.9
Balsam-pear (bitter gourd), pods, cooked, boiled, drained, without salt	0.84	0.18	19	2.32
Bamboo shoots, raw	2.6	0.3	27	3
Bamboo shoots, cooked, boiled, drained, without salt	1.53	0.22	12	0.92
Bamboo shoots, canned, drained solids	1.72	0.4	19	1.82
Beans, kidney, mature seeds, sprouted, raw	4.2	0.5	29	4.1
Beans, kidney, mature seeds, sprouted, cooked, boiled, drained, without salt	4.83	0.58	33	4.72
Lima beans, immature seeds, raw	6.84	0.86	113	15.27

Food Name ---> per 100 g	Protein (g)	Fat (g)	Calories	Net Carb (g)
Lima beans, immature seeds, cooked, boiled, drained, without salt	6.81	0.32	123	18.24
Lima beans, immature seeds, canned, regular pack, solids and liquids	4.07	0.29	71	9.73
Lima beans, immature seeds, frozen, fordhook, unprepared	6.4	0.35	106	14.33
Lima beans, immature seeds, frozen, fordhook, cooked, boiled, drained, without salt	6.07	0.34	103	14.02
Lima beans, immature seeds, frozen, baby, unprepared	7.59	0.44	132	19.14
Lima beans, immature seeds, frozen, baby, cooked, boiled, drained, without salt	6.65	0.3	105	14.65
Mung beans, mature seeds, sprouted, raw	3.04	0.18	30	4.14
Mung beans, mature seeds, sprouted, cooked, boiled, drained, without salt	2.03	0.09	21	3.39
Mung beans, mature seeds, sprouted, cooked, stir-fried	4.3	0.21	50	8.69
Beans, navy, mature seeds, sprouted, raw	6.15	0.7	67	13.05
Beans, navy, mature seeds, sprouted, cooked, boiled, drained, without salt	7.07	0.81	78	15.01
Beans, pinto, immature seeds, frozen, unprepared	9.8	0.5	170	26.8
Beans, pinto, immature seeds, frozen, cooked, boiled, drained, without salt	9.31	0.48	162	25.47
Beans, shellie, canned, solids and liquids	1.76	0.19	30	2.79
Beans, snap, green, raw	1.83	0.22	31	4.27
Beans, snap, green, cooked, boiled, drained, without salt	1.89	0.28	35	4.68
Beans, snap, green, canned, regular pack, solids and liquids	0.72	0.17	15	1.77
Beans, snap, green, canned, regular pack, drained solids	1.12	0.46	22	2.42
Beans, snap, canned, all styles, seasoned, solids and liquids	0.83	0.2	16	1.99
Beans, snap, green, frozen, all styles, unprepared	1.79	0.21	39	4.94
Beans, snap, green, frozen, cooked, boiled, drained without salt	1.49	0.17	28	3.45
Beans, snap, green, frozen, all styles, microwaved	1.98	0.41	40	3.58
Beans, snap, green, microwaved	2.31	0.5	39	3.01
Beets, raw	1.61	0.17	43	6.76
Beets, cooked, boiled, drained	1.68	0.18	44	7.96
Beets, canned, regular pack, solids and liquids	0.73	0.09	30	5.94
Beets, canned, drained solids	0.91	0.14	31	5.41

Food Name ---> per 100 g	Protein (g)	Fat (g)	Calories	Net Carb (g)
Beet greens, raw	2.2	0.13	22	0.63
Beet greens, cooked, boiled, drained, without salt	2.57	0.2	27	2.56
Broadbeans, immature seeds, raw	5.6	0.6	72	7.5
Broadbeans, immature seeds, cooked, boiled, drained, without salt	4.8	0.5	62	6.5
Broccoli, raw	2.82	0.37	34	4.04
Broccoli, cooked, boiled, drained, without salt	2.38	0.41	35	3.88
Broccoli, frozen, chopped, unprepared	2.81	0.29	26	1.78
Broccoli, frozen, chopped, cooked, boiled, drained, without salt	3.1	0.12	28	2.35
Broccoli, frozen, spears, unprepared	3.06	0.34	29	2.35
Broccoli, frozen, spears, cooked, boiled, drained, without salt	3.1	0.11	28	2.36
Broccoli raab, raw	3.17	0.49	22	0.15
Broccoli raab, cooked	3.83	0.52	33	0.32
Brussels sprouts, raw	3.38	0.3	43	5.15
Brussels sprouts, cooked, boiled, drained, without salt	2.55	0.5	36	4.5
Brussels sprouts, frozen, unprepared	3.78	0.41	41	4.06
Brussels sprouts, frozen, cooked, boiled, drained, without salt	3.64	0.39	42	4.22
Burdock root, raw	1.53	0.15	72	14.04
Burdock root, cooked, boiled, drained, without salt	2.09	0.14	88	19.35
Butterbur, (fuki), raw	0.39	0.04	14	3.61
Butterbur, cooked, boiled, drained, without salt	0.23	0.02	8	2.16
Butterbur, canned	0.11	0.13	3	0.38
Cabbage, raw	1.28	0.1	25	3.3
Cabbage, cooked, boiled, drained, without salt	1.27	0.06	23	3.61
Cabbage, red, raw	1.43	0.16	31	5.27
Cabbage, red, cooked, boiled, drained, without salt	1.51	0.09	29	4.34
Cabbage, savoy, raw	2	0.1	27	3
Cabbage, savoy, cooked, boiled, drained, without salt	1.8	0.09	24	2.61
Cabbage, chinese (pak-choi), raw	1.5	0.2	13	1.18
Cabbage, chinese (pak-choi), cooked, boiled, drained, without salt	1.56	0.16	12	0.78
Cabbage, kimchi	1.1	0.5	15	0.8

Food Name ---> per 100 g	Protein (g)	Fat (g)	Calories	Net Carb (g)
Cabbage, chinese (pe-tsai), raw	1.2	0.2	16	2.03
Cabbage, chinese (pe-tsai), cooked, boiled, drained, without salt	1.5	0.17	14	0.71
Cardoon, raw	0.7	0.1	17	2.47
Cardoon, cooked, boiled, drained, without salt	0.76	0.11	22	3.63
Carrots, raw	0.93	0.24	41	6.78
Carrots, cooked, boiled, drained, without salt	0.76	0.18	35	5.22
Carrots, canned, regular pack, solids and liquids	0.58	0.14	23	3.57
Carrots, canned, regular pack, drained solids	0.64	0.19	25	4.04
Carrots, frozen, unprepared	0.78	0.46	36	4.6
Carrots, frozen, cooked, boiled, drained, without salt	0.58	0.68	37	4.43
Cassava, raw	1.36	0.28	160	36.26
Cauliflower, raw	1.92	0.28	25	2.97
Cauliflower, cooked, boiled, drained, without salt	1.84	0.45	23	1.81
Cauliflower, frozen, unprepared	2.01	0.27	24	2.38
Cauliflower, frozen, cooked, boiled, drained, without salt	1.61	0.22	19	1.05
Celeriac, raw	1.5	0.3	42	7.4
Celeriac, cooked, boiled, drained, without salt	0.96	0.19	27	4.7
Celery, raw	0.69	0.17	16	1.37
Celery, cooked, boiled, drained, without salt	0.83	0.16	18	2.4
Celtuce, raw	0.85	0.3	18	1.95
Chard, swiss, raw	1.8	0.2	19	2.14
Chard, swiss, cooked, boiled, drained, without salt	1.88	0.08	20	2.03
Chayote, fruit, raw	0.82	0.13	19	2.81
Chayote, fruit, cooked, boiled, drained, without salt	0.62	0.48	24	2.29
Chicory, witloof, raw	0.9	0.1	17	0.9
Chicory greens, raw	1.7	0.3	23	0.7
Chicory roots, raw	1.4	0.2	72	16.01
Chives, raw	3.27	0.73	30	1.85
Chrysanthemum, garland, raw	3.36	0.56	24	0.02
Chrysanthemum, garland, cooked, boiled, drained, without salt	1.64	0.09	20	2.01
Collards, raw	3.02	0.61	32	1.42

Food Name ---> per 100 g	Protein (g)	Fat (g)	Calories	Net Carb (g)
Collards, cooked, boiled, drained, without salt	2.71	0.72	33	1.65
Collards, frozen, chopped, unprepared	2.69	0.37	33	2.86
Collards, frozen, chopped, cooked, boiled, drained, without salt	2.97	0.41	36	4.3
Coriander (cilantro) leaves, raw	2.13	0.52	23	0.87
Corn, sweet, yellow, raw	3.27	1.35	86	16.7
Corn, sweet, yellow, cooked, boiled, drained, without salt	3.41	1.5	96	18.58
Corn, sweet, yellow, canned, brine pack, regular pack, solids and liquids	1.95	0.77	61	12.16
Corn, sweet, yellow, canned, whole kernel, drained solids	2.29	1.22	67	12.34
Corn, sweet, yellow, canned, cream style, regular pack	1.74	0.42	72	16.93
Corn, sweet, yellow, canned, vacuum pack, regular pack	2.41	0.5	79	17.44
Corn, sweet, yellow, canned, drained solids, rinsed with tap water	2.18	1.43	74	11.32
Corn, sweet, yellow, frozen, kernels cut off cob, unprepared	3.02	0.78	88	18.61
Corn, sweet, yellow, frozen, kernels cut off cob, boiled, drained, without salt	2.55	0.67	81	16.9
Corn, sweet, yellow, frozen, kernels on cob, unprepared	3.28	0.78	98	20.7
Corn, sweet, yellow, frozen, kernels on cob, cooked, boiled, drained, without salt	3.11	0.74	94	19.53
Corn, yellow, whole kernel, frozen, microwaved	3.62	1.42	131	23.27
Corn with red and green peppers, canned, solids and liquids	2.33	0.55	75	18.17
Cornsalad, raw	2	0.4	21	3.6
Cowpeas (blackeyes), immature seeds, raw	2.95	0.35	90	13.83
Cowpeas (blackeyes), immature seeds, cooked, boiled, drained, without salt	3.17	0.38	97	15.32
Cowpeas (blackeyes), immature seeds, frozen, unprepared	8.98	0.7	139	20.13
Cowpeas (blackeyes), immature seeds, frozen, cooked, boiled, drained, without salt	8.49	0.66	132	17.36
Cowpeas, young pods with seeds, raw	3.3	0.3	44	6.2
Cowpeas, young pods with seeds, cooked, boiled, drained, without salt	2.6	0.3	34	7
Yardlong bean, raw	2.8	0.4	47	8.35
Yardlong bean, cooked, boiled, drained, without salt	2.53	0.1	47	9.18
Cowpeas, leafy tips, raw	4.1	0.25	29	4.82

Food Name ---> per 100 g	Protein (g)	Fat (g)	Calories	Net Carb (g)
Cowpeas, leafy tips, cooked, boiled, drained, without salt	4.67	0.1	22	2.8
Cress, garden, raw	2.6	0.7	32	4.4
Cress, garden, cooked, boiled, drained, without salt	1.9	0.6	23	3.1
Cucumber, with peel, raw	0.65	0.11	15	3.13
Cucumber, peeled, raw	0.59	0.16	12	1.46
Dandelion greens, raw	2.7	0.7	45	5.7
Dandelion greens, cooked, boiled, drained, without salt	2	0.6	33	3.5
Eggplant, raw	0.98	0.18	25	2.88
Eggplant, cooked, boiled, drained, without salt	0.83	0.23	35	6.23
Edamame, frozen, unprepared	11.22	4.73	109	2.81
Edamame, frozen, prepared	11.91	5.2	121	3.71
Endive, raw	1.25	0.2	17	0.25
Escarole, cooked, boiled, drained, no salt added	1.15	0.18	19	0.27
Garlic, raw	6.36	0.5	149	30.96
Ginger root, raw	1.82	0.75	80	15.77
Gourd, white-flowered (calabash), raw	0.62	0.02	14	2.89
Gourd, white-flowered (calabash), cooked, boiled, drained, without salt	0.6	0.02	15	2.49
Gourd, dishcloth (towelgourd), raw	1.2	0.2	20	3.25
Gourd, dishcloth (towelgourd), cooked, boiled, drained, without salt	0.66	0.34	56	11.44
Drumstick leaves, raw	9.4	1.4	64	6.28
Drumstick leaves, cooked, boiled, drained, without salt	5.27	0.93	60	9.15
Hyacinth-beans, immature seeds, raw	2.1	0.2	46	5.89
Hyacinth-beans, immature seeds, cooked, boiled, drained, without salt	2.95	0.27	50	9.2
Jerusalem-artichokes, raw	2	0.01	73	15.84
Jew's ear, (pepeao), raw	0.48	0.04	25	6.75
Pepeao, dried	4.82	0.44	298	81.03
Jute, potherb, raw	4.65	0.25	34	5.8
Jute, potherb, cooked, boiled, drained, without salt	3.68	0.2	37	5.29
Kale, raw	4.28	0.93	49	5.15

Food Name ---> per 100 g	Protein (g)	Fat (g)	Calories	Net Carb (g)
Kale, cooked, boiled, drained, without salt	1.9	0.4	28	3.63
Kale, frozen, unprepared	2.66	0.46	28	2.9
Kale, frozen, cooked, boiled, drained, without salt	2.84	0.49	30	3.23
Kanpyo, (dried gourd strips)	8.58	0.56	258	55.23
Mushrooms, shiitake, raw	2.24	0.49	34	4.29
Mushrooms, Chanterelle, raw	1.49	0.53	38	3.06
Mushrooms, morel, raw	3.12	0.57	31	2.3
Kohlrabi, raw	1.7	0.1	27	2.6
Kohlrabi, cooked, boiled, drained, without salt	1.8	0.11	29	5.59
Mushrooms, portabella, grilled	3.28	0.58	29	2.24
Lambsquarters, raw	4.2	0.8	43	3.3
Lambsquarters, cooked, boiled, drained, without salt	3.2	0.7	32	2.9
Leeks, (bulb and lower leaf-portion), raw	1.5	0.3	61	12.35
Leeks, (bulb and lower leaf-portion), cooked, boiled, drained, without salt	0.81	0.2	31	6.62
Lentils, sprouted, raw	8.96	0.55	106	22.14
Lentils, sprouted, cooked, stir-fried, without salt	8.8	0.45	101	21.25
Lettuce, butterhead (includes boston and bibb types), raw	1.35	0.22	13	1.13
Lettuce, cos or romaine, raw	1.23	0.3	17	1.19
Lettuce, iceberg (includes crisphead types), raw	0.9	0.14	14	1.77
Lettuce, green leaf, raw	1.36	0.15	15	1.57
Lotus root, raw	2.6	0.1	74	12.33
Lotus root, cooked, boiled, drained, without salt	1.58	0.07	66	12.92
Lettuce, red leaf, raw	1.33	0.22	16	1.36
Mountain yam, hawaii, raw	1.34	0.1	67	13.8
Mountain yam, hawaii, cooked, steamed, without salt	1.73	0.08	82	20
Mushrooms, white, raw	3.09	0.34	22	2.26
Mushrooms, white, cooked, boiled, drained, without salt	2.17	0.47	28	3.09
Mushrooms, white, stir-fried	3.58	0.33	26	2.24
Mushrooms, canned, drained solids	1.87	0.29	25	2.69
Mushrooms, portabella, raw	2.11	0.35	22	2.57
Mushrooms, brown, italian, or crimini, raw	2.5	0.1	22	3.7

Food Name ---> per 100 g	Protein (g)	Fat (g)	Calories	Net Carb (g)
Mushrooms, shiitake, stir-fried	3.45	0.35	39	4.08
Mushrooms, shiitake, dried	9.58	0.99	296	63.87
Mushrooms, shiitake, cooked, without salt	1.56	0.22	56	12.29
Mustard greens, raw	2.86	0.42	27	1.47
Mustard greens, cooked, boiled, drained, without salt	2.56	0.47	26	2.51
Mustard greens, frozen, unprepared	2.49	0.27	20	0.11
Mustard greens, frozen, cooked, boiled, drained, without salt	2.27	0.25	19	0.31
Mustard spinach, (tendergreen), raw	2.2	0.3	22	1.1
Mustard spinach, (tendergreen), cooked, boiled, drained, without salt	1.7	0.2	16	0.8
New Zealand spinach, raw	1.5	0.2	14	1
New Zealand spinach, cooked, boiled, drained, without salt	1.3	0.17	12	0.73
Okra, raw	1.93	0.19	33	4.25
Okra, cooked, boiled, drained, without salt	1.87	0.21	22	2.01
Okra, frozen, unprepared	1.69	0.25	30	4.43
Okra, frozen, cooked, boiled, drained, without salt	1.63	0.24	29	4.31
Onions, raw	1.1	0.1	40	7.64
Onions, cooked, boiled, drained, without salt	1.36	0.19	44	8.75
Onions, dehydrated flakes	8.95	0.46	349	74.08
Onions, canned, solids and liquids	0.85	0.09	19	2.82
Onions, yellow, sauteed	0.95	10.8	132	6.16
Onions, frozen, chopped, unprepared	0.79	0.1	29	5.02
Onions, frozen, chopped, cooked, boiled, drained, without salt	0.77	0.1	28	4.79
Onions, frozen, whole, unprepared	0.89	0.06	35	6.75
Onions, frozen, whole, cooked, boiled, drained, without salt	0.71	0.05	28	5.3
Onions, spring or scallions (includes tops and bulb), raw	1.83	0.19	32	4.74
Onions, young green, tops only	0.97	0.47	27	3.94
Onions, welsh, raw	1.9	0.4	34	4.1
Onions, sweet, raw	0.8	0.08	32	6.65
Onion rings, breaded, par fried, frozen, unprepared	3.15	14.1	258	28.73
Onion rings, breaded, par fried, frozen, prepared, heated in oven	4.14	14.3	276	31.59

Food Name ---> per 100 g	Protein (g)	Fat (g)	Calories	Net Carb (g)
Parsley, fresh	2.97	0.79	36	3.03
Parsnips, raw	1.2	0.3	75	13.09
Parsnips, cooked, boiled, drained, without salt	1.32	0.3	71	13.41
Peas, edible-podded, raw	2.8	0.2	42	4.95
Peas, edible-podded, boiled, drained, without salt	3.27	0.23	42	4.25
Peas, edible-podded, frozen, unprepared	2.8	0.3	42	4.1
Peas, edible-podded, frozen, cooked, boiled, drained, without salt	3.5	0.38	52	5.92
Peas, green, raw	5.42	0.4	81	8.75
Peas, green, cooked, boiled, drained, without salt	5.36	0.22	84	10.13
Peas, green, canned, regular pack, solids and liquids	3.01	0.48	58	7.3
Peas, green (includes baby and lesuer types), canned, drained solids, unprepared	4.47	0.8	68	6.46
Peas, green, canned, seasoned, solids and liquids	3.09	0.27	50	7.25
Peas, green, canned, drained solids, rinsed in tap water	4.33	0.95	71	11.82
Peas, green, frozen, unprepared	5.22	0.4	77	9.12
Peas, green, frozen, cooked, boiled, drained, without salt	5.15	0.27	78	9.76
Peas, mature seeds, sprouted, raw	8.8	0.68	124	27.11
Peas, mature seeds, sprouted, cooked, boiled, drained, without salt	7.05	0.51	98	17.08
Peas and carrots, canned, regular pack, solids and liquids	2.17	0.27	38	6.48
Peas and carrots, frozen, unprepared	3.4	0.47	53	7.75
Peas and carrots, frozen, cooked, boiled, drained, without salt	3.09	0.42	48	7.02
Peas and onions, canned, solids and liquids	3.28	0.38	51	6.27
Peas and onions, frozen, unprepared	3.98	0.32	70	10.01
Peas and onions, frozen, cooked, boiled, drained, without salt	2.54	0.2	45	6.43
Peppers, hot chili, green, canned, pods, excluding seeds, solids and liquids	0.9	0.1	21	3.8
Peppers, sweet, green, raw	0.86	0.17	20	2.94
Peppers, sweet, green, cooked, boiled, drained, without salt	0.92	0.2	28	5.5
Peppers, sweet, green, canned, solids and liquids	0.8	0.3	18	2.7
Peppers, sweet, green, frozen, chopped, unprepared	1.08	0.21	20	2.85

Food Name ---> per 100 g	Protein (g)	Fat (g)	Calories	Net Carb (g)
Peppers, sweet, green, frozen, chopped, boiled, drained, without salt	0.95	0.18	18	3
Peppers, sweet, green, sauteed	0.78	11.85	127	2.42
Pigeonpeas, immature seeds, raw	7.2	1.64	136	18.78
Pigeonpeas, immature seeds, cooked, boiled, drained, without salt	5.96	1.36	111	15.29
Poi	0.38	0.14	112	26.83
Pokeberry shoots, (poke), raw	2.6	0.4	23	2
Pokeberry shoots, (poke), cooked, boiled, drained, without salt	2.3	0.4	20	1.6
Potatoes, flesh and skin, raw	2.05	0.09	77	15.39
Potatoes, russet, flesh and skin, raw	2.14	0.08	79	16.77
Potatoes, white, flesh and skin, raw	1.68	0.1	69	13.31
Potatoes, red, flesh and skin, raw	1.89	0.14	70	14.2
Potatoes, Russet, flesh and skin, baked	2.63	0.13	97	19.14
Potatoes, white, flesh and skin, baked	2.1	0.15	94	18.98
Potatoes, red, flesh and skin, baked	2.3	0.15	89	17.79
Potatoes, french fried, crinkle or regular cut, salt added in processing, frozen, as purchased	2.34	4.99	150	21.96
Potatoes, french fried, crinkle or regular cut, salt added in processing, frozen, oven-heated	2.51	5.13	166	25.2
Potatoes, roasted, salt added in processing, frozen, unprepared	2.22	1.81	130	23.55
Potatoes, raw, skin	2.57	0.1	58	9.94
Potatoes, baked, flesh, without salt	1.96	0.1	93	20.05
Potatoes, baked, skin, without salt	4.29	0.1	198	38.16
Potatoes, boiled, cooked in skin, flesh, without salt	1.87	0.1	87	18.33
Potatoes, boiled, cooked in skin, skin, without salt	2.86	0.1	78	13.91
Potatoes, boiled, cooked without skin, flesh, without salt	1.71	0.1	86	18.21
Potatoes, microwaved, cooked in skin, flesh, without salt	2.1	0.1	100	21.68
Potatoes, microwaved, cooked in skin, skin, without salt	4.39	0.1	132	24.13
Potatoes, hash brown, home-prepared	3	12.52	265	31.91
Potatoes, mashed, home-prepared, whole milk and margarine added	1.96	4.2	113	15.44
Potatoes, scalloped, home-prepared with butter	2.87	3.68	88	8.88

Food Name ---> per 100 g	Protein (g)	Fat (g)	Calories	Net Carb (g)
Potatoes, au gratin, home-prepared from recipe using butter	5.06	7.59	132	9.47
Potatoes, canned, solids and liquids	1.2	0.11	44	8.49
Potatoes, canned, drained solids	1.41	0.21	60	11.31
Potatoes, mashed, dehydrated, flakes without milk, dry form	8.34	0.41	354	74.57
Potatoes, mashed, dehydrated, prepared from flakes without milk, whole milk and butter added	1.77	5.13	97	10.07
Potatoes, mashed, dehydrated, granules without milk, dry form	8.22	0.54	372	78.41
Potatoes, mashed, dehydrated, prepared from granules without milk, whole milk and butter added	2.05	4.96	108	12.16
Potatoes, mashed, dehydrated, granules with milk, dry form	10.9	1.1	357	71.1
Potatoes, mashed, dehydrated, prepared from granules with milk, water and margarine added	2.13	4.8	116	14.83
Potatoes, au gratin, dry mix, unprepared	8.9	3.7	314	70.21
Potatoes, au gratin, dry mix, prepared with water, whole milk and butter	2.3	4.12	93	11.94
Potatoes, scalloped, dry mix, unprepared	7.77	4.59	358	65.33
Potatoes, scalloped, dry mix, prepared with water, whole milk and butter	2.12	4.3	93	11.67
Potatoes, hash brown, frozen, plain, unprepared	2.06	0.62	82	16.32
Potatoes, hash brown, frozen, plain, prepared, pan fried in canola oil	2.65	11.59	219	25.31
Potatoes, hash brown, frozen, with butter sauce, unprepared	1.87	6.66	135	15.38
Potatoes, hash brown, frozen, with butter sauce, prepared	2.46	8.79	178	20.33
Potatoes, french fried, shoestring, salt added in processing, frozen, as purchased	2.16	6.24	167	23.29
Potatoes, french fried, shoestring, salt added in processing, frozen, oven-heated	2.9	6.76	199	28.86
Potatoes, o'brien, frozen, unprepared	1.83	0.14	76	15.57
Potatoes, o'brien, frozen, prepared	2.22	13.21	204	20.16
Potato puffs, frozen, unprepared	1.93	8.71	178	22.5
Potato puffs, frozen, oven-heated	2.13	9.05	192	25.29
Potatoes, frozen, whole, unprepared	2.38	0.16	78	16.27
Potatoes, frozen, whole, cooked, boiled, drained, without salt	1.98	0.13	65	13.12

Food Name ---> per 100 g	Protein (g)	Fat (g)	Calories	Net Carb (g)
Potatoes, french fried, all types, salt added in processing, frozen, unprepared	2.24	4.66	147	22.91
Potatoes, french fried, all types, salt added in processing, frozen, home-prepared, oven heated	2.75	5.48	158	23.55
Potatoes, french fried, cottage-cut, salt not added in processing, frozen, as purchased	2.42	5.78	153	20.98
Potatoes, french fried, cottage-cut, salt not added in processing, frozen, oven-heated	3.44	8.2	218	30.83
Potatoes, frozen, french fried, par fried, extruded, unprepared	2.83	14.95	260	27.25
Potatoes, frozen, french fried, par fried, extruded, prepared, heated in oven, without salt	3.55	18.71	333	36.48
USDA Commodity, Potato wedges, frozen	2.7	2.2	123	23.5
Potatoes, french fried, steak fries, salt added in processing, frozen, as purchased	2.19	3.39	133	21.61
Potatoes, french fried, steak fries, salt added in processing, frozen, oven-heated	2.57	3.76	152	24.38
Potato flour	6.9	0.34	357	77.2
Potato salad, home-prepared	2.68	8.2	143	9.87
Pumpkin flowers, raw	1.03	0.07	15	3.28
Pumpkin flowers, cooked, boiled, drained, without salt	1.09	0.08	15	2.4
Pumpkin leaves, raw	3.15	0.4	19	2.33
Pumpkin leaves, cooked, boiled, drained, without salt	2.72	0.22	21	0.69
Pumpkin, raw	1	0.1	26	6
Pumpkin, cooked, boiled, drained, without salt	0.72	0.07	20	3.8
Pumpkin, canned, without salt	1.1	0.28	34	5.19
Pumpkin pie mix, canned	1.09	0.13	104	18.09
Purslane, raw	2.03	0.36	20	3.39
Purslane, cooked, boiled, drained, without salt	1.49	0.19	18	3.55
Radishes, raw	0.68	0.1	16	1.8
Radishes, oriental, raw	0.6	0.1	18	2.5
Radishes, oriental, cooked, boiled, drained, without salt	0.67	0.24	17	1.83
Radishes, oriental, dried	7.9	0.72	271	39.47
Rutabagas, raw	1.08	0.16	37	6.32
Rutabagas, cooked, boiled, drained, without salt	0.93	0.18	30	5.04

Food Name ---> per 100 g	Protein (g)	Fat (g)	Calories	Net Carb (g)
Salsify, (vegetable oyster), raw	3.3	0.2	82	15.3
Salsify, cooked, boiled, drained, without salt	2.73	0.17	68	12.26
Sauerkraut, canned, solids and liquids	0.91	0.14	19	1.38
Seaweed, agar, raw	0.54	0.03	26	6.25
Seaweed, irishmoss, raw	1.51	0.16	49	10.99
Seaweed, kelp, raw	1.68	0.56	43	8.27
Seaweed, laver, raw	5.81	0.28	35	4.81
Sesbania flower, raw	1.28	0.04	27	6.73
Sesbania flower, cooked, steamed, without salt	1.14	0.05	22	5.23
Soybeans, green, raw	12.95	6.8	147	6.85
Soybeans, green, cooked, boiled, drained, without salt	12.35	6.4	141	6.85
Soybeans, mature seeds, sprouted, raw	13.09	6.7	122	8.47
Soybeans, mature seeds, sprouted, cooked, steamed	8.47	4.45	81	5.73
Soybeans, mature seeds, sprouted, cooked, stir-fried	13.1	7.1	125	8.6
Spinach, raw	2.86	0.39	23	1.43
Spinach, cooked, boiled, drained, without salt	2.97	0.26	23	1.35
Spinach, canned, regular pack, solids and liquids	2.11	0.37	19	1.32
Spinach, canned, regular pack, drained solids	2.81	0.5	23	1
Spinach, frozen, chopped or leaf, unprepared	3.63	0.57	29	1.31
Spinach, frozen, chopped or leaf, cooked, boiled, drained, without salt	4.01	0.87	34	1.1
Squash, summer, crookneck and straightneck, raw	1.01	0.27	19	2.88
Squash, summer, crookneck and straightneck, cooked, boiled, drained, without salt	1.04	0.39	23	2.69
Squash, summer, crookneck and straightneck, canned, drained, solid, without salt	0.61	0.07	13	1.56
Squash, summer, crookneck and straightneck, frozen, unprepared	0.83	0.14	20	3.6
Squash, summer, crookneck and straightneck, frozen, cooked, boiled, drained, without salt	1.28	0.2	25	4.14
Squash, summer, scallop, raw	1.2	0.2	18	2.64
Squash, summer, scallop, cooked, boiled, drained, without salt	1.03	0.17	16	1.4
Squash, summer, zucchini, includes skin, raw	1.21	0.32	17	2.11

Food Name ---> per 100 g	Protein (g)	Fat (g)	Calories	Net Carb (g)
Squash, summer, zucchini, includes skin, cooked, boiled, drained, without salt	1.14	0.36	15	1.69
Squash, summer, zucchini, includes skin, frozen, unprepared	1.16	0.13	17	2.28
Squash, summer, zucchini, includes skin, frozen, cooked, boiled, drained, without salt	1.15	0.13	17	2.26
Squash, summer, zucchini, italian style, canned	1.03	0.11	29	6.85
Squash, winter, acorn, raw	0.8	0.1	40	8.92
Squash, winter, acorn, cooked, baked, without salt	1.12	0.14	56	10.18
Squash, winter, acorn, cooked, boiled, mashed, without salt	0.67	0.08	34	6.19
Squash, winter, butternut, raw	1	0.1	45	9.69
Squash, winter, butternut, cooked, baked, without salt	0.9	0.09	40	7.29
Squash, winter, butternut, frozen, unprepared	1.76	0.1	57	13.11
Squash, winter, butternut, frozen, cooked, boiled, without salt	1.23	0.07	39	10.05
Squash, winter, hubbard, raw	2	0.5	40	4.8
Squash, winter, hubbard, baked, without salt	2.48	0.62	50	5.91
Squash, winter, hubbard, cooked, boiled, mashed, without salt	1.48	0.37	30	3.56
Squash, winter, spaghetti, raw	0.64	0.57	31	5.41
Squash, winter, spaghetti, cooked, boiled, drained, or baked, without salt	0.66	0.26	27	5.06
Succotash, (corn and limas), raw	5.03	1.02	99	15.79
Succotash, (corn and limas), cooked, boiled, drained, without salt	5.07	0.8	115	19.88
Succotash, (corn and limas), canned, with cream style corn	2.64	0.54	77	14.61
Succotash, (corn and limas), canned, with whole kernel corn, solids and liquids	2.6	0.49	63	11.38
Succotash, (corn and limas), frozen, unprepared	4.31	0.89	93	15.94
Succotash, (corn and limas), frozen, cooked, boiled, drained, without salt	4.31	0.89	93	15.85
Swamp cabbage, (skunk cabbage), raw	2.6	0.2	19	1.04
Swamp cabbage (skunk cabbage), cooked, boiled, drained, without salt	2.08	0.24	20	1.8
Sweet potato leaves, raw	2.49	0.51	42	3.52
Sweet potato leaves, cooked, steamed, without salt	2.18	0.34	41	5.48
Sweet potato, raw, unprepared	1.57	0.05	86	17.12

Food Name ---> per 100 g	Protein (g)	Fat (g)	Calories	Net Carb (g)
Sweet potato, cooked, baked in skin, flesh, without salt	2.01	0.15	90	17.41
Sweet potato, cooked, boiled, without skin	1.37	0.14	76	15.22
Sweet potato, canned, vacuum pack	1.65	0.2	91	19.32
Sweet potato, canned, mashed	1.98	0.2	101	21.49
Sweet potato, frozen, unprepared	1.71	0.18	96	20.52
Sweet potato, frozen, cooked, baked, without salt	1.71	0.12	100	21.6
Taro, raw	1.5	0.2	112	22.36
Taro, cooked, without salt	0.52	0.11	142	29.5
Taro leaves, raw	4.98	0.74	42	3
Taro leaves, cooked, steamed, without salt	2.72	0.41	24	2.02
Taro shoots, raw	0.92	0.09	11	2.32
Taro shoots, cooked, without salt	0.73	0.08	14	3.2
Taro, tahitian, raw	2.79	0.97	44	6.91
Taro, tahitian, cooked, without salt	4.16	0.68	44	6.85
Tomatoes, green, raw	1.2	0.2	23	4
Tomatoes, red, ripe, raw, year round average	0.88	0.2	18	2.69
Tomatoes, red, ripe, cooked	0.95	0.11	18	3.31
Tomatoes, red, ripe, canned, packed in tomato juice	0.79	0.25	16	1.57
Tomatoes, red, ripe, canned, stewed	0.91	0.19	26	5.19
Tomatoes, red, ripe, canned, with green chilies	0.69	0.08	15	3.62
Tomato juice, canned, with salt added	0.85	0.29	17	3.13
Tomato products, canned, paste, without salt added	4.32	0.47	82	14.81
Tomato products, canned, puree, without salt added	1.65	0.21	38	7.08
Tomato powder	12.91	0.44	302	58.18
Tomato products, canned, sauce	1.2	0.3	24	3.81
Tomato products, canned, sauce, with mushrooms	1.45	0.13	35	6.93
Tomato products, canned, sauce, with onions	1.56	0.19	42	8.14
Tomato products, canned, sauce, with herbs and cheese	2.13	1.93	59	8.04
Tomato products, canned, sauce, with onions, green peppers, and celery	0.94	0.74	41	7.37
Tomato products, canned, sauce, with tomato tidbits	1.32	0.39	32	5.69
Tree fern, cooked, without salt	0.29	0.07	40	7.28

Food Name ---> per 100 g	Protein (g)	Fat (g)	Calories	Net Carb (g)
Turnips, raw	0.9	0.1	28	4.63
Turnips, cooked, boiled, drained, without salt	0.71	0.08	22	3.06
Turnips, frozen, unprepared	1.04	0.16	16	1.14
Turnips, frozen, cooked, boiled, drained, without salt	1.53	0.24	23	2.35
Turnip greens, raw	1.5	0.3	32	3.93
Turnip greens, cooked, boiled, drained, without salt	1.14	0.23	20	0.86
Turnip greens, canned, solids and liquids	1.36	0.3	14	0.72
Turnip greens, frozen, unprepared	2.47	0.31	22	1.17
Turnip greens, frozen, cooked, boiled, drained, without salt	3.35	0.42	29	1.58
Turnip greens and turnips, frozen, unprepared	2.46	0.19	21	0.99
Turnip greens and turnips, frozen, cooked, boiled, drained, without salt	2.99	0.38	35	1.75
Vegetable juice cocktail, canned	0.93	0.31	22	3.37
Vegetables, mixed, canned, solids and liquids	1.42	0.25	36	3.33
Vegetables, mixed, canned, drained solids	2.59	0.25	49	6.26
Vegetables, mixed, frozen, unprepared	3.33	0.52	72	9.47
Vegetables, mixed, frozen, cooked, boiled, drained, without salt	2.86	0.15	65	8.69
Vegetable juice cocktail, low sodium, canned	0.91	0.32	19	3.33
Vinespinach, (basella), raw	1.8	0.3	19	3.4
Waterchestnuts, chinese, (matai), raw	1.4	0.1	97	20.94
Waterchestnuts, chinese, canned, solids and liquids	0.88	0.06	50	9.8
Watercress, raw	2.3	0.1	11	0.79
Waxgourd, (chinese preserving melon), raw	0.4	0.2	13	0.1
Waxgourd, (chinese preserving melon), cooked, boiled, drained, without salt	0.4	0.2	14	2.04
Winged beans, immature seeds, raw	6.95	0.87	49	4.31
Winged beans, immature seeds, cooked, boiled, drained, without salt	5.31	0.66	38	3.21
Winged bean leaves, raw	5.85	1.1	74	14.1
Winged bean tuber, raw	11.6	0.9	148	28.1
Yam, raw	1.53	0.17	118	23.78
Yam, cooked, boiled, drained, or baked, without salt	1.49	0.14	116	23.58

Food Name ---> per 100 g	Protein (g)	Fat (g)	Calories	Net Carb (g)
Yambean (jicama), raw	0.72	0.09	38	3.92
Yambean (jicama), cooked, boiled, drained, without salt	0.72	0.09	38	8.82
Beets, harvard, canned, solids and liquids	0.84	0.06	73	15.68
Beets, pickled, canned, solids and liquids	0.8	0.08	65	15.48
Borage, raw	1.8	0.7	21	3.06
Borage, cooked, boiled, drained, without salt	2.09	0.81	25	3.55
Chives, freeze-dried	21.2	3.5	311	38.09
Dock, raw	2	0.7	22	0.3
Dock, cooked, boiled, drained, without salt	1.83	0.64	20	0.33
Eppaw, raw	4.6	1.8	150	31.68
Drumstick pods, raw	2.1	0.2	37	5.33
Drumstick pods, cooked, boiled, drained, without salt	2.09	0.19	36	3.98
Kale, scotch, raw	2.8	0.6	42	6.62
Kale, scotch, cooked, boiled, drained, without salt	1.9	0.41	28	4.43
Leeks, (bulb and lower-leaf portion), freeze-dried	15.2	2.1	321	64.25
Parsley, freeze-dried	31.3	5.2	271	9.68
Beans, mung, mature seeds, sprouted, canned, drained solids	1.4	0.06	12	1.34
Peppers, jalapeno, canned, solids and liquids	0.92	0.94	27	2.14
Peppers, sweet, green, freeze-dried	17.9	3	314	47.4
Radishes, white icicle, raw	1.1	0.1	14	1.23
Shallots, freeze-dried	12.3	0.5	348	65
Squash, summer, all varieties, raw	1.21	0.18	16	2.25
Squash, summer, all varieties, cooked, boiled, drained, without salt	0.91	0.31	20	2.91
Squash, winter, all varieties, raw	0.95	0.13	34	7.09
Squash, winter, all varieties, cooked, baked, without salt	0.89	0.35	37	6.05
Sweet potato, canned, syrup pack, solids and liquids	0.98	0.2	89	18.43
Sweet potato, canned, syrup pack, drained solids	1.28	0.32	108	22.36
Tomato products, canned, sauce, spanish style	1.44	0.27	33	5.84
Beans, pinto, mature seeds, sprouted, raw	5.25	0.9	62	11.6
Beans, pinto, mature seeds, sprouted, cooked, boiled, drained, without salt	1.86	0.32	22	4.1

Food Name ---> per 100 g	Protein (g)	Fat (g)	Calories	Net Carb (g)
Carrot juice, canned	0.95	0.15	40	8.48
Corn pudding, home prepared	4.42	5.04	131	15.77
Potatoes, mashed, home-prepared, whole milk added	1.91	0.57	83	16.07
Spinach souffle	7.89	12.95	172	5.2
Sweet potato, cooked, candied, home-prepared	0.89	3.54	164	30.02
Tomatoes, red, ripe, cooked, stewed	1.96	2.68	79	11.35
Seaweed, agar, dried	6.21	0.3	306	73.18
Seaweed, spirulina, raw	5.92	0.39	26	2.02
Seaweed, spirulina, dried	57.47	7.72	290	20.3
Seaweed, wakame, raw	3.03	0.64	45	8.64
Peppers, hot chili, green, raw	2	0.2	40	7.96
Potatoes, o'brien, home-prepared	2.35	1.28	81	15.47
Potato pancakes	6.08	14.76	268	24.51
Potatoes, baked, flesh and skin, without salt	2.5	0.13	93	18.95
Potatoes, microwaved, cooked in skin, flesh and skin, without salt	2.44	0.1	105	21.94
Radish seeds, sprouted, raw	3.81	2.53	43	3.6
Shallots, raw	2.5	0.1	72	13.6
Carrot, dehydrated	8.1	1.49	341	55.97
Tomatoes, crushed, canned	1.64	0.28	32	5.39
Tomatoes, orange, raw	1.16	0.19	16	2.28
Tomatoes, yellow, raw	0.98	0.26	15	2.28
Arrowroot, raw	4.24	0.2	65	12.09
Chrysanthemum leaves, raw	3.36	0.56	24	0.01
Amaranth leaves, cooked, boiled, drained, with salt	2.11	0.18	21	4.11
Arrowhead, cooked, boiled, drained, with salt	4.49	0.1	78	16.14
Artichokes, (globe or french), cooked, boiled, drained, with salt	2.89	0.34	51	5.69
Artichokes, (globe or french), frozen, cooked, boiled, drained, with salt	3.11	0.5	45	4.58
Asparagus, cooked, boiled, drained, with salt	2.4	0.22	22	2.11
Asparagus, canned, no salt added, solids and liquids	1.8	0.18	15	1.48
Asparagus, frozen, cooked, boiled, drained, with salt	2.95	0.42	18	0.32

Food Name ---> per 100 g	Protein (g)	Fat (g)	Calories	Net Carb (g)
Balsam-pear (bitter gourd), leafy tips, cooked, boiled, drained, with salt	3.6	0.2	32	4.26
Balsam-pear (bitter gourd), pods, cooked, boiled, drained, with salt	0.84	0.18	19	2.32
Bamboo shoots, cooked, boiled, drained, with salt	1.53	0.22	11	0.52
Beans, kidney, mature seeds, sprouted, cooked, boiled, drained, with salt	4.83	0.58	33	4.72
Lima beans, immature seeds, cooked, boiled, drained, with salt	6.81	0.32	123	18.34
Lima beans, immature seeds, canned, no salt added, solids and liquids	4.07	0.29	71	9.73
Lima beans, immature seeds, frozen, baby, cooked, boiled, drained, with salt	6.65	0.3	105	14.65
Lima beans, immature seeds, frozen, fordhook, cooked, boiled, drained, with salt	6.07	0.34	103	14.02
Mung beans, mature seeds, sprouted, cooked, boiled, drained, with salt	2.03	0.09	19	2.8
Beans, navy, mature seeds, sprouted, cooked, boiled, drained, with salt	7.07	0.81	78	15.01
Beans, pinto, immature seeds, frozen, cooked, boiled, drained, with salt	9.31	0.48	162	25.47
Beans, pinto, mature seeds, sprouted, cooked, boiled, drained, with salt	1.86	0.32	20	3.5
Beans, snap, yellow, raw	1.82	0.12	31	3.73
Beans, snap, green, cooked, boiled, drained, with salt	1.89	0.28	35	4.68
Beans, snap, yellow, cooked, boiled, drained, without salt	1.89	0.28	35	4.58
Beans, snap, yellow, cooked, boiled, drained, with salt	1.89	0.28	35	4.58
Beans, snap, green, canned, no salt added, solids and liquids	0.8	0.1	15	2
Beans, snap, yellow, canned, regular pack, solids and liquids	0.8	0.1	15	2
Beans, snap, yellow, canned, no salt added, solids and liquids	0.8	0.1	15	2
Beans, snap, green, canned, no salt added, drained solids	1.12	0.46	22	2.42
Beans, snap, yellow, frozen, all styles, unprepared	1.8	0.21	33	4.78
Beans, snap, green, frozen, cooked, boiled, drained, with salt	1.49	0.17	28	3.45
Beans, snap, yellow, frozen, cooked, boiled, drained, without salt	1.49	0.17	28	3.45
Beans, snap, yellow, frozen, cooked, boiled, drained, with salt	1.49	0.17	28	3.45

Food Name ---> per 100 g	Protein (g)	Fat (g)	Calories	Net Carb (g)
Beets, cooked, boiled. drained, with salt	1.68	0.18	44	7.96
Beets, canned, no salt added, solids and liquids	0.8	0.07	28	5.37
Beet greens, cooked, boiled, drained, with salt	2.57	0.2	27	2.56
Borage, cooked, boiled, drained, with salt	2.09	0.81	25	3.55
Broadbeans, immature seeds, cooked, boiled, drained, with salt	4.8	0.5	62	10.1
Broccoli, leaves, raw	2.98	0.35	28	2.76
Broccoli, flower clusters, raw	2.98	0.35	28	2.76
Broccoli, stalks, raw	2.98	0.35	28	5.24
Broccoli, cooked, boiled, drained, with salt	2.38	0.41	35	3.88
Broccoli, frozen, chopped, cooked, boiled, drained, with salt	3.1	0.12	28	2.35
Broccoli, frozen, spears, cooked, boiled, drained, with salt	3.1	0.11	28	2.35
Brussels sprouts, cooked, boiled, drained, with salt	2.55	0.5	36	4.5
Brussels sprouts, frozen, cooked, boiled, drained, with salt	3.64	0.39	42	4.22
Burdock root, cooked, boiled, drained, with salt	2.09	0.14	88	19.35
Butterbur, cooked, boiled, drained, with salt	0.23	0.02	8	2.16
Cabbage, common (danish, domestic, and pointed types), freshly harvest, raw	1.21	0.18	24	3.07
Cabbage, common (danish, domestic, and pointed types), stored, raw	1.21	0.18	24	3.07
Cabbage, common, cooked, boiled, drained, with salt	1.27	0.06	23	3.61
Cabbage, red, cooked, boiled, drained, with salt	1.51	0.09	29	4.34
Cabbage, savoy, cooked, boiled, drained, with salt	1.8	0.09	24	2.61
Cabbage, chinese (pak-choi), cooked, boiled, drained, with salt	1.56	0.16	12	0.78
Cabbage, chinese (pe-tsai), cooked, boiled, drained, with salt	1.5	0.17	14	0.71
Cardoon, cooked, boiled, drained, with salt	0.76	0.11	20	3.04
Carrots, cooked, boiled, drained, with salt	0.76	0.18	35	5.22
Carrots, canned, no salt added, solids and liquids	0.59	0.14	23	3.56
Carrots, canned, no salt added, drained solids	0.64	0.19	25	4.04
Carrots, frozen, cooked, boiled, drained, with salt	0.58	0.68	37	4.43
Cauliflower, cooked, boiled, drained, with salt	1.84	0.45	23	1.81
Cauliflower, frozen, cooked, boiled, drained, with salt	1.61	0.22	17	0.46
Celeriac, cooked, boiled, drained, with salt	0.96	0.19	27	5.9

Food Name ---> per 100 g	Protein (g)	Fat (g)	Calories	Net Carb (g)
Celery, cooked, boiled, drained, with salt	0.83	0.16	18	2.4
Chard, swiss, cooked, boiled, drained, with salt	1.88	0.08	20	2.03
Chayote, fruit, cooked, boiled, drained, with salt	0.62	0.48	22	1.7
Chrysanthemum, garland, cooked, boiled, drained, with salt	1.64	0.09	20	2.01
Collards, cooked, boiled, drained, with salt	2.71	0.72	33	1.65
Collards, frozen, chopped, cooked, boiled, drained, with salt	2.97	0.41	36	4.3
Corn, sweet, yellow, cooked, boiled, drained, with salt	3.41	1.5	96	18.58
Corn, sweet, yellow, canned, no salt added, solids and liquids	1.95	0.77	61	12.16
Corn, sweet, yellow, canned, cream style, no salt added	1.74	0.42	72	16.93
Corn, sweet, yellow, canned, vacuum pack, no salt added	2.41	0.5	79	17.44
Corn, sweet, yellow, frozen, kernels, cut off cob, boiled, drained, with salt	2.55	0.67	79	16.31
Corn, sweet, yellow, frozen, kernels on cob, cooked, boiled, drained, with salt	3.11	0.74	94	19.53
Cowpeas (blackeyes), immature seeds, cooked, boiled, drained, with salt	3.17	0.38	94	14.73
Cowpeas (blackeyes), immature seeds, frozen, cooked, boiled, drained, with salt	8.49	0.66	131	17.1
Cowpeas, young pods with seeds, cooked, boiled, drained, with salt	2.6	0.3	34	7
Cowpeas, leafy tips, cooked, boiled, drained, with salt	4.67	0.1	22	2.8
Cress, garden, cooked, boiled, drained, with salt	1.9	0.6	23	3.1
Dandelion greens, cooked, boiled, drained, with salt	2	0.6	33	3.5
Eggplant, cooked, boiled, drained, with salt	0.83	0.23	33	5.64
Gourd, white-flowered (calabash), cooked, boiled, drained, with salt	0.6	0.02	13	1.9
Gourd, dishcloth (towelgourd), cooked, boiled, drained, with salt	0.66	0.34	54	10.85
Drumstick leaves, cooked, boiled, drained, with salt	5.27	0.93	60	9.15
Drumstick pods, cooked, boiled, drained, with salt	2.09	0.19	36	3.98
Hyacinth-beans, immature seeds, cooked, boiled, drained, with salt	2.95	0.27	50	9.2
Jute, potherb, cooked, boiled, drained, with salt	3.68	0.2	37	5.29
Kale, cooked, boiled, drained, with salt	1.9	0.4	28	3.63

Food Name ---> per 100 g	Protein (g)	Fat (g)	Calories	Net Carb (g)
Kale, frozen, cooked, boiled, drained, with salt	2.84	0.49	30	3.23
Kale, scotch, cooked, boiled, drained, with salt	1.9	0.41	28	5.62
Kohlrabi, cooked, boiled, drained, with salt	1.8	0.11	29	5.59
Lambsquarters, cooked, boiled, drained, with salt	3.2	0.7	32	2.9
Leeks, (bulb and lower leaf-portion), cooked, boiled, drained, with salt	0.81	0.2	31	6.62
Lotus root, cooked, boiled, drained, with salt	1.58	0.07	66	12.92
Mushrooms, white, cooked, boiled, drained, with salt	2.17	0.47	28	3.09
Mushrooms, shiitake, cooked, with salt	1.56	0.22	56	12.29
Mustard greens, cooked, boiled, drained, with salt	2.56	0.47	26	2.51
Mustard greens, frozen, cooked, boiled, drained, with salt	2.27	0.25	19	0.31
Mustard spinach, (tendergreen), cooked, boiled, drained, with salt	1.7	0.2	16	0.8
New zealand spinach, cooked, boiled, drained, with salt	1.3	0.17	12	0.73
Okra, cooked, boiled, drained, with salt	1.87	0.21	22	2.01
Okra, frozen, cooked, boiled, drained, with salt	1.63	0.24	34	4.31
Onions, cooked, boiled, drained, with salt	1.36	0.19	42	8.16
Onions, frozen, chopped, cooked, boiled, drained, with salt	0.77	0.1	26	4.3
Onions, frozen, whole, cooked, boiled, drained, with salt	0.71	0.05	26	4.71
Parsnips, cooked, boiled, drained, with salt	1.32	0.3	71	13.01
Peas, edible-podded, cooked, boiled, drained, with salt	3.27	0.23	40	3.66
Peas, edible-podded, frozen, cooked, boiled, drained, with salt	3.5	0.38	50	5.33
Peas, green, cooked, boiled, drained, with salt	5.36	0.22	84	10.13
Peas, green, canned, no salt added, solids and liquids	3.19	0.3	53	6.45
Peas, green, canned, no salt added, drained solids	4.42	0.35	69	8.48
Peas, green, frozen, cooked, boiled, drained, with salt	5.15	0.27	78	9.76
Peas, mature seeds, sprouted, cooked, boiled, drained, with salt	7.05	0.51	98	17.08
Peas and carrots, canned, no salt added, solids and liquids	2.17	0.27	38	5.18
Peas and carrots, frozen, cooked, boiled, drained, with salt	3.09	0.42	48	7.02
Peas and onions, frozen, cooked, boiled, drained, with salt	2.54	0.2	45	6.43
Peppers, hot chili, red, raw	1.87	0.44	40	7.31

Food Name ---> per 100 g	Protein (g)	Fat (g)	Calories	Net Carb (g)
Peppers, hot chili, red, canned, excluding seeds, solids and liquids	0.9	0.1	21	3.8
Peppers, sweet, red, raw	0.99	0.3	31	3.93
Peppers, sweet, green, cooked, boiled, drained, with salt	0.92	0.2	26	4.91
Peppers, sweet, red, cooked, boiled, drained, without salt	0.92	0.2	28	5.5
Peppers, sweet, red, cooked, boiled, drained, with salt	0.92	0.2	26	4.91
Peppers, sweet, green, frozen, chopped, cooked, boiled, drained, with salt	0.95	0.18	16	2.41
Pigeonpeas, immature seeds, cooked, boiled, drained, with salt	5.96	1.36	111	15.29
Pokeberry shoots, (poke), cooked, boiled, drained, with salt	2.3	0.4	20	1.6
Potatoes, baked, flesh and skin, with salt	2.5	0.13	93	18.95
Potatoes, baked, flesh, with salt	1.96	0.1	93	20.05
Potatoes, baked, skin only, with salt	4.29	0.1	198	38.16
Potatoes, boiled, cooked in skin, flesh, with salt	1.87	0.1	87	18.13
Potatoes, boiled, cooked in skin, skin, with salt	2.86	0.1	78	13.9
Potatoes, boiled, cooked without skin, flesh, with salt	1.71	0.1	86	18.01
Potatoes, microwaved, cooked, in skin, flesh and skin, with salt	2.44	0.1	105	21.94
Potatoes, microwaved, cooked in skin, flesh, with salt	2.1	0.1	100	21.68
Potatoes, microwaved, cooked, in skin, skin with salt	4.39	0.1	132	24.13
Potatoes, frozen, whole, cooked, boiled, drained, with salt	1.98	0.13	63	12.53
Potatoes, frozen, french fried, par fried, cottage-cut, prepared, heated in oven, with salt	3.44	8.2	218	30.83
Potatoes, french fried, all types, salt not added in processing, frozen, oven-heated	2.66	5.22	172	26.11
Potatoes, french fried, all types, salt not added in processing, frozen, as purchased	2.24	4.66	150	22.91
Potatoes, au gratin, home-prepared from recipe using margarine	5.06	7.59	132	9.47
Potatoes, scalloped, home-prepared with margarine	2.87	3.68	88	8.88
Pumpkin, cooked, boiled, drained, with salt	0.72	0.07	18	3.21
Pumpkin, canned, with salt	1.1	0.28	34	5.19
Pumpkin, flowers, cooked, boiled, drained, with salt	1.09	0.08	15	2.28
Pumpkin leaves, cooked, boiled, drained, with salt	2.72	0.22	21	0.69

Food Name ---> per 100 g	Protein (g)	Fat (g)	Calories	Net Carb (g)
Purslane, cooked, boiled, drained, with salt	1.49	0.19	18	3.55
Radishes, oriental, cooked, boiled, drained, with salt	0.67	0.24	17	1.83
Rutabagas, cooked, boiled, drained, with salt	0.93	0.18	30	5.04
Salsify, cooked, boiled, drained, with salt	2.73	0.17	68	12.26
Soybeans, green, cooked, boiled, drained, with salt	12.35	6.4	141	6.85
Spinach, cooked, boiled, drained, with salt	2.97	0.26	23	1.35
Spinach, canned, no salt added, solids and liquids	2.11	0.37	19	0.72
Spinach, frozen, chopped or leaf, cooked, boiled, drained, with salt	4.01	0.87	34	1.1
Squash, summer, all varieties, cooked, boiled, drained, with salt	0.91	0.31	20	2.91
Squash, summer, crookneck and straightneck, cooked, boiled, drained, with salt	1.04	0.39	19	2.69
Squash, summer, crookneck and straightneck, frozen, cooked, boiled, drained, with salt	1.28	0.2	25	4.14
Squash, summer, scallop, cooked, boiled, drained, with salt	1.03	0.17	16	1.4
Squash, summer, zucchini, includes skin, cooked, boiled, drained, with salt	1.14	0.36	15	1.69
Squash, summer, zucchini, includes skin, frozen, cooked, boiled, drained, with salt	1.15	0.13	14	1.67
Squash, winter, all varieties, cooked, baked, with salt	0.89	0.35	37	6.05
Squash, winter, acorn, cooked, baked, with salt	1.12	0.14	56	10.18
Squash, winter, acorn, cooked, boiled, mashed, with salt	0.67	0.08	34	6.19
Squash, winter, butternut, cooked, baked, with salt	0.9	0.09	40	7.29
Squash, winter, butternut, frozen, cooked, boiled, with salt	1.23	0.07	39	10.04
Squash, winter, hubbard, baked, with salt	2.48	0.62	50	5.91
Squash, winter, hubbard, cooked, boiled, mashed, with salt	1.48	0.37	30	3.56
Squash, winter, spaghetti, cooked, boiled, drained, or baked, with salt	0.66	0.26	27	5.06
Succotash, (corn and limas), cooked, boiled, drained, with salt	5.07	0.8	111	24.37
Succotash, (corn and limas), frozen, cooked, boiled, drained, with salt	4.31	0.89	93	15.85
Swamp cabbage (skunk cabbage), cooked, boiled, drained, with salt	2.08	0.24	20	1.8
Sweet potato leaves, cooked, steamed, with salt	2.18	0.34	35	5.48

Food Name ---> per 100 g	Protein (g)	Fat (g)	Calories	Net Carb (g)
Sweet potato, cooked, baked in skin, flesh, with salt	2.01	0.15	92	17.41
Sweet potato, cooked, boiled, without skin, with salt	1.37	0.14	76	15.22
Sweet potato, frozen, cooked, baked, with salt	1.71	0.12	100	21.6
Taro, cooked, with salt	0.52	0.11	142	29.5
Taro, leaves, cooked, steamed, with salt	2.72	0.41	24	1.89
Taro, shoots, cooked, with salt	0.73	0.08	14	3.19
Taro, tahitian, cooked, with salt	4.16	0.68	44	6.85
Tomatoes, red, ripe, cooked, with salt	0.95	0.11	18	3.31
Tomatoes, red, ripe, canned, packed in tomato juice, no salt added	0.79	0.25	16	1.57
Tomato juice, canned, without salt added	0.85	0.29	17	3.13
Tomato products, canned, puree, with salt added	1.65	0.21	38	7.08
Turnips, cooked, boiled, drained, with salt	0.71	0.08	22	3.06
Turnips, frozen, cooked, boiled, drained, with salt	1.53	0.24	21	1.73
Turnip greens, cooked, boiled, drained, with salt	1.14	0.23	20	0.86
Turnip greens, frozen, cooked, boiled, drained, with salt	3.35	0.42	29	1.58
Turnip greens and turnips, frozen, cooked, boiled, drained, with salt	2.99	0.38	34	1.64
Vegetables, mixed, frozen, cooked, boiled, drained, with salt	2.86	0.15	60	8.69
Waxgourd, (chinese preserving melon), cooked, boiled, drained, with salt	0.4	0.2	11	1.45
Winged bean, immature seeds, cooked, boiled, drained, with salt	5.31	0.66	37	3.21
Yam, cooked, boiled, drained, or baked, with salt	1.49	0.14	114	23.09
Yambean (jicama), cooked, boiled, drained, with salt	0.72	0.09	36	8.23
Yardlong bean, cooked, boiled, drained, with salt	2.53	0.1	47	9.17
Corn, sweet, white, raw	3.22	1.18	86	16.32
Corn, sweet, white, cooked, boiled, drained, without salt	3.34	1.41	97	19.01
Corn, sweet, white, cooked, boiled, drained, with salt	3.34	1.41	97	19.01
Corn, sweet, white, canned, whole kernel, regular pack, solids and liquids	1.95	0.5	64	13.71
Corn, sweet, white, canned, whole kernel, no salt added, solids and liquids	1.95	0.5	64	14.71

Food Name ---> per 100 g	Protein (g)	Fat (g)	Calories	Net Carb (g)
Corn, sweet, white, canned, whole kernel, drained solids	2.32	1.37	71	12.76
Corn, sweet, white, canned, cream style, regular pack	1.74	0.42	74	17.42
Corn, sweet, white, canned, cream style, no salt added	1.74	0.42	72	16.93
Corn, sweet, white, canned, vacuum pack, regular pack	2.41	0.5	79	17.44
Corn, sweet, white, canned, vacuum pack, no salt added	2.41	0.5	79	17.44
Corn, sweet, white, frozen, kernels cut off cob, unprepared	3.02	0.77	88	17.83
Corn, sweet, white, frozen, kernels cut off cob, boiled, drained, without salt	2.75	0.43	80	17.16
Corn, sweet, white, frozen, kernels cut off cob, boiled, drained, with salt	2.75	0.43	80	17.16
Corn, sweet, white, frozen, kernels on cob, unprepared	3.28	0.78	98	20.7
Corn, sweet, white, frozen, kernels on cob, cooked, boiled, drained, without salt	3.11	0.74	94	20.23
Corn, sweet, white, frozen, kernels on cob, cooked, boiled, drained, with salt	3.11	0.74	94	19.53
Peppers, sweet, red, canned, solids and liquids	0.8	0.3	18	2.7
Peppers, sweet, red, frozen, chopped, unprepared	1.08	0.21	20	2.85
Peppers, sweet, red, frozen, chopped, boiled, drained, without salt	0.95	0.18	16	2.51
Peppers, sweet, red, frozen, chopped, boiled, drained, with salt	0.95	0.18	16	2.51
Peppers, sweet, red, sauteed	1.04	12.75	133	4.77
Sesbania flower, cooked, steamed, with salt	1.14	0.05	21	5.1
Soybeans, mature seeds, sprouted, cooked, steamed, with salt	8.47	4.45	81	5.73
Soybeans, mature seeds, sprouted, cooked, stir-fried, with salt	13.1	7.1	125	8.6
Dock, cooked, boiled, drained, with salt	1.83	0.64	20	2.93
Lentils, sprouted, cooked, stir-fried, with salt	8.8	0.45	101	21.25
Mountain yam, hawaii, cooked, steamed, with salt	1.73	0.08	82	19.99
Tree fern, cooked, with salt	0.29	0.07	40	7.08
Potatoes, mashed, prepared from granules, without milk, whole milk and margarine	2.05	4.93	108	12.2
Potatoes, mashed, dehydrated, prepared from flakes without milk, whole milk and margarine added	1.9	5.6	113	12.72
Peppers, sweet, red, freeze-dried	17.9	3	314	47.4
Beans, snap, yellow, canned, regular pack, drained solids	1.15	0.1	20	3.2

Food Name ---> per 100 g	Protein (g)	Fat (g)	Calories	Net Carb (g)
Beans, snap, yellow, canned, no salt added, drained solids	1.15	0.1	20	3.2
Potatoes, mashed, home-prepared, whole milk and butter added	1.86	4.22	113	15.31
Catsup	1.04	0.1	101	27.1
Mushrooms, brown, italian, or crimini, exposed to ultraviolet light, raw	2.5	0.1	22	3.7
Pickles, cucumber, dill or kosher dill	0.5	0.3	12	1.41
Mushroom, white, exposed to ultraviolet light, raw	3.09	0.34	22	2.26
Mushrooms, portabella, exposed to ultraviolet light, grilled	3.28	0.58	29	2.24
Pickles, cucumber, sweet (includes bread and butter pickles)	0.58	0.41	91	20.15
Pickles, cucumber, sour	0.33	0.2	11	1.06
Pimento, canned	1.1	0.3	23	3.2
Pickle relish, hot dog	1.5	0.46	91	21.85
Pickle relish, sweet	0.37	0.47	130	33.96
Pickles, cucumber, sour, low sodium	0.33	0.2	11	1.06
Pickles, cucumber, dill, reduced sodium	0.5	0.3	12	1.41
Pickles, cucumber, sweet, low sodium (includes bread and butter pickles)	0.37	0.26	122	32.63
Catsup, low sodium	1.04	0.1	101	27.1
Mushrooms, enoki, raw	2.66	0.29	37	5.11
Peppers, sweet, yellow, raw	1	0.21	27	5.42
Radicchio, raw	1.43	0.25	23	3.58
Squash, zucchini, baby, raw	2.71	0.4	21	2.01
Tomatillos, raw	0.96	1.02	32	3.94
Tomatoes, sun-dried	14.11	2.97	258	43.46
Tomatoes, sun-dried, packed in oil, drained	5.06	14.08	213	17.53
Fennel, bulb, raw	1.24	0.2	31	4.2
Pickle relish, hamburger	0.63	0.54	129	31.28
Arugula, raw	2.58	0.66	25	2.05
Carrots, baby, raw	0.64	0.13	35	5.34
Hearts of palm, canned	2.52	0.62	28	2.22
Peppers, hot chile, sun-dried	10.58	5.81	324	41.16

Food Name ---> per 100 g	Protein (g)	Fat (g)	Calories	Net Carb (g)
Nopales, raw	1.32	0.09	16	1.13
Nopales, cooked, without salt	1.35	0.05	15	1.28
Cauliflower, green, raw	2.95	0.3	31	2.89
Cauliflower, green, cooked, no salt added	3.04	0.31	32	2.98
Cauliflower, green, cooked, with salt	3.04	0.31	32	2.98
Broccoli, chinese, cooked	1.14	0.72	22	1.31
Cabbage, napa, cooked	1.1	0.17	12	2.23
Lemon grass (citronella), raw	1.82	0.49	99	25.31
Beans, fava, in pod, raw	7.92	0.73	88	10.13
Grape leaves, raw	5.6	2.12	93	6.31
Grape leaves, canned	4.27	1.97	69	1.81
Pepper, banana, raw	1.66	0.45	27	1.95
Peppers, serrano, raw	1.74	0.44	32	3
Peppers, ancho, dried	11.86	8.2	281	29.82
Peppers, jalapeno, raw	0.91	0.37	29	3.7
Peppers, chili, green, canned	0.72	0.27	21	2.9
Peppers, hungarian, raw	0.8	0.41	29	5.7
Peppers, pasilla, dried	12.35	15.85	345	24.33
Pickles, chowchow, with cauliflower onion mustard, sweet	1.5	0.9	121	25.14
Epazote, raw	0.33	0.52	32	3.64
Fireweed, leaves, raw	4.71	2.75	103	8.62
Malabar spinach, cooked	2.98	0.78	23	0.61
Mushrooms, oyster, raw	3.31	0.41	33	3.79
Fungi, Cloud ears, dried	9.25	0.73	284	2.91
Mushrooms, straw, canned, drained solids	3.83	0.68	32	2.14
Wasabi, root, raw	4.8	0.63	109	15.74
Yautia (tannier), raw	1.46	0.4	98	22.13
Mushrooms, white, microwaved	3.91	0.46	35	3.54
Mushrooms, maitake, raw	1.94	0.19	31	4.27
Broccoli, chinese, raw	1.2	0.76	30	2.07
Fiddlehead ferns, raw	4.55	0.4	34	5.54

Food Name ---> per 100 g	Protein (g)	Fat (g)	Calories	Net Carb (g)
Fiddlehead ferns, frozen, unprepared	4.31	0.35	34	5.74
Mushrooms, portabella, exposed to ultraviolet light, raw	2.11	0.35	22	2.57
CAMPBELL'S, Tomato juice	0.82	0	21	3.32
CAMPBELL'S, Tomato juice, low sodium	0.82	0	21	3.32
CAMPBELL'S, V8 Vegetable Juice, Organic V8	0.41	0	20	3.73
CAMPBELL'S, Organic Tomato juice	0.82	0	21	3.32
HEALTHY REQUEST Tomato juice	0.82	0	21	3.73
CAMPBELL'S, V8 100% Vegetable Juice	0.82	0	21	3.32
CAMPBELL'S, V8 Vegetable Juice, Essential Antioxidants V8	0.82	0	21	3.73
CAMPBELL'S, V8 Vegetable Juice, Calcium Enriched V8	0.82	0	21	3.73
CAMPBELL'S, V8 Vegetable Juice, Low Sodium V8	0.82	0	21	3.32
CAMPBELL'S, V8 Vegetable Juice, Spicy Hot V8	0.82	0	21	3.32
PACE, Jalapenos Nacho Sliced Peppers	0	0	13	0.03
PACE, Diced Green Chilies	0	0	27	3.37
CAMPBELL'S, V8 60% Vegetable Juice, V8 V-Lite	0.41	0	14	2.48
CAMPBELL'S, V8 Vegetable Juice, Low Sodium Spicy Hot	0.82	0	21	3.73
CAMPBELL'S, V8 Vegetable Juice, High Fiber V8	0.82	0	25	3.29
Seaweed, Canadian Cultivated EMI-TSUNOMATA, dry	15.34	1.39	259	9.54
Seaweed, Canadian Cultivated EMI-TSUNOMATA, rehydrated	1.86	0.17	31	1.12
Potatoes, hash brown, refrigerated, unprepared	1.75	0.08	84	17.36
Potatoes, hash brown, refrigerated, prepared, pan-fried in canola oil	3.24	10.3	242	30.39
Sweet Potatoes, french fried, frozen as packaged, salt added in processing	2.16	8.92	182	29.88
Sweet Potatoes, french fried, crosscut, frozen, unprepared	1.7	11.1	209	22.12
Sweet Potato puffs, frozen, unprepared	1.36	3.58	161	28.82
Potatoes, yellow fleshed, roasted, salt added in processing, frozen, unprepared	1.99	1.85	119	20.84
Potatoes, yellow fleshed, french fried, frozen, unprepared	2.47	5.84	162	22.81
Potatoes, yellow fleshed, hash brown, shredded, salt added in processing, frozen, unprepared	2.04	0.07	81	15.98
Potatoes, french fried, wedge cut, frozen, unprepared	2.56	7.47	166	19.82

Food Name ---> per 100 g	Protein (g)	Fat (g)	Calories	Net Carb (g)
Potatoes, french fried, steak cut, salt not added in processing, frozen, unprepared	2.4	3.42	138	21.91
Potatoes, french fried, cross cut, frozen, unprepared	2.7	10	193	20.65
Vegetable smoothie, NAKED JUICE, KALE BLAZER	0.8	0.07	28	6.3
Ginger root, pickled, canned, with artificial sweetener	0.33	0.1	20	2.23
Peppers, hot pickled, canned	0.8	0.4	22	1.96
Vegetable juice, BOLTHOUSE FARMS, DAILY GREENS	0.49	0.04	31	6.93
Potatoes, mashed, ready-to-eat	1.97	5.01	106	11.39
Radishes, hawaiian style, pickled	1.1	0.3	28	3
Cabbage, japanese style, fresh, pickled	1.6	0.1	30	2.57
Cabbage, mustard, salted	1.1	0.1	28	2.53
Eggplant, pickled	0.9	0.7	49	7.27
Tomato sauce, canned, no salt added	1.2	0.3	24	3.81
Potatoes, canned, drained solids, no salt added	1.4	0.2	62	11.2
Vegetables, mixed (corn, lima beans, peas, green beans, carrots) canned, no salt added	1.4	0.2	37	4.21
Tomato and vegetable juice, low sodium	0.6	0.1	22	3.79
Turnip greens, canned, no salt added	1.36	0.3	19	1.51
Hearts of palm, raw	2.7	0.2	115	24.11
Yeast extract spread	23.88	0.9	185	13.92
Celery flakes, dried	11.3	2.1	319	35.9

Online tools

We have developed some useful, easy-to-use and powerful tool in our website: https://easyketodiet.net

You can find the following tools:
- Keto Calculator, for the calculation of your TDEE and your daily macros
  - https://www.easyketodiet.net/advanced-keto-calculator/

- Glycemic Index Counter:
  - https://www.easyketodiet.net/glycemic-index-counter/

- Keto Carb Counter
  - https://www.easyketodiet.net/keto-carb-counter/

Made in the USA
Columbia, SC
12 November 2020

24377454R00286